Health Management

Health Management

Edited by **Felix Rohmer**

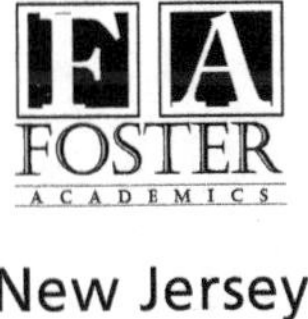

New Jersey

Published by Foster Academics,
61 Van Reypen Street,
Jersey City, NJ 07306, USA
www.fosteracademics.com

Health Management
Edited by Felix Rohmer

International Standard Book Number: 978-1-63242-222-4 (Hardback)

Printed in the United States of America.

Contents

Preface

This book aims to highlight the current researches and provides a platform to further the scope of innovations in this area. This book is a product of the combined efforts of many researchers and scientists, after going through thorough studies and analysis from different parts of the world. The objective of this book is to provide the readers with the latest information of the field.

Researchers and doctors, as well as managers of healthcare units face new challenges: escalating validity and authenticity of clinical trials, efficiently disseminating medical products, managing hospitals and clinics flexibly, and supervising treatment processes effectively. The advancement in our understanding of health management guarantees exceptional potential in terms of describing the causes of diseases and useful treatment. However, improved capabilities generate new issues. The objective of this book is to bring forth issues concerning health management in a way that would be pleasing for scholars and practitioners.

I would like to express my sincere thanks to the authors for their dedicated efforts in the completion of this book. I acknowledge the efforts of the publisher for providing constant support. Lastly, I would like to thank my family for their support in all academic endeavors.

Editor

General Issues

1

Human Walking Analysis, Evaluation and Classification Based on Motion Capture System

Bofeng Zhang[1], Susu Jiang[1], Ke Yan[1] and Daming Wei[1,2]
[1]*School of Computer Engineering and Science, Shanghai University*
[2]*Professor Emeritus, The University of Aizu, Fukushima,*
[1]*P. R. of China*
[2]*Japan*

1. Introduction

Gait analysis is the systematic study of human walking. It is helpful in the medical management of those diseases which affect the locomotion systems. Recently, the gait motion capture systems are becoming widely used by doctors and physical therapists for kinematics analysis and biomechanics and motion capture research, sports medicine and physical therapy, including human gait analysis and injury rehabilitation. This chapter describes some new progress on human walking analysis that our group made in the past few years based on motion capture system.

Generally, ageing causes many changes to neuromuscular system of a human being, for an example, his walking capabilities degenerate by ageing. Because these changes sometimes result in an increase the number of falls during daily walking, especially after the age of 75, it is very important to study the age related changes in the walking gait of elderly subjects. Many researchers studied stability of human walking gait and it was quoted that human walking gait stability decreases with age increasing the risk of falls in elderly people.

Many studies have been reported about the change in the kinematics parameters with age (Arif et al., 2004). This paper only focuses on the progress of walking modeling and walking stability. Especially, in order to simplify the method of data acquisition, this paper suggests process of reduction on dynamic stability features through feature selection. That will help us analyze stability in a more clear way.

1.1 Background of walking model

Various methods are used to overcome the difficulties imposed by the extraction of human gait features. Two approaches are being used for human gait analysis: model-based and non-model-based methods.

The non-model-based method is applied in image-based gait analysis (marker-less analysis). Feature correspondence between successive frames is based upon prediction, velocity, shape, texture and colour. Small motion between consecutive frames is the main assumption, whereby feature correspondence is conducted using various geometric constraints.

For the first one, a priori shape model is established to match real data to this predefined model, and thereby extracting the corresponding features once the best match is obtained. Stick models and volumetric models are the most commonly used methods. The model-

based approach is the most popular method being used for human motion analysis due to its advantages. It can extract detailed and accurate motion data.
Nash (Nash et al., 1998) proposed a parametric gait model consisting of a pair of articulated lines, jointed at the hip to extract moving articulated objects from a temporal sequence of images. Pendulum model was used to extract and describes human gait for recognition automatically (Cunado et al., 2003). The human leg was modelled as two pendulums joined in series. Zhang (Zhang et al., 2004) proposed a model-based approach to gait recognition by employing a 5-link biped locomotion human model. Akita (Akita, 1984) proposed a model consisting of six segments comprising of two arms, two legs, the torso and the head. Lee (Lee, 2003) suggested a 7-ellipse model, to describe a representation of gait appearance for the purpose of person identification and classification. A 2D stick figure model, which composed of 7 segments, was used to represent the human body, and joint angles and angular velocities are calculated to describe the gait motion (Yoo et la., 2002). Guo (Guo et al., 1994) represented the human body structure in the silhouette by a stick figure model which had 10 sticks articulated with six joints. Cheng (Cheng & Moura, 1998) represented the human body as a stick figure which was considered to be composed of 12 rigid parts. Dockstader (Dockstader et al, 2002) suggested the use of a hierarchical, structural model of the human body which had 15 points. Rohr (Rohr, 1994) proposed a volumetric model for the analysis of human motion, using 14 elliptical cylinders to model the human body. Karaulova (Karaulova et al., 2000) have used the stick figure model to build a novel hierarchical model of human dynamics represented using hidden Markov models.

1.2 Background of walking stability

Theoretically, human walking has rigid periodicity so the next step should repeat the first step strictly. That is to say, all steps must be consistent completely and have no any deference at all. In fact, there is no normal walking pattern and the walking pattern varies from person to person. These walking patterns are considered to be stable until and unless there is an evidence of fall of the person. During walking, human tries to generate periodic series of motions. But due to the physiological limitations, these motions do not re-main exactly periodic but contains some variability or randomness in it. He/she does not try to correct this variability or randomness of these motions if it remains within stability limits. This variability present in the walking patterns is due to not only internal perturbation but also due to external perturbations. The amount of variability present in the walking pattern reflects the quality of neuromuscular control of the human being.
There are many researches which are related to human walking stability. Corriveau et al compare the postural stability of elderly stroke patients with those of healthy elderly people using the distance between the centre of pressure (COP) and the centre of mass (COM) in terms of root mean square. Statistical significance of the COP-COM variable was larger in the stroke group than in healthy subjects, in both the anteroposterior (AP) and mediolateral (ML) directions (Corriveau et al., 2004).
Effect of age on the variability or irregularity of the acceleration of COM in ML, vertical and AP directions is analyzed by Arif et al, using approximate entropy technique for young and elderly subjects of subjects (Arif et al., 2004).
Literature (Hylton et al., 2003) tried to evaluate acceleration patterns at the head and pelvis in young and older subjects when walking on a level and an irregular walking surface. The subjects are two groups, 30 young people aged 22–39 years (mean 29.0, SD 4.3), and 30 older people with a low risk of falling aged 75–85 years (mean 79.0, SD 3.0).

The maximum Floquet multipliers (FM) are used to measure orbital stability of upper body in difference walking speed (Marin et al., 2006). Orbital stability changed very little with speed. The general purpose of (Kavanagh, 2006) is to examine factors that may influence acceleration features of the upper body during walking.

Balance in quiet upright stance, which was studied by (Stirling & Zakynthinaki, 2004), does not imply motionless stability, in fact a ML and AP body sway occurs. Almost 95% of the anterior-posterior sway happens around the ankle and the hip axis.

Sutherland et al investigated the development of mature walking in children of age from one to seven years old (Sutherland et al., 1980). The objective of literature (PH. Chou, 2003) was to investigate the gait maturation of Taiwan children. Elderly subjects exhibits gait pattern characterized by reduced velocity, shorter step length and increased step timing variability (Hylton et al., 2003). It is mentioned that elderly people reduce their walking speed to improve their walking stability in the literature.

While many walking stability indices have been proposed, there is still no commonly accepted way to define, much less quantify, locomotors stability.

1.3 Background of walking symmetry

The concept of gait symmetry itself is no acceptable unified definition, more often many people's research assumes that the normal gait is symmetric, which is to simplify data collection and analysis of gait. In fact gait symmetry was only evaluated with a small number of biomechanical studies that used quantitative data of the two lower limbs. In addition, the gait symmetry was not actually carried out enough exploration. It is because there is no participation of a considerable more number of test objects. One hand, the gait parameter of information provided is the effects of the movement not the reasons of the movement. This may also affect explaining the behaviour of the lower limbs. The other hand, the gait symmetry is not clearly defined, and the use only single gait parameters or a simple statistical method to compare which has made study of gait symmetry been more limited.

Maybe it stands to reason that a healthy man or woman has left leg and right leg symmetrically, and normal gait seems symmetric with ones right-side and left-side. What about the walking stability or dynamic balance if there is not so symmetric? Can we get some quantity or relationship of symmetry and balance?

Gait symmetry is multifaceted. Normal walking seems right-left symmetry because normal people walk with their right foot and left foot. The ability of maintaining balance is essential to keep normal walking. Poor balance is an independent risk factor for falling, so anything that improves balance can have a positive effect on safety and function after stroke. Balance is described as the ability to maintain or move within a weight-bearing posture without falling. We have not found any trends study relating to walking stability and symmetry of human gait. And the trends indicated what meanings.

Yang in his doctoral thesis paper (Yang, 2001) proposed the symmetry indicators of step length and stride length, to describe the step in the role of gait symmetry. But phase symmetry and the step length symmetry are not fully reflects the characteristics of gait, especially the joint angle in the role of symmetry.

2. Modeling assumptions and theoretical framework

Walking is a complex dynamic activity. A good human model for gait analysis should be simple, but extensive enough to capture the dynamics of most walkers.

Almost existing models, which have from 2 segments to more than 15 segments, have two pitfalls. Firstly, they paid more attention to the sagittal plane, and overlook the other two planes, transverse plane and frontal plane. Secondly, it is not enough to describe the particularity of the feet. Most of them regarded the foot as a point. Thus, it is difficult to decide the gait cycle, such as initial heel contact, heel rise, and toe off. So a new walking model, so called Fourteen-Linkage (FL) model, is proposed.

2.1 Fourteen-linkage model

DEFINITION 1. (Fourteen-Linkage Model) We suggest a walking model, which is a collection of 19 points, 14 segments and 12 joints, used to specify the position and the configuration of a human body, as shown in Fig. 1.

Position describes the location of a body segment or joint in space, measured in meters. In FL model, the 19 points can be decided by the 30 markers we measured from motion capture system. The relationships between the model and markers are also shown in Fig. 1(a).

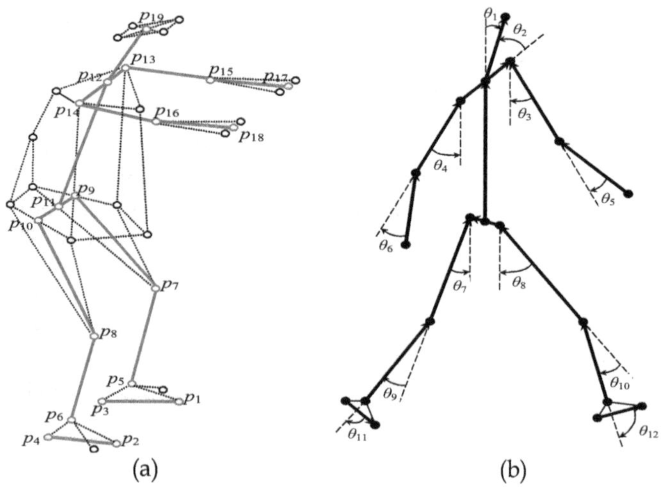

Fig. 1. Fourteen-linkage (FL) Model

Body segments are considered to be rigid bodies for the purposes of describing the motion of the body. 14 segments are composed of these points, such as head (S_1), shoulder (S_2), left and right upper-arms (S_3, S_4), left and right forearms (S_5, S_6), trunk (S_7), pelvis (S_8), left and right thighs (S_9, S_{10}), left and right shanks (S_{11}, S_{12}), and left and right feet (S_{13}, S_{14}).

12 joints between adjacent segments are composed of these segments, such as head-trunk (θ_1), head-shoulder (θ_2), shoulder (θ_3, θ_4), elbows (θ_5, θ_6), hips (θ_7, θ_8), knees (θ_9, θ_{10}), ankles (θ_{11}, θ_{12}), see Fig. 1(b).

2.2 Definitions of walking stability

In human movement, kinematics is the study of the positions, angles, velocities, and accelerations of body segments and joints during motion.

FL model M consists of displacement P, segment angle Φ, joint angle Θ, and their velocity V and acceleration A, angular velocity Ω and angular acceleration Λ at time t, represented as 9-tuple as Equation (1).

$$\begin{aligned} M = [&P(t), \Phi(t), \Theta(t), \\ &V(t), \Omega_\Phi(t), \Omega_\Theta(t), \\ &A(t), \Lambda_\Phi(t), \Lambda_\Theta(t)] \end{aligned} \tag{1}$$

where

$$P(t) = \left[p_1, p_2, p_3, \cdots, p_{19}\right]^T$$

$$\Phi(t) = \left[\varphi_1, \varphi_2, \varphi_3, \cdots, \varphi_{14}\right]^T$$

$$\Theta(t) = \left[\theta_1, \theta_2, \theta_3, \cdots, \theta_{12}\right]^T$$

$$V(t) = \left[v_1, v_2, v_3, \cdots, v_{19}\right]^T$$

$$\Omega_\Phi(t) = \left[\omega_{\varphi 1}, \omega_{\varphi 2}, \omega_{\varphi 3}, \cdots, \omega_{\varphi 14}\right]^T$$

$$\Omega_\Theta(t) = \left[\omega_{\theta 1}, \omega_{\theta 2}, \omega_{\theta 3}, \cdots, \omega_{\theta 12}\right]^T$$

$$A(t) = \left[a_1, a_2, a_3, \cdots, a_{19}\right]^T$$

$$\Lambda_\Phi(t) = \left[a_{\varphi 1}, a_{\varphi 2}, a_{\varphi 3}, \cdots, a_{\varphi 14}\right]^T$$

$$\Lambda_\Theta(t) = \left[a_{\theta 1}, a_{\theta 2}, a_{\theta 3}, \cdots, a_{\theta 12}\right]^T$$

Segment angle, as shown in Equation (2), is the angle of the projections of segment with the coordinate axes. It consists of the angles between projections in transverse plane, frontal plane and sagittal plane with axis X, Y and Z respectively, see Fig. 2.

$$\varphi = (\varphi_x, \varphi_y, \varphi_z) \tag{2}$$

Note that it is an absolute measure, meaning that it changes according to the orientation of the body.

Joint angle is the angle between the two segments on either side of the joint. It is defined as Equation (3).

$$\theta = (\theta_{xoy}, \theta_{yoz}, \theta_{zox}, \theta_s) \tag{3}$$

where θ_s is the joint angle in space, and θ_{xoy}, θ_{yoz}, θ_{zox} are the projections of joint angle in transverse plane, frontal plane and sagittal plane respectively. Since joint angle θ_s is relative to the segment angles, it doesn't change with the body orientation.

Velocity may be linear (change in displacement) or angular (change in angle). Normally, velocity is derived from displacement or angle data by the process of differentiation. Acceleration is change in velocity. Again, it may be linear (change in linear velocity) or angular (change in angular velocity). Acceleration, too, is usually calculated from the displacement data by differentiating twice. It can also be measured directly by an accelerometer.

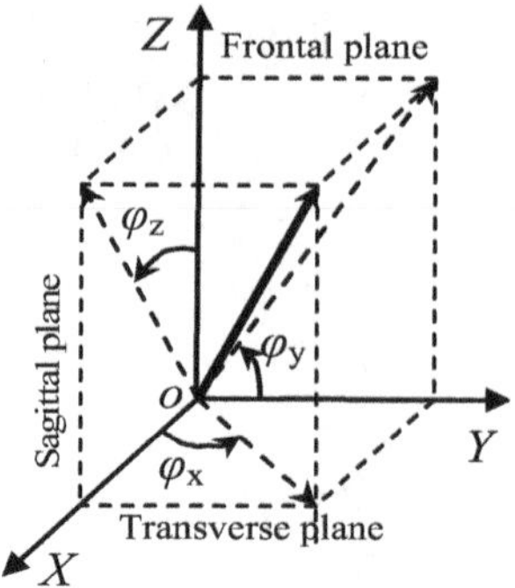

Fig. 2. Segment angle

2.3 Definitions of walking symmetry

For walking symmetry, only consider the bilateral of positions, segments and joints on both sides of human body. In FL-Model, there are 8 points, 5 segments and 5 joint angles unilateral met this condition. These attributes are all three-dimensional data. They are motion data and its velocity and acceleration of {Knee, Ankle, Heel, Toe, Shoulder, Elbow, Wrist, Hip}, Segment Angle and its velocity and acceleration of {Thigh, Shank, Foot, Upper-arm, Forearm}, Joint Angle and its velocity and acceleration of {Hip, Knee, Ankle, Shoulder, Elbow}. These attributes can also be expressed with $p_{1\sim10}$, $p_{13\sim18}$, $\varphi_{3\sim6}$, $\varphi_{9\sim14}$, $\theta_{3\sim12}$, as shown in Fig. 1.

3. Walking data preprocessing

Data preprocessing is an important issue for data analysis, as real-world data tend to be incomplete, noisy, and inconsistent. Data preprocessing includes data cleaning, data integration, data transformation, and data reduction. Although numerous methods of data preprocessing have been developed, data preprocessing remains an active area of research, due to the huge amount inconsistent or dirty data and the complexity of the problem. Before we talk about the methods of walking data preprocessing, let us have a look at walking data measuring.

3.1 Walking data measuring

There are many measurements of human gait, such as basic data (spatial and temporal data), kinematics (displacement, velocity and acceleration data), kinetics (force and moment data), electromyography (electrical activity of lower limb muscles), and image and graphics (individual silhouette images, monocular, image sequence, video). We adopt the kinematical approach in modeling the human movements.

Two kinds of data, motion data and acceleration data are measured using two different systems. The Motion data are gotten from motion capture system (Vicon MX System by OMG Plc), while acceleration data are obtained by a 3-axis accelerometer.

The providers walk along 5m straight line in level plane 3 times at them natural normal walking speeds. 30 markers are attached to the body, as shown in Fig. 3. Fig. 4 shows a snapshot of data acquisition using a motion capture system in the University of Aizu, Fukushima, Japan. The highlights show markers on human body.

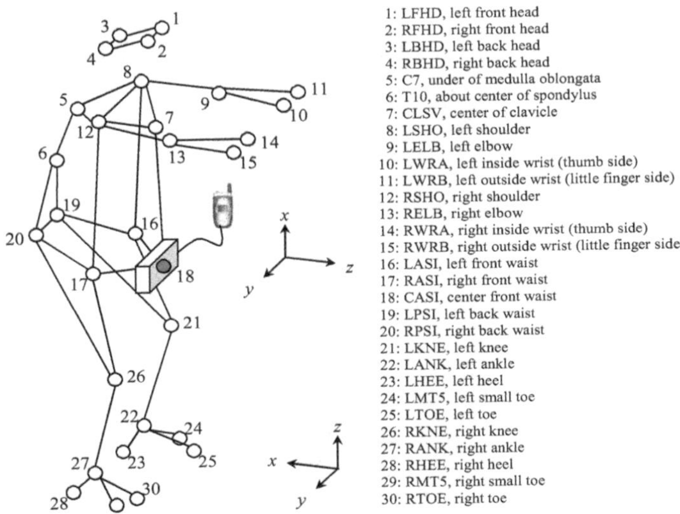

Fig. 3. Markers attached to the body

The motion capture system can detect the three dimensions displacement data at tree directions: anterior-posterior, left-right, and superior-inferior. The sampling rate of motion data is 120Hz.

At the same time, a tri-axial accelerometer unit is mounted with CASI, the same point as marker 18, see Fig. 3. The accelerometer is connected with a mobile phone to save the acceleration data. After that the data can be transferred to computer. Acceleration data are also collected in three dimensions as same as motion data, including the gravity acceleration. But the directions are not same. The sampling rate of acceleration data is 90Hz. To calibrate the accelerometer, before each testing session, it was placed with each of the orthogonal axes vertically, to estimate the ±1g values.

By the way, a movie is taken by a video camera while he/she is walking. 44 normal persons from 20 to 69 year old are measured. These subjects are classified into 5 groups (20+, 30+, 40+, 50+, and 60+) by the age.

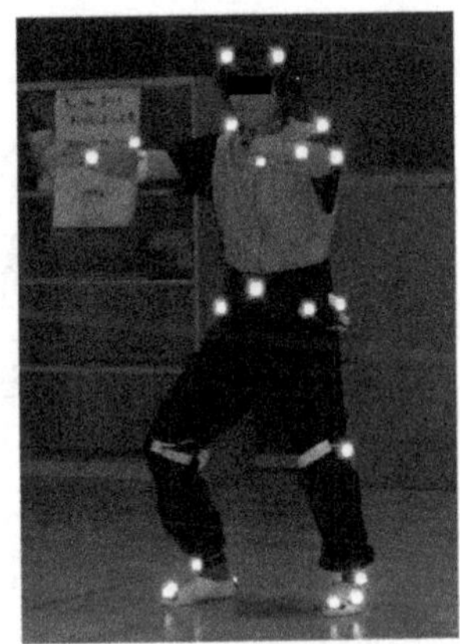

Fig. 4. A snapshot of data acquisition using a motion capture system

3.2 Data cleaning

Data cleaning attempts to fill in missing values, smooth out noise, and correct inconsistencies in the data.

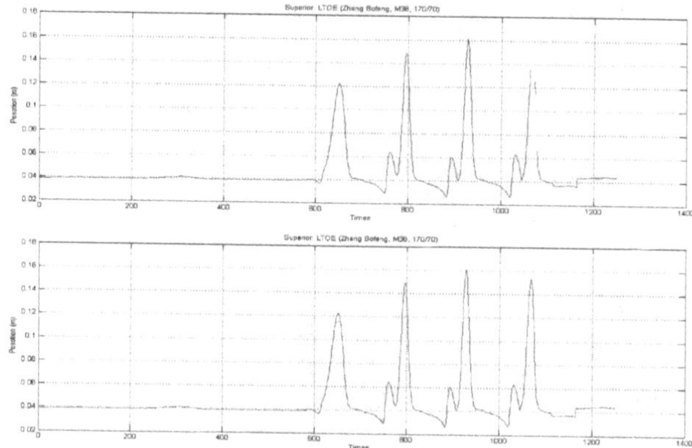

Fig. 5. Interpolation of missing data in left toe

3.2.1 Missing data

In the walking data measured by the motion capture systems, there are some missing data because the system can not detect the markers at a moment. Many interpolation methods could be used, such as nearest neighbor interpolation, linear interpolation, cubic spline interpolation, piecewise cubic Hermite interpolation and *N*-th degree polynomial interpolation. We choose the spline method to interpolate the missing data because the cubic spline interpolation is a piecewise continuous curve, passing through each of the values in the source data. An example is shown in Fig. 5.

3.2.2 Noisy data

In acceleration data, there are many noisy data, as shown in Fig. 6. We should try to identify and cut these noisy data from the source data.

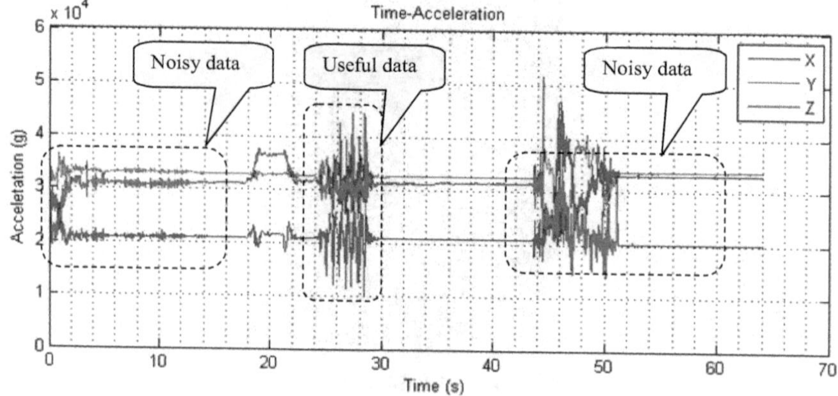

Fig. 6. The noisy data in acceleration data

And there are some noisy data in motion data caused by vibration. Since the walking signal resides in the low frequency range, it is easily affected by interference from other signal and noise sources. Butterworth low-pass filter is used to reduce noise by passing signal which frequency below twice walking cadence. Some examples are shown in Fig. 7 to Fig. 8.

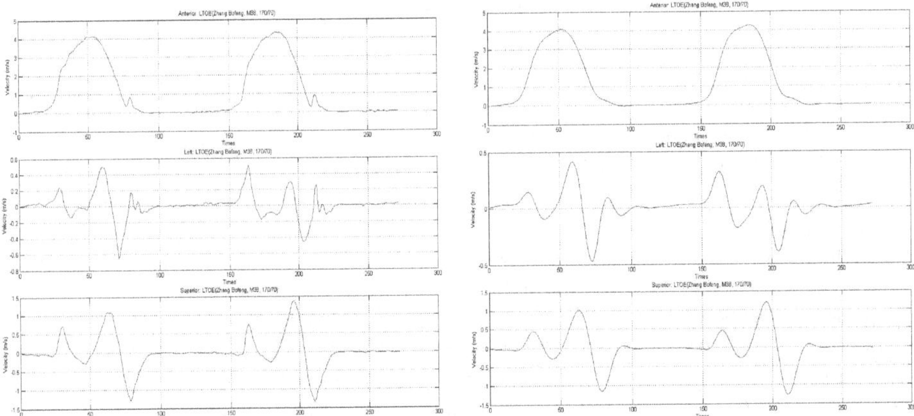

Fig. 7. Velocity data of left toe (No filtering & Filtering)

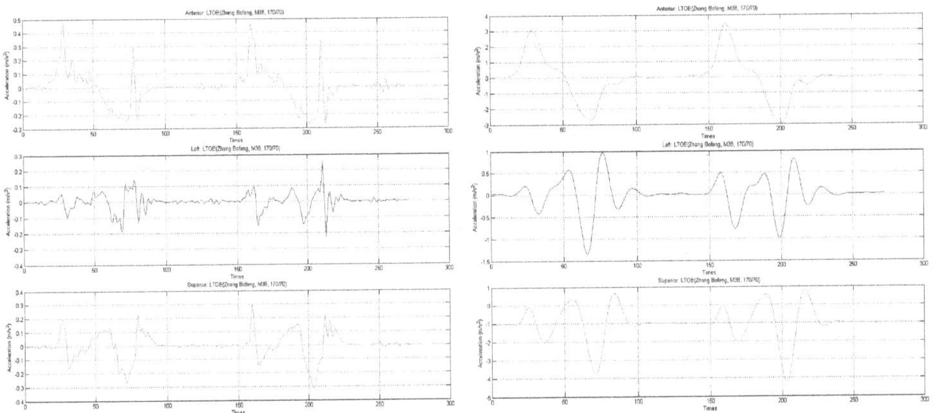

Fig. 8. Acceleration data of left toe (No filtering & Filtering)

3.2.3 Inconsistent data

Because of the faults of the measure systems, one marker can be identified as two or more. In the source file, there is more than one column to store them. So these inconsistent data must be processed by the mean methods, see Equation (4).

$$\begin{cases} \overline{x} = \dfrac{1}{N}\sum_{i=1}^{N} x_i \\ \overline{y} = \dfrac{1}{N}\sum_{i=1}^{N} y_i \\ \overline{z} = \dfrac{1}{N}\sum_{i=1}^{N} z_i \end{cases} \tag{4}$$

3.3 Data transformation

Data transformation converts the data into appropriate forms for analysis further. The coordinate of acceleration data is not parallel the space coordinate because the accelerometer is set up obliquely, so we need to normalize the coordinate.

3.3.1 Calibration

The aim of calibration is to transform raw data to acceleration of gravity (g). The standard of vibration amplitude is maintained in terms of electrical output of reference accelerometer corresponding to a known value of displacement. Acceleration singles are sampled at 90Hz using purpose-written software and saved on computer for subsequent analysis. To calibrate the accelerations before each testing session, they ware placed with each of the orthogonal axes vertically, first pointing up, then down, which enabled the device to be statically calibrated to estimate the ±1g values. An example is shown in Fig. 9.

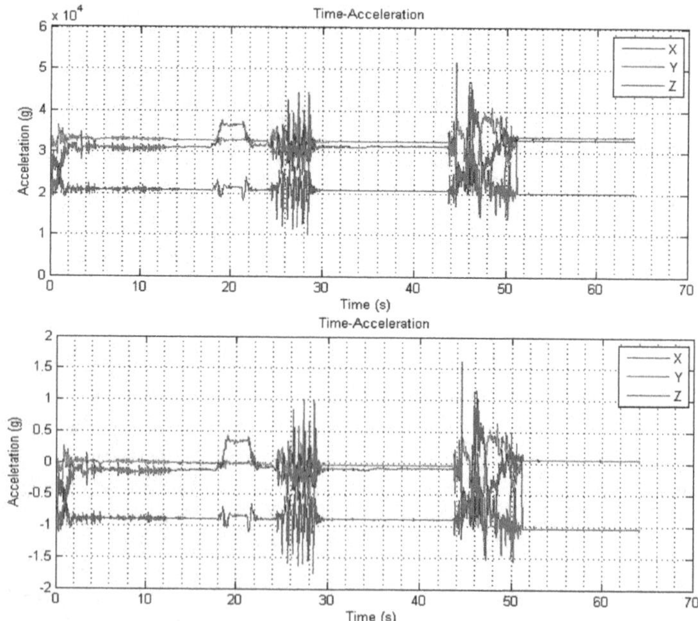

Fig. 9. Calibration of acceleration data

3.3.2 Adjusting acceleration data

Theoretically, the means of X and Y should be '0', that of Z should be '-1'. But actually, it is not true. The coordinate of acceleration data is not parallel with the space coordinate because the accelerometer is set up in gradient, see Fig. 10 so we need to adjust the coordinate.

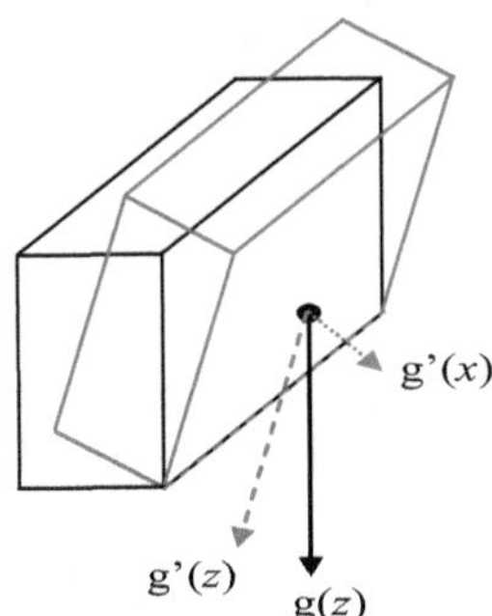

Fig. 10. The accelerometer set up in gradient

The method of adjusting is to rotate the accelerometer in correct position, as shown in Fig. 11. Adjusting rule is that the means of X and Y should be '0'. Firstly, calculate rotation matrix R with Homogeneous Coordinate used Equation (5), and then adjust the acceleration data to vertical position by Equation (6).

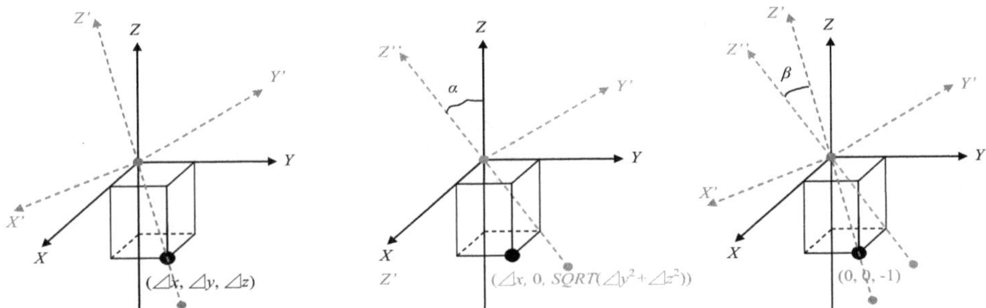

Fig. 11. Title of figure, left justified

$$R = R_x \times R_y = \begin{bmatrix} 1 & 0 & 0 & 0 \\ 0 & \cos(\alpha) & \sin(\alpha) & 0 \\ 0 & -\sin(\alpha) & \cos(\alpha) & 0 \\ 0 & 0 & 0 & 1 \end{bmatrix} \times \begin{bmatrix} \cos(\beta) & 0 & -\sin(\beta) & 0 \\ 0 & 1 & 0 & 0 \\ \sin(\beta) & 0 & \cos(\beta) & 0 \\ 0 & 0 & 0 & 1 \end{bmatrix} \tag{5}$$

$$A' = AxR \tag{6}$$

An example of adjusting is shown in Fig. 12.

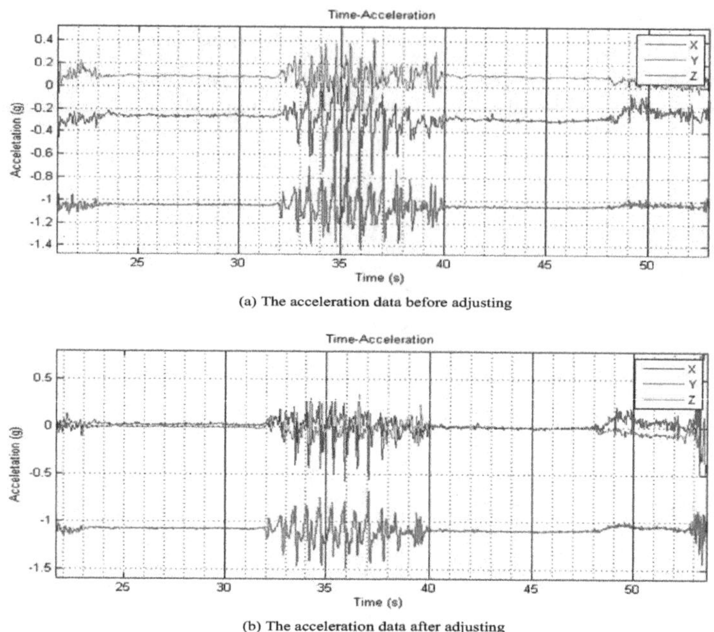

(a) The acceleration data before adjusting

(b) The acceleration data after adjusting

Fig. 12. An example of adjusting result

3.4 Data integration

Data integration combines data from multiple sources to form a coherent data store. Metadata, correlation analysis, data conflict detection, and the resolution of semantic heterogeneity contribute toward smooth data integration.

3.4.1 Converting the coordinates

The coordinate of acceleration data is different from that of motion data, so we should match the acceleration data and motion data in the same coordinates. We define the coordinates, as shown in Fig. 13, x: anterior, y: left, z: superior.

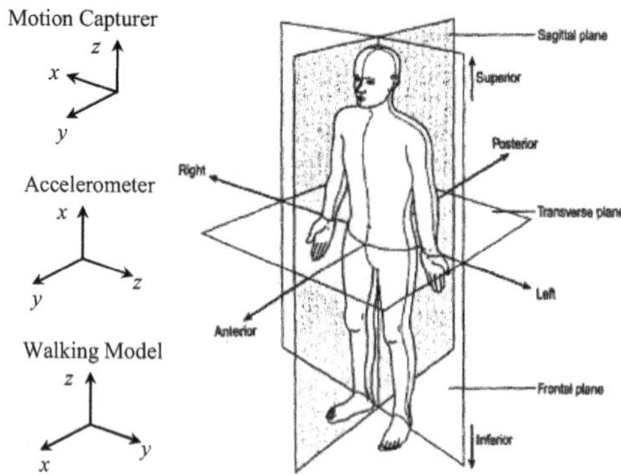

Fig. 13. Converting the coordinates

3.4.2 Aligning the acceleration data with the motion data

The acceleration data and motion data come from different systems, the sampling rates are different, the time of starting measurement are not same, as shown in Fig. 14

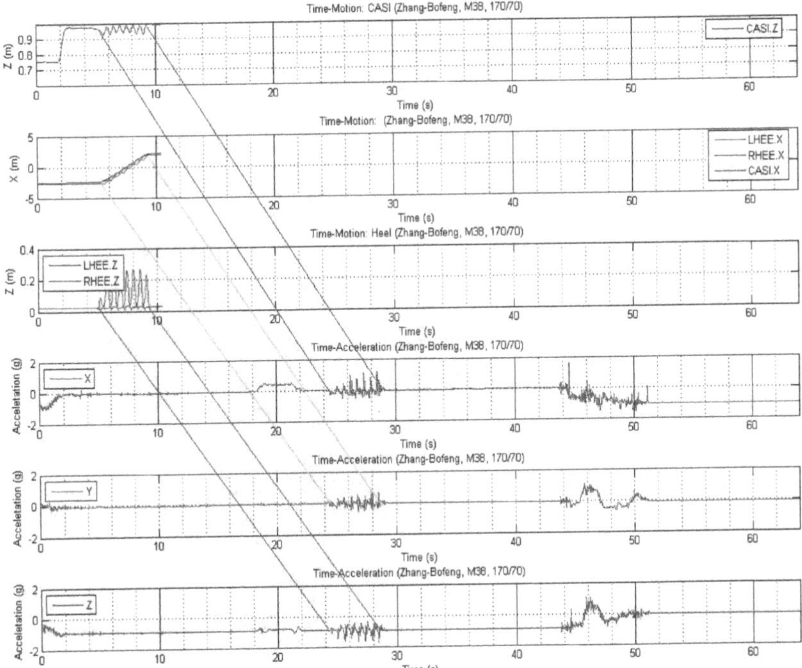

Fig. 14. Title of figure, left justified

so we must find which point of motion data is correlative with which point in acceleration data. The aligning method has two steps.

1. Computing the acceleration with motion data by Equation (7), as shown in Fig. 15.

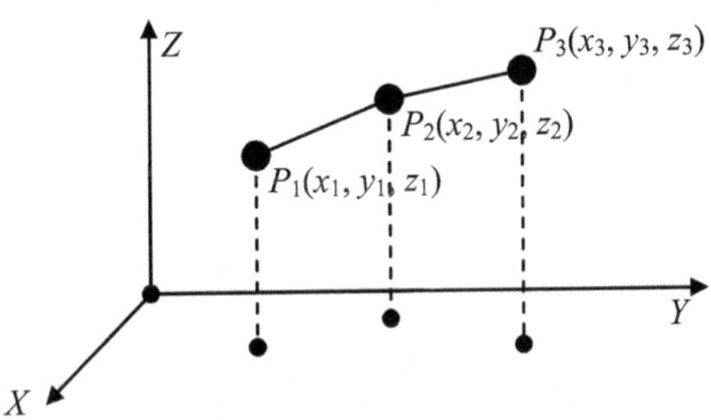

Fig. 15. Computing acceleration with motion data

$$\begin{cases} a_i(x) = \dfrac{x_{i+2} - 2x_{i+1} + x_i}{\Delta t^2} \\ a_i(y) = \dfrac{y_{i+2} - 2y_{i+1} + y_i}{\Delta t^2} \quad (i = 1, N-2) \\ a_i(z) = \dfrac{z_{i+2} - 2z_{i+1} + z_i}{\Delta t^2} \end{cases} \tag{7}$$

2. Comparing the acceleration between the computing data and accelerometer data by minimum of relativity. The result of aligning is shown in Fig. 16.

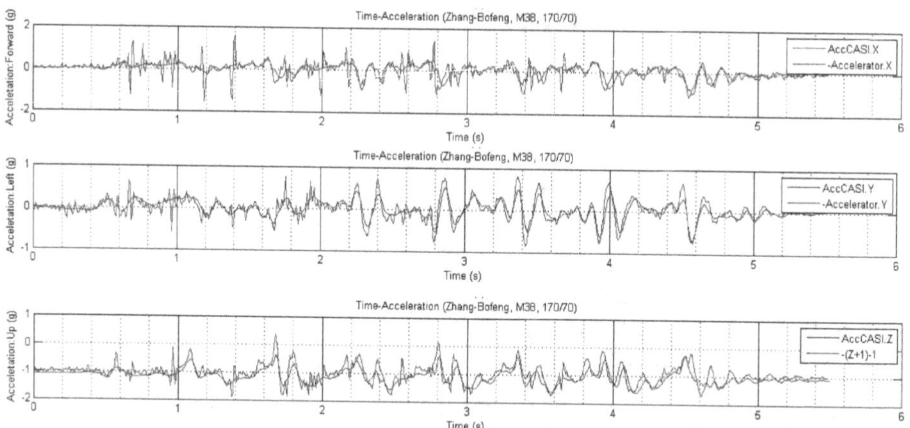

Fig. 16. The result of aligning motion data and acceleration data

3.5 Data reduction

Data reduction techniques can be used to obtain a reduced representation of the data while minimizing the loss of information content. To obtain a reduced representation of the data set, such as speed, average span, frequency, and so on, data reduction techniques can be applied, for examples, aggregation operations and conception hierarchy generation. We propose a hierarchical structure shown in Fig. 17.

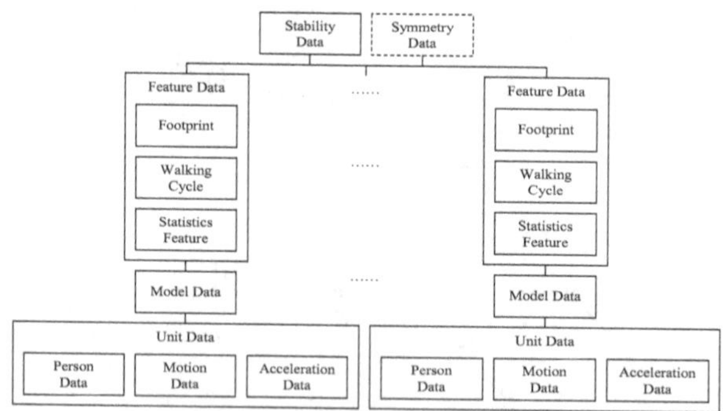

Fig. 17. The hierarchical structure of walking data

4. Walking stability analysis

Although there is now a wealth of literature pertaining to the maintenance of stability when standing, there is a relative paucity of information regarding the biomechanics and physiology of walking stability. Various models are currently in development, but a unified model of walking stability does not exist yet. Unlike standing, the balance of walking is a kind of dynamic balance (Menz, 2000).

Standard deviation is used to define the variability or randomness of the walking pattern. Less the amount of variability means better neuromuscular control and walking stability. We extract a set of hierarchical features from FL model, such as walking cycle features, footprint features.

4.1 Footprint stability

Footprint analysis is a typical method of walking research as shown in Fig. 18.

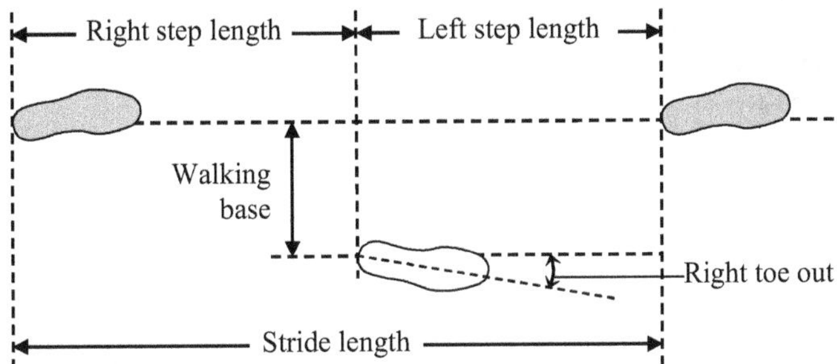

Fig. 18. Features of footprint stability

4.1.1 Definition of footprint stability

DEFINITION 2. (Footprint Stability) Footprint stability is described by the variability of the footprint stability features. We extract some of the stability features of footprint F_S *(F)*, such as the variability of cycle time f1, left step length f2, right step length f3, speed f4, walking base f5, left toe out f6, and right toe out f7, as shown in Equation (8).

$$F_S(F) = \sum_{i=1}^{7} \delta(f_i) / \mu(f_i) \tag{8}$$

where $\delta(f_i)$ is the standard deviation of the feature f_i, and $\mu(f_i)$ is the mathematical expectation of the feature f_i.

4.1.2 Effects of aging on footprint stability

Now, the variability of the footprint features per decade of age is calculated, as shown in Table 1.

The footprint variability in last row of Table 1 is sum of the above items. It can be seen that the variability is increasing with the age, see Fig. 19. That is to say, the footprint stability is declined with the age, and especially there is a dramatic increasing over 50 years old. But the twenties are exceptional, maybe because the twenties walk more springily than the elders.

Age	20+	30+	40+	50+	60+
CycleTime	0.0437	0.0293	0.0333	0.0464	0.0716
LStepLength	0.0825	0.0779	0.0568	0.0766	0.0811
RStepLength	0.0645	0.0790	0.1099	0.0586	0.0645
Speed	0.0833	0.0736	0.0819	0.0709	0.0880
WalkingBase	0.1783	0.1721	0.1495	0.1269	0.1343
LToeOut	0.4047	0.1579	0.2407	0.2383	1.3606
RToeOut	0.3246	0.2175	0.3473	0.5013	1.0242
$F_S(F)$	1.1817	0.8073	1.0195	1.1190	2.8243

Table 1. Variability of footprint features

4.2 Cycle stability

The gait cycle is defined as the time interval between two successive occurrences of one of the repetitive events of walking. The detection of the human gait period can provide important information to determine the positions of the human body.

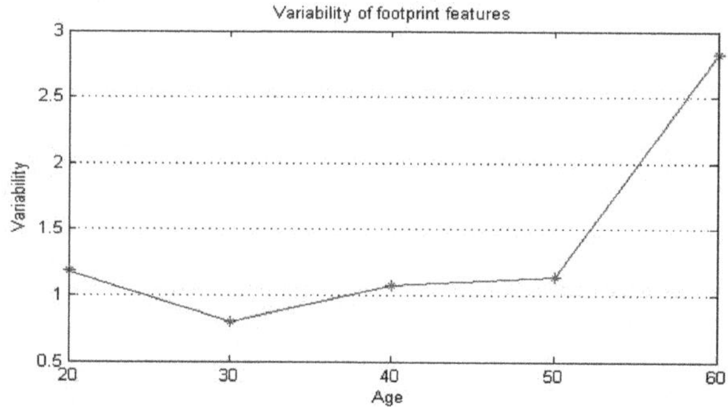

Fig. 19. Footprint stability with age

4.2.1 Definition of cycle stability

DEFINITION 3. (Cycle Stability) Cycle stability is described by the variability of the cycle stability features. The cycle stability $F_S(C)$ is defined as Equation (9).

$$F_S(C) = \sum_{i=1}^{7} \delta(c_i) / \mu(f_4) \tag{9}$$

where $\delta(c_i)$ is the standard deviation of the time when event i occurs, c_i = {LTO, LFA, LTV, LIC, RTO, RFA, RTV}, and $\mu(f_4)$ is the mathematical expectation of the speed f_4.

Generally, 7 events are used to identify major events during the walking cycle (Whittle, 2007). For the symmetry of left side and right side, 10 events are employed in this paper, as shown in Fig. 20.

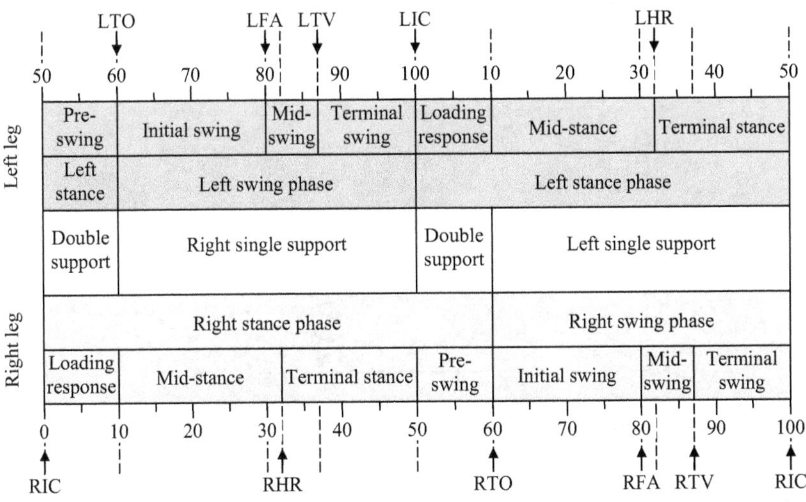

Fig. 20. Walking cycle in normal gait

Such as
RIC = right foot initial contact;
LTO = left toe off;
LFA = left foot adjacent to right foot;
RHR = right heel rise;
LTV = left tibia vertical;
LIC = left foot initial contact;
RTO = right toe off;
RFA = right foot adjacent to left foot;
LHR = left heel rise;
RTV = right tibia vertical.

4.2.2 Effects of aging on cycle stability

Table 2 shows the variability of walking cycle features per decade of age.

Age	20+	30+	40+	50+	60+
RIC	0.0000	0.0000	0.0000	0.0000	0.0000
LTO	1.6664	1.2287	1.2272	0.9334	1.2268
LFA	1.2846	1.7323	1.3302	1.0199	1.1198
LTV	1.6354	1.8543	1.4046	1.2759	0.9008
LIC	1.2822	1.0320	1.0900	0.9751	0.7036
RTO	1.3563	1.2323	1.2866	0.7376	0.8605
RFA	0.9731	1.3764	1.4480	1.0737	0.8847
RTV	1.0459	1.2067	1.3846	1.3705	1.0909
$F_S(C)$	9.2440	9.6627	9.1713	7.3861	6.7870

Table 2. Variability of walking cycle features

Fig. 21 shows that the cycle variability is declined with the age almost. This is not same as a common assumption. The reason is that the elder walking more rigidly and inflexibly.

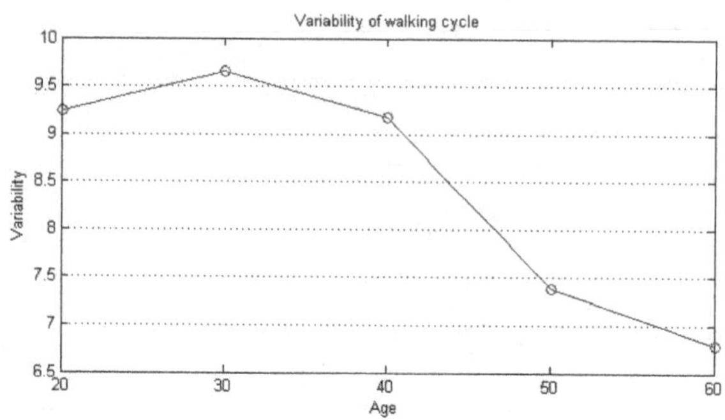

Fig. 21. Cycle stability with age

4.3 Orbital stability

Orbital stability defines how purely periodic systems respond to small perturbations discretely after one complete cycle (i.e. one stride) and may be better suited to study strongly periodic movements like walking (Marin, 2006).

4.3.1 Definition of orbital stability

DEFINITION 4. (Orbital Stability) Orbital stability is described by the variability of the orbital stability features. The orbital stability $F_S(O)$ of lower limbs is composed of three parts, position stability $F_S(P)$, segment stability $F_S(S)$ and Joint stability $F_S(J)$, as shown in Equation (10).

$$F_S(O) = F_S(P) + F_S(S) + F_S(J) \tag{10}$$

where position stability $F_S(P)$ is defined by standard deviation of the maximums and minimums of displacement, velocity and acceleration (knees, heels, and toes), as shown in Equation (11).

$$\begin{aligned} F_S(P) = &\delta[\vee(p_i(Z))] + \delta[\vee(v_i(Z))] + \delta[\vee(A_i(Z))] \\ &+\delta[\wedge(p_i(Z))] + \delta[\wedge(v_i(Z))] + \delta[\wedge(A_i(Z))] \\ &(i = 1 \sim 4,7,8) \end{aligned} \tag{11}$$

$\vee(x)$ and $\wedge(x)$ are the maximum and minimum value of x respectively.

Segment stability $F_S(S)$ is defined by standard deviation of the maximums and minimums of segment angle, angular velocity and angular acceleration (thighs, shanks and feet), as shown in Equation (12).

$$\begin{aligned} F_S(S) = &\delta[\vee(\varphi_i(Z))] + \delta[\vee(\omega_{\varphi i}(Z))] + \delta[\vee(\alpha_{\varphi i}(Z))] \\ &+\delta[\wedge(\varphi_i(Z))] + \delta[\wedge(\omega_{\varphi i}(Z))] + \delta[\wedge(\alpha_{\varphi i}(Z))] \\ &(i = 9 \sim 14) \end{aligned} \tag{12}$$

Joint stability $F_S(J)$ is defined by standard deviation of the maximums and minimums of displacement, velocity and acceleration (hips, knees and ankles), as shown in Equation (13).

$$\begin{aligned} F_S(J) &= \delta[\vee(\theta_i(Z))] + \delta[\vee(\omega_{\theta i}(Z))] + \delta[\vee(\alpha_{\theta i}(Z))] \\ &+ \delta[\wedge(\theta_i(Z))] + \delta[\wedge(\omega_{\theta i}(Z))] + \delta[\wedge(\alpha_{\theta i}(Z))] \\ &(i = 7 \sim 12) \end{aligned} \tag{13}$$

Thus, the orbital stability of lower limbs includes 108 indexes. For examples, Fig.22 and Fig. 23 show the joint angles of hips (θ_7, θ_8), knees (θ_9, θ_{10}) and ankles (θ_{11}, θ_{12}) in sagittal plane during a single walking cycle, their angular velocity ($\omega_{\theta 9}$, $\omega_{\theta 10}$, $\omega_{\theta 11}$, $\omega_{\theta 12}$) and angular acceleration ($a_{\theta 9}$, $a_{\theta 10}$, $a_{\theta 11}$, $a_{\theta 12}$) respectively.

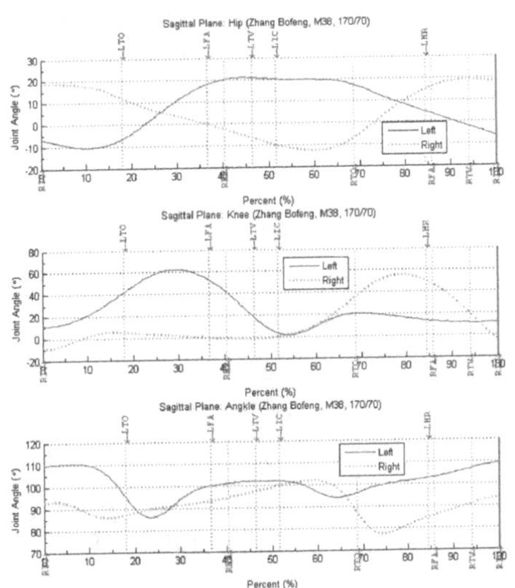

Fig. 22. Joint angles

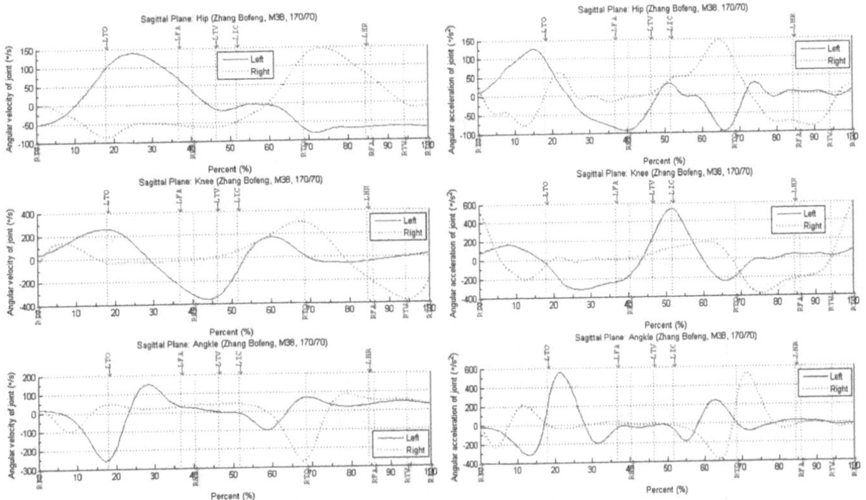

Fig. 23. Angular velocity and acceleration of joint

4.3.2 Outlier analysis in orbital stability

Because of the errors of computing, maybe there are few outliers in the features of orbital stability. For an example, the last 3 cycles of the displacement of right hip (p10) at vertical is shown in Fig. 25. There is an outlier in the last cycle, the left maximum point should be found instead of the right maximum point.

There are a variety of outlier detection approaches from several areas, including statistics, machine learning, and data mining. A kind of proximity-based outlier detection approach, called distance to k-nearest neighbor, is used to find the outliers in orbital stability. This approach is more general and more easily applied than statistical approached, since it is easier to determine a meaningful proximity measure for a data set than to determine its statistics distribution.

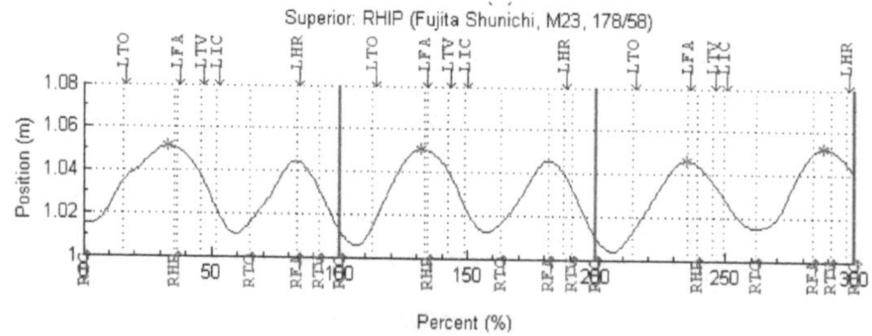

Fig. 24. Last 3 cycles of the displacement of right hip (p10) at vertical

Fig. 25 shows the outliers in the displacement of right hip (p10). The points with a circle are the outlier point. The outlier score of an object is given by the distance to its k-nearest neighbor, using a value of k = 5.

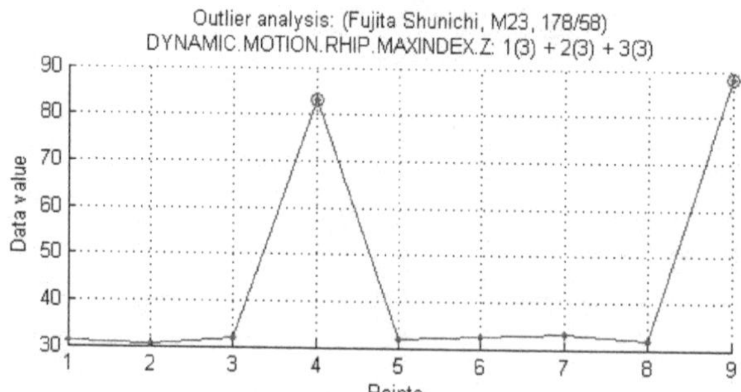

Fig. 25. Outliers in the displacement of right hip

4.3.3 Effects of aging on orbital stability

After analysis all subjects between 20 to 70 years old, the item results of orbital stability are shown in Fig. 26. The position stability $F_S(P)$, segment stability $F_S(S)$, joint stability $F_S(J)$ and the whole orbital stability are in shown in Fig. 27. It is observed that, although each of orbital variability does not increase strictly with age, the variability of orbital features increases with age generally. As persons grow old, the orbital stability is becoming weakly.

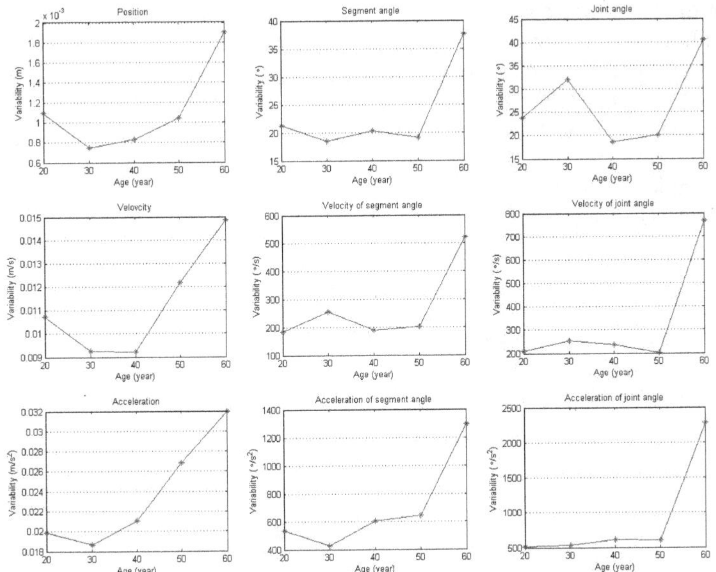

Fig. 26. Each item of orbital stability with age

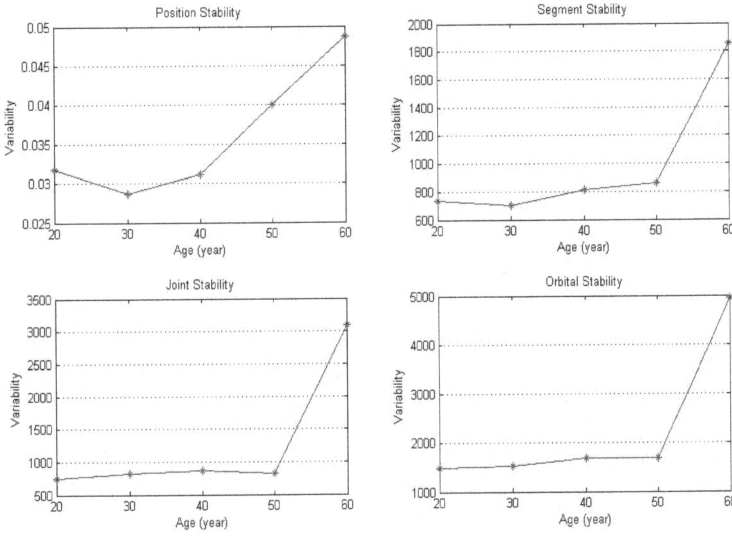

Fig. 27. Position stability, segment stability and joint stability, and orbital stability with age

4.4 Dynamic stability based on dynamic time warping (DTW)

Dynamic stability is the main reason for leading to falls for people, especially for elders. This section discusses age influence on dynamic stability based on dynamic time warping.

4.4.1 Definition of dynamic stability

Subject's walking is one kind of periodic movements and the same events will happen during different walking cycles, so the similarity of the data between adjacent cycles to assess subject's walking stability.

This paper used dynamic time warping (DTW) to calculate this similarity, which is a method for flexible pattern-matching scheme. It translates, compress and expands a pair of patterns so similar features within the two patterns are matched (Li, 2003). Fig. 28 and Equation (14) show details.

$$D(S_i) = \frac{\sum_{j=1}^{n-1} DTW(\theta_j, \theta_{j+1})}{n-1} (n > 1) \tag{14}$$

where D is the number of walking cycles, $D(S_i)$ is the average of similarity at feature S_i.

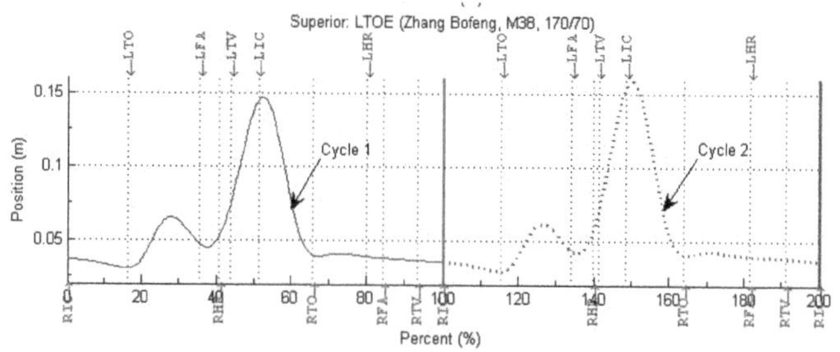

(a) The source data of left toe at superior

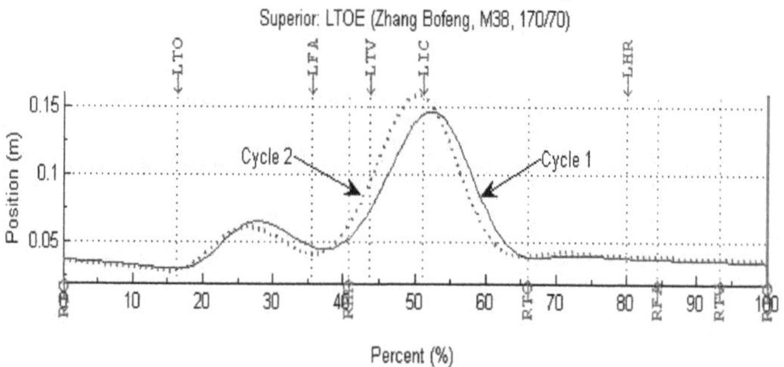

(b) Compare between two adjacent cycles

Fig. 28. Similarity between two adjacent cycles by DTW

4.4.2 Extracting of dynamic stability features

According to FL model, it's easy to get corresponding position, velocity and acceleration motion data of 19 points. Therefore, 19×3=57 features are extracted to describe human dynamic stability.

4.4.3 Effects of aging on dynamic stability

Equation (15) calculates the sum of single feature value by age.

$$S(A_k, S_i) = \frac{1}{m \times l_k} \sum_{j=1}^{m} D_j(S_i) \tag{15}$$

where m is the number of subjects in the same age class, l_k is the average leg length of subjects in the same age class, $D_j(S_i)$ is similarity value of the selected feature i by Equation (14), is a single stability value of the same feature i in the same age class A_k, and k is the number of age class.

According to Equation (14), similarity value of all selected features in the same age group was calculated by age.

$$F(A_k) = \sum_{i=1}^{p} S(A_k, S_i) \tag{16}$$

where p is the number of features, in this case, p is equal to 32, and k is equal to 5.

Fig. 29 shows trend on the change of dynamic stability.

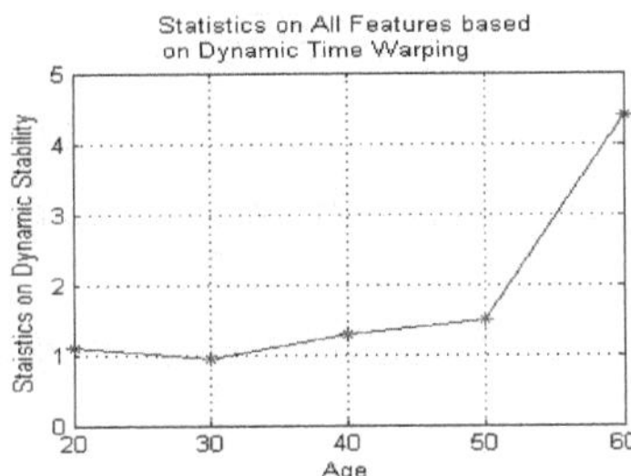

Fig. 29. Statistic on stability of all dynamic features

This figure tells us that if all dynamic features are employed to do statistics on such kind of stability, the dynamic stability is decreasing with ageing except the twenties. It seems that all of those features are desirable.

4.5 Feature selection on dynamic stability

The previous section did statistic on all 57 dynamic stability. To reduce the computational complexity, and more importantly, to get more important and contributing features, this paper did feature selection on those 57 dynamic features. On the one hand, it could simplify the method of data acquisition; On the other hand, it is more persuasive by analyzing those selected features.

This section ties to find the best features reflecting the relationship between age and walking stability among those 57 ones, which include 2^{57}-1 different kinds of feature combination. A classic method of feature selection, which is the cooperation of adaptive genetic algorithm and support vector machine, was used to do it.

4.5.1 Improved crossover operation

In order to avoid that better solutions with high fitness disappear in a standard genetic algorithm although the algorithm is accommodated again and again. This paper proposed a formulation to adjust crossover probability (p_c) between average fitness and maximum fitness, as shown in Equation (17).

$$p_c^i = \begin{cases} p_c^{i-1} * \dfrac{f' - f_{avg}}{f_{\max} - f_{avg}}, f' \geq f_{avg} \\ p_c^{i-1} * \dfrac{f_{avg} - f'}{f_{\max} - f_{avg}}, f' \prec f_{avg} \end{cases} \quad (17)$$

where f_{max} is the maximum fitness of current population, f_{avg} is the average fitness of current population, f' is the larger fitness between two individuals in crossover operation.

4.5.2 Improved mutation operation

Just as crossover operation, there are the same problems with mutation operation.
If probability of mutation (p_m) is undersize, new individual can't be generated easily, inversely, genetic algorithm will be a pure searching process.
To solve this problem, this paper improved it as shown in Equation (18).

$$p_m^i = \begin{cases} p_m^{i-1} * \dfrac{f - f_{avg}}{f_{\max} - f_{avg}}, f \geq f_{avg} \\ p_m^{i-1} * \dfrac{f_{avg} - f}{f_{\max} - f_{avg}}, f \prec f_{avg} \end{cases} \quad (18)$$

where f is the fitness of individual going to mutate. All other parameters have the same meaning as Equation (17).

4.5.3 Improved support vector machine (SVM)

According to information of age classification, SVM was used to separate datasets and assess fitness of specific feature combination during feature selection. This paper improves SVM in two parts: classification balancing and evaluation.
A conventional SVM is to build a decision function $f_c(x)$ for each class C. Then use Equation (19) as the predicted class label.

$$d(x) = \arg\max(f_c(x)) \quad (19)$$

However, this equation may fail to work in some skewed inseparable distribution. Therefore, it's improved as Equation (20), which suggests a function $p_c(f)$ to balance values of $f_c(x)$ in Equation (19).

$$d(x) = \arg\max(p_c(f_c(x))) \quad (20)$$

Another problem is about evaluation. Generally, correctness is calculated by *correctNumber/totalNumber*, but it does not fit well to skewed distributions. It's improved as Equation (21) described.

$$F(M,b,\vec{w}) = 1 - (1-b) \times \sum_{i=1}^{n} \frac{e_i}{m} - U \quad (21)$$

$$U = \begin{cases} 0, & \sum_{i=1}^{n} e_i = 0 \\ b \times \dfrac{\max\limits_{0 \le i \le n} \dfrac{e_i w_i}{c_i}}{\max\limits_{0 \le i \le n} w_i} \times \dfrac{\sum_{i=1}^{n} \left| \dfrac{e_i w_i}{c_i} - \varsigma \right|}{n\varsigma}, & otherwise \end{cases}$$

where M is the confusion matrix, b is a coefficient that balances the total correctness and the balance achievement, $\bar{w}$ is the importance weight between classes, n is the number of classes, e_i is the sum of non-diagonal entries of i-th row of M, m is the sum of all entries of M, namely total number of patterns, $\sum_{i=1}^{n} w_i = n$, ς is the average value of $e_i w_i / c_i$.

4.5.4 Selected stable features

After 18 generations of GA, 32 walking stability features were selected with classification correctness from 89.4% to 94.7%.

To compare number of markers between before and after feature selection, those 32 features are marked with 14 red markers, as shown in Fig. 30. It means that there is (30-14)/30=53.3% reduction on markers, which could simplify equipment to a large extent.

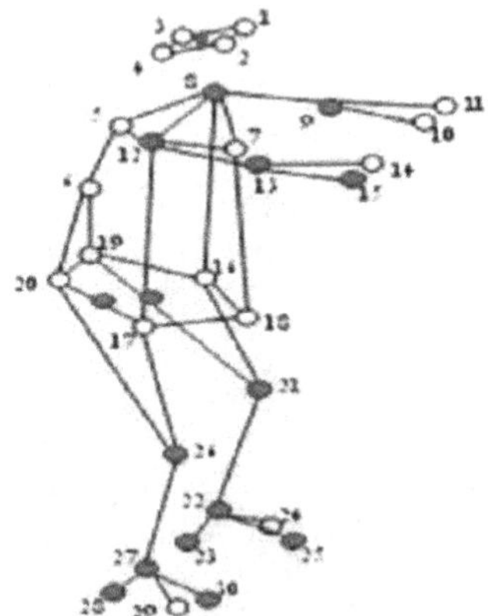

Fig. 30. Red markers corresponding to selected features

4.5.5 Effects of aging on dynamic stability after feature selection

Fig. 30 told us that the selected markers are almost symmetrical. To increase the symmetry, other three features are added, such as LHIP in position, RELB in velocity, RSHO and LELB in acceleration. Table 3 shows these fours features with gray background in details.

The difference between this method and previous one is the number of dynamic features. Therefore, the same statistic method will be applied on this one. Another, the similarity calculated by DTW is used to assess the stability of specific dynamic feature. Because DTW doesn't care about the data unite, all features from position, velocity and acceleration will be counted together.

Age	20+	30+	40+	50+	60+
Position					
LHIP	0.0001	0.0000	0.0001	0.0001	0.0003
RHIP	0.0001	0.0001	0.0001	0.0001	0.0003
CENT	0.0001	0.0000	0.0001	0.0001	0.0003
LKNE	0.0002	0.0005	0.0001	0.0006	0.0003
RKNE	0.0002	0.0002	0.0001	0.0004	0.0013
LANK	0.0012	0.0010	0.0001	0.0001	0.0009
RANK	0.0013	0.0006	0.0001	0.0001	0.0005
LHEE	0.0028	0.0027	0.0001	0.0002	0.0013
RHEE	0.0027	0.0018	0.0000	0.0001	0.0011
LTOE	0.0004	0.0001	0.0001	0.0001	0.0002
RTOE	0.0004	0.0002	0.0001	0.0001	0.0002
Velocity					
LELB	0.0125	0.0023	0.0122	0.0046	0.0055
RELB	0.0111	0.0030	0.0080	0.0039	0.0055
CENT	0.0021	0.0009	0.0016	0.0018	0.0024
LKNE	0.0109	0.0077	0.0038	0.0035	0.0066
RKNE	0.0109	0.0076	0.0024	0.0034	0.0054
LANK	0.0563	0.0405	0.0088	0.0091	0.0495
RANK	0.0678	0.0318	0.0594	0.0062	0.1520
LHEE	0.1522	0.1369	0.0055	0.0200	0.0775
RHEE	0.1447	0.0892	0.0073	0.0847	0.0662
LTOE	0.0336	0.0135	0.0067	0.0079	0.0158
RTOE	0.0400	0.0201	0.0129	0.0569	0.0204
Acceleration					
LSHO	0.0071	0.0030	0.0041	0.0061	0.0037
RSHO	0.0071	0.0033	0.0047	0.0054	0.0035
NECK	0.0062	0.0028	0.0038	0.0051	0.0031
LELB	0.0162	0.0046	0.0230	0.0080	0.0069
RELB	0.0137	0.0045	0.0094	0.0080	0.0077
CENT	0.0059	0.0029	0.0054	0.0349	0.0449
LKNE	0.0293	0.0179	0.0214	0.0119	0.0161
RKNE	0.0299	0.0187	0.0095	0.0136	0.0204
LANK	0.0765	0.0505	0.0342	0.0432	0.0562
RANK	0.0915	0.0544	0.4998	0.0270	2.2505
LHEE	0.1604	0.1196	0.0812	0.0901	0.0887
RHEE	0.1662	0.1154	0.0477	0.2507	0.0980
LTOE	0.1567	0.0687	0.0274	0.2517	0.0965
RTOE	0.2266	0.1225	0.0816	0.2483	0.1541
$F(A_k)$	**1.5449**	**0.9497**	**1.0028**	**1.0980**	**3.2639**

Table 3. Selected features in three types

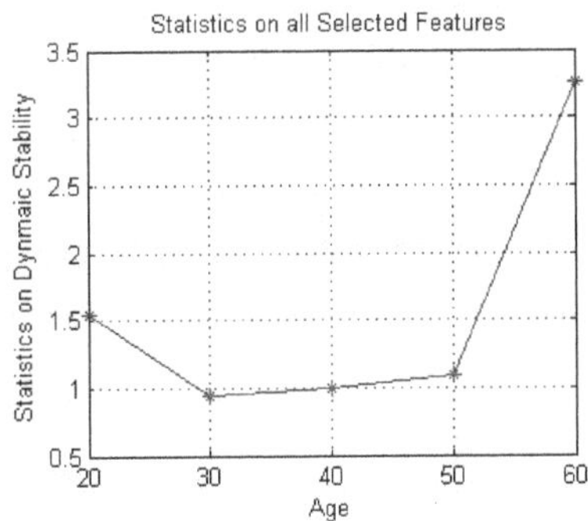

Fig. 31. Statistic on stability of selected dynamic features

As a response to the assumption that elder the person is, less stable his gait is. This method assesses walking stability by searching the best contributing features and doing statistics on them. The result shows that walking stability truly becomes worse as ageing except the group of twenties.

5. Walking symmetry analysis

Gait symmetry analysis is a part of normal gait analysis. Our research is based on the Fourteen-Linkage Walking Model of human. The detail of this model can be seen in chapter 2. We all know, gait symmetry reflects the general characteristics of human walk gait, and it is an important indicator to assess the function of the human walk. Especially in the human aging process the recession of brain and central nervous system and physiological function will affect the lower limb gait of left or right side, and lead gait mutation.

5.1 Footprint symmetry

Here, we mainly aim to investigate the footprint properties of the left and right foot. See Fig.32, the symmetric properties were step length and toe out angle of two feet.

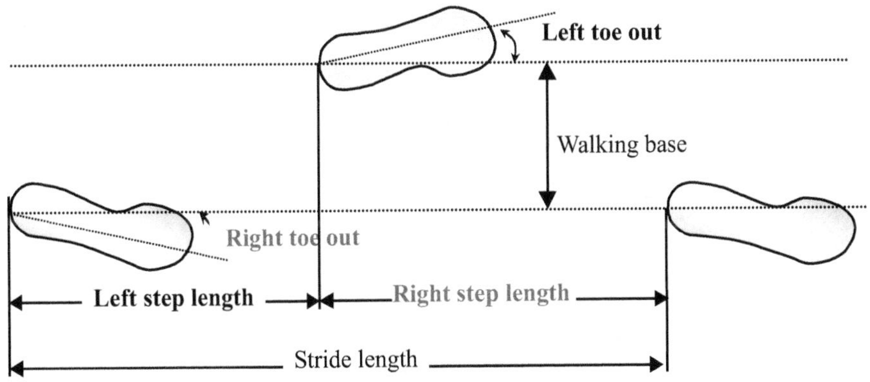

Fig. 32. Features of footprint for symmetry analysis

Besides step length and toe out angle, we also consider step factor and walk ratio.
Step factor is the value of step length divided by leg length.
Walk ratio is the value of step length divided by step rate and step rate is the number of steps per minute someone walks.

5.1.1 Definition of footprint symmetry

DEFINITION 5. (Footprint Symmetry) Footprint symmetry is described by the difference of the bilateral footprint features. We extract some symmetrical features of footprint as *S(F)*, which contains the difference of Step length about two feet, the difference of Toe out angle of right foot and left foot, the difference of bilateral Step factor and the difference of bilateral Walk ratio, as shown in Equation (22).

$$S(F) = \sum_{i=1}^{4} | \delta(LA_i) / \mu(LA_i) - \delta(RA_i) / \mu(RA_i) | \tag{22}$$

Here $\delta(A_i)$ is the standard deviation of the feature A_i, and $\mu(A_i)$ is the mathematical expectation of the feature A_i. A_i is the element of {LStepLength, RStepLength; LToeout, RToeout; LStepFactor, RStepFactor; LWalkRatio, RWalkRatio}.
The δ/μ of footprint bilateral features per decade of age is calculated, shown as the upper part in Table 4. The last row of Table 4 is the *S(F)* of above items.

5.1.2 Effects of aging on footprint symmetry

It can be seen that the variation of footprint feature is mostly less than 0.02 excepted on feature *Toeout* as shown in Fig. 33.

Age	20+	30+	40+	50+	60+
S(StepLength)	0.01818	0.00865	0.00238	0.01286	0.00210
S(Toeout)	0.01660	0.04051	0.04079	0.16155	0.05628
S(StepFactor)	0.01803	0.00859	0.00247	0.01157	0.00298
S(WalkRatio)	0.00814	0.01854	0.00939	0.00293	0.00638
S(F)	**0.06095**	**0.0763**	**0.05504**	**0.18892**	**0.06774**

Table 4. Variation of footprint features

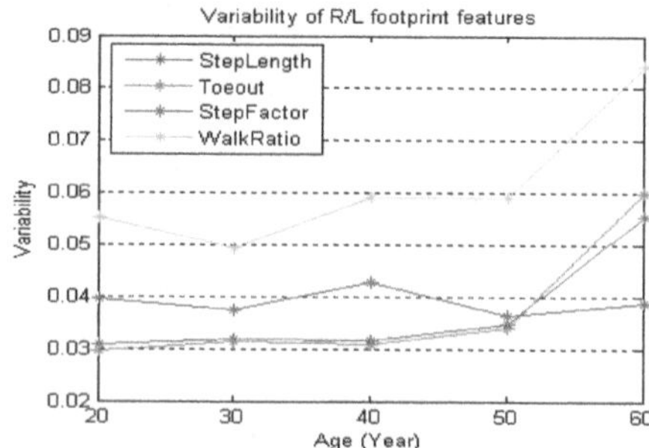

Fig. 33. Variation of footprint features

5.2 Cycle symmetry

This section shows the main characteristics of the symmetry of the gait cycles. As movement of two legs turns symmetrically, the ten tags of walking cycle (see Fig. 20) in fact is a symmetrical composition of 5 keywords in one side, they are TO, FA, TV, IC, HR.

5.2.1 Definition of cycle symmetry

DEFINITION 6. (Cycle Symmetry) Cycle symmetry is described by the variability of the cycle symmetric features. The cycle symmetry $S(C)$ is defined as Equation (23).

$$\mathbf{S(C)} = \sum_{i=1}^{4} \left| \delta(LC_i) / \mu(LC_i) - \delta(RC_i) / \mu(RC_i) \right| / \mu(S_i) \tag{23}$$

Here $\delta(C_i)$ is the standard deviation of the feature C_i and $\mu(C_i)$ is its mathematical expectation, and $\mu(S_i)$ is the mathematical expectation of the feature Speed. LC_i or RC_i is the element of {LTO, RTO; LHR, RHR; LFA, RFA; LTV, RTV}. Since the use of the relative value of sagittal plane, so the IC in here is meaningless.

5.2.2 Effects of aging on cycle symmetry

Here described left and right foot gait cycle symmetrical properties change with aging groups. We calculated the δ/μ on average speed of every decade of age, as shown in Table 5.

Age	20+	30+	40+	50+	60+
S(TO)	*0.05567*	*0.10183*	*0.04917*	*0.03336*	*0.05064*
S(FA)	*0.01323*	*0.01264*	*0.0179*	*0.01706*	*0.01161*
S(HR)	*0.03106*	*0.01222*	*0.03407*	*0.01832*	*0.02689*
S(TV)	*0.00201*	*0.03435*	*0.01366*	*0.01486*	*0.00648*
S(C)	**0.10198**	**0.16104**	**0.11479**	**0.08359**	**0.09562**

Table 5. Variation of cycle features

Also the last line of Table 5 is the different value of feet around the corresponding cycle time points. It can be seen that the variation of cycle feature of every group is less 0.20, but the variety has no obvious trend as shown in Fig. 34.

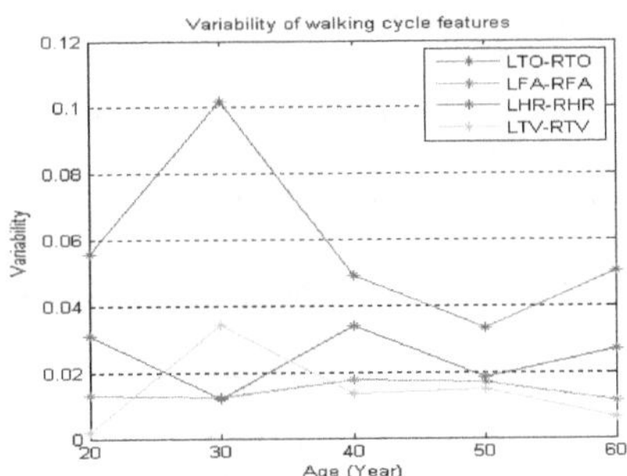

Fig. 34. Variation of cycle feature

5.3 Orbital symmetry

Orbital symmetry is described by the variability of the locus of symmetric points of body, in particular in the sagittal plane. Before doing calculation, we must do some adjustment about

dynamic data of right side and left side. Adjustment method is to move the left side data ahead about half stride cycle. That is, we let the LIC to match the RIC. The first removal data may put to last part according to stride cycle, or be doffed and then we got three steps bilateral data.
It is clearly that selected features of symmetry may as indicators for evaluation of a person's gait. According to our work, the indices of motion data may be an immediate measure for quantification dynamic gait symmetry. The indices of up-body even the arm can be used as a factor to qualify the symmetry of human walking. The symmetry of gait should include footprint, cycle and dynamic data.
Normal walking does not need consider anything, but walking is very complex control, including central command, physical balance and coordination control, involving segments about feet, ankle, knee, hip, torso, neck, shoulder, arm and joint coordination. Any aspect of the disorder may affect gait symmetry, and some abnormalities may be compensatory or conceal. Pathological gait is often characterized by asymmetry, the selected frequencies of the movements of the limbs may deviate considerably from their eigenfrequencies and symmetry may be abandoned (Murray, 1967).

5.4 Dynamic symmetry based on dynamic time warping

In theory, the dynamic symmetry of gait is described by the properties which dynamic changed. These dynamic properties consist of three parts: position point symmetry, segment angle symmetry and joints angle symmetry.

5.4.1 Definition of dynamic symmetry

Theoretically, dynamic symmetry is described by the variability of the walking symmetric bilateral features. The dynamic symmetry is also composed of three parts, position symmetry *S(Mo)*, segment symmetry *S(SA)* and Joint symmetry *S(JA)*, as Equation (24).

$$S(D) = S(Mo) + S(SA) + S(JA) \tag{24}$$

Here, $S(Mo) = \sum_{i=1}^{8}\Delta\left(LP(t)_i, RP(t)_i\right)$, $S(SA) = \sum_{i=1}^{5}\Delta\left(L\Phi(t)_i, R\Phi(t)_i\right)$, $S(JA) = \sum_{i=1}^{5}\Delta\left(L\Theta(t)_i, R\Theta(t)_i\right)$.

And LP(t)∈{ p1, p3, p5, p7, p9, p13, p15, p17 }, RP(t)∈{ p2, p4, p6, p8, p10, p14, p16, p18 }, LΦ(t)∈{ φ3, φ5, φ9, φ11, φ13 }, RΦ(t)∈{ φ4, φ6, φ10, φ12, φ14 }, LΘ(t)∈{ θ3, θ5, θ7, θ9, θ11 }, RΘ(t)∈{ θ4, θ6, θ8, θ10, θ12 }.
The symbol *Δ* in the formulas will be described in next section. It is the DTW algorithm used to calculate the distance of two sequences with different length of them. Here consider all the symmetry properties included on upper body and lower body is want given the general definition of gait dynamic symmetry.
Considering 3-dimension, add $d=\{x, y, z\}$ to Equation (24), then we got Equation (25).

$$S_d(D) = S_d(Mo) + S_d(SA) + S_d(JA) \tag{25}$$

Here *Mo* means motion data which has 8 attributes, *SA* means Segment Angle data and *JA* means Joint Angle data, they both have 5 attributes. There is a total of 18 attributes.
Actually, we use the index like $S_x(Mo)$, $S_y(Mo)$, $S_z(Mo)$ and $S_x(SA)$, $S_y(SA)$, $S_z(SA)$ and $S_x(JA)$, $S_y(JA)$, $S_z(JA)$, not the $S_d(D)$.
The dynamic walking symmetry also has velocity and acceleration data. We got attributes as follow: $VMo \subset V(t)$, $VSA \subset \Omega\Phi(t)$, $VJA \subset \Omega\Theta(t)$, $AMo \subset A(t)$, $ASA \subset \Lambda\Phi(t)$, $AJA \subset \Lambda\Theta(t)$.
Then, we also can do calculation with three velocity equations.

Similarly, it can easily be listed out three acceleration formulas. Thus, we have three sets of attributes, each containing 18 attributes. So, considering three directions, the dynamic symmetry may include 3×18×3=162 indexes.

5.4.2 Effects of aging on dynamic symmetry

We use DTW algorithm to calculate the discrepancy between right data and left data on all attributes of all tested persons. The example of calculated result is shown as Fig. 35. We can see that somebody was more asymmetry than others on this attribute, for example number 2 and number 11 in Z direction.

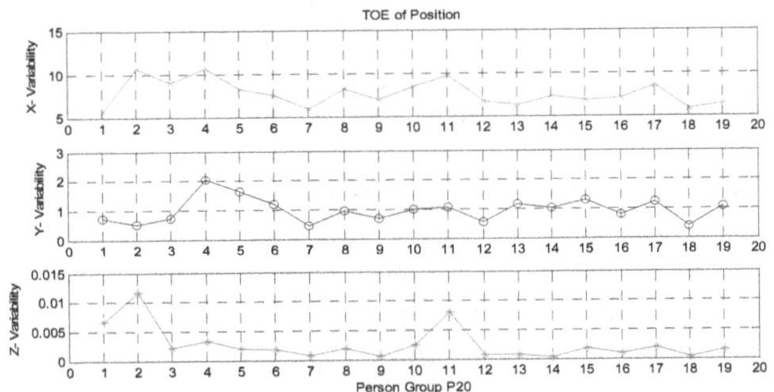

Fig. 35. Example of calculated result on one attribute

A total of 162 attribute needs for a similar calculation, to get the related discrepant values like Fig. 35. These results were used to do statistical analysis about gait symmetry.

5.5 Feature selection on dynamic symmetry

The dynamic symmetry is concerned with some direction features more meaningfully. Also some features did not reflect out gait characteristics goodly. Therefore, it is necessary in a large number of features to make a choice.

The existing gait symmetry indicators more used in accordance with the swing phase and stance phase, then neglected bilateral discrepancy of these phase while them were divided from cycles, thereby reducing the sensitivity of indicators.

We analyzed all results of the calculations and found that the dynamic symmetry is concerned with some direction indicators more meaningfully. Also some indicators did not reflect out gait characteristics goodly. Therefore, it is necessary in a large number of indicators to make a choice. In other words, it must do some feature selection.

Human walking is a complex procedure with both limb position variability and limb motion. When quantifying symmetry of walking gait, the used parameters and calculations should be chosen carefully (Karaharju-Huisnan, 2001)

5.5.1 Selected symmetric features

Although the tested persons are all healthy and walking with normal gait, but the individual may have a great difference in gait symmetry. So the general average method may result in larger bias, then it can think over use standard deviation.

Consider the three dimensional direction respectively, the gait symmetry data can available in three matrices. Then the rows of the matrix are the various attributes, and columns correspond

to the tested persons of gait symmetry data. In this way we get three 54×n matrices and n is person number. The original data come from the calculation results of bilateral discrepancy about symmetric attributes, and the calculation method was described in above sections.
For every attribute, that is the row of the matrix here, it can use the function *fa* to calculate the minimal rate of discrepant value.

$$fa = \frac{\bar{A} - A_{\min}}{A_{\max} - A_{\min}} \tag{26}$$

Here A also expresses the discrepant value on attribute A of all persons. So $\bar{A}$ is the average value of all tested persons on attribute A, the A_{min} is the minimum value of the row, and the A_{max} is the maximum value evidently.
It is clear, attribute A is the element of the set which includes all symmetric attributes about 8 position items, 5 segment angle items, 5 joint angle items and their velocity and acceleration data.
The following table shows the comparable rates on Z direction, or namely sagittal direction.

	SHO	ELB	WRI	HIP	KNE	ANK	HEE	TOE
Mo	0.166	0.157	**0.030**	**0.033**	0.113	**0.073**	0.151	0.180
VMo	0.408	0.177	**0.059**	**0.029**	0.453	**0.063**	0.289	0.292
AMo	0.266	0.305	**0.042**	**0.024**	0.262	**0.046**	0.292	0.176

Table 6. Position attributes with velocity and acceleration

	UPPERAR	FOREAR	THIGH	SHANK	FOOT
SA	0.191	**0.048**	**0.034**	**0.079**	0.132
VSA	0.147	0.109	**0.038**	**0.046**	0.225
ASA	0.220	**0.043**	**0.039**	**0.032**	0.168

Table 7. Segment angle attributes with velocity and acceleration

	SHOULDER	ELBOW	HIP	KNEE	ANKLE
JA	0.213	0.124	**0.031**	0.144	0.109
VJA	0.172	0.280	0.133	**0.069**	0.247
AJA	**0.046**	**0.042**	**0.037**	**0.048**	**0.031**

Table 8. Joint angle attributes with velocity and acceleration

There are 24 attributes in Table 6 to Table 8, and their rate less than 0.1 (see bold). In other words, these attributes have expressed better gait symmetry in this database. Also it can do same work on other two directions.
These attributes can be selected out for future testing a person whether or not symmetrical of his gait.

5.5.2 Clustering on symmetry features for classification

We use dynamic time warping (DTW) algorithm to calculate the similarity between bilateral symmetric attributes. Consider the three dimensional direction respectively, the gait symmetry data can available in three matrices. Then the rows of the matrix are the various attributes, and columns correspond to the tested persons of gait symmetry data. In this way we get three 54xn matrices (assumed we have n valid test persons). The matrices data come from the calculation results of bilateral discrepancy about symmetric attributes.

Now we plan to do some clustering analysis, we need an algorithm which is no high cost on machine, but better on efficiency. Since there is a lot of clustering algorithms, for the sake of quickly carry out research and obtain some results, we have chosen the affinity propagation clustering algorithm APCLUSTER (Frey & Dueck, 2007). The reason for using this algorithm is that it not only can do clustering on data but also can pass the original information rather than random values into the clustering processing, and meanwhile the algorithm has good performance and efficiency.

Using the APCLUSTER algorithm, we have done all the attributes clustering analysis in collusion with age or height or weight and so on. But in order to facilitate description, the following example is mainly discussed on age and gait symmetric data of sagittal direction. In addition, here we had 48 valid test objects, that is to say n=48.

Before the data entry the clustering algorithm function for computing, we also need to normalize the data, so that the two vectors may in the same range, and then the output graphics could be easier to see clearly with the clustering results. The normalizing ways and means are as follows.

$$x_i' = \frac{x_i - \min A}{\max A - \min A} \tag{27}$$

In the Equation (27), the A is a vector and x_i is its element. The *minA* is the minimum element of the vector and evidently the *maxA* is the maximum element of the vector. We get normalized element data as x_i'. That is, the original vector is $A = (x_1, x_2, ..., x_n)$, and then the normalized vector is $A' = (x_1', x_2', ..., x_n')$.

Here are some examples of clustering of symmetric attributes. One clustering result is shown in Fig. 36. The inputs of the clustering algorithm are two vectors, one is the test person's gait kinetic data of Position Elbow and another is the corresponding age data.

In terms of our Fourteen-Linkage walking model, there are 54 symmetric attributes in one direction and they can be done clustering analysis. So there are 162 attributes in all for three directions. For each gait symmetric attribute to do clustering, the original symmetry data must be normalized to a vector. Take test person's age data to a vector, and take their gait data of one symmetric attribute to another vector. So the horizontal axis is normalized age data, and the vertical axis is normalized data of the symmetric attribute.

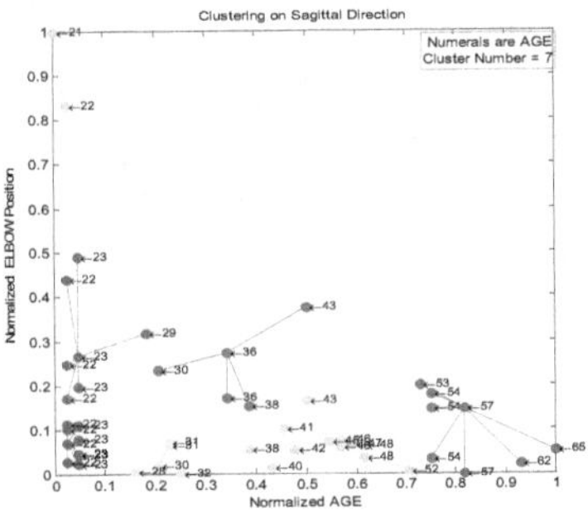

Fig. 36. Clustering on Position Elbow and Age

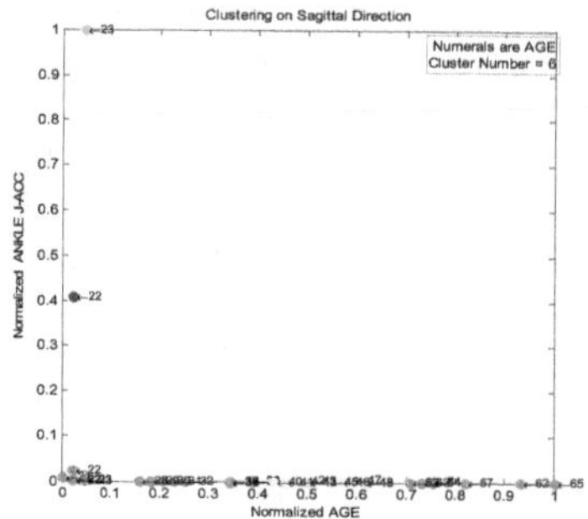

(a) Clustering on Acc of Joint Ankle and Age

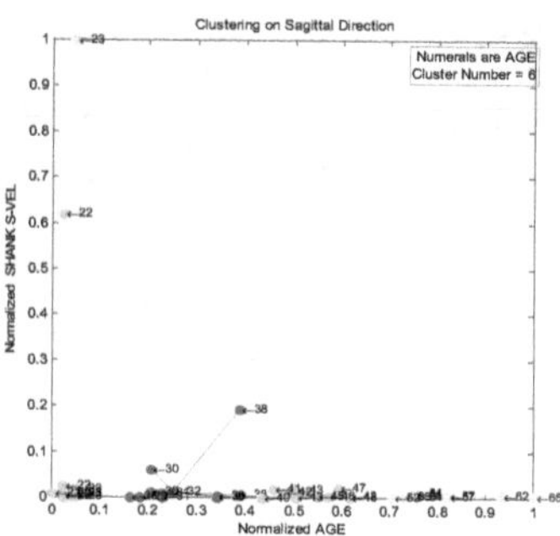

(b) Clustering on Vel of Segment Shank and Age

Fig. 37. More examples of clustering

For all the clustering results how to evaluate them. We used the following formula to calculate a mean square error. The formula is as follows.

$$SA = \frac{1}{m}\sum_{i=1}^{m}\left(\frac{1}{n_i}\sum_{j=1}^{n_i} D\left(G_i(j) - C_i\right)\right) \tag{28}$$

Here m is the number of clustering centres or number of clustering groups, n_i is the number of members of each group, and C_i is the clustering centre of group i, while $G_i(j)$ denoted the member-point of the group i.

The distance calculation in the Equation (28) can use the Euclid's, such as the Equation (36).

$$D_1\left(G_i(j) - C_i\right) = \sqrt[2]{\left(x_{G_i(j)} - x_{c_i}\right)^2 + \left(y_{G_i(j)} - y_{c_i}\right)^2} \tag{29}$$

Of course, the distance can be calculated using other methods, such as the absolute value of errors. This will be discussed later.

Use the Equation (28) with (29), we have calculated the values of all the clustering, choose the smallest ten values of the clustering attributes, and listed in Table 9.

Attributes of Z-dir	No.	SA using D_1	Clustering
THIGH S-ACC	1	0.035657274	6
HIP J-ACC	2	0.035669813	6
ANKLE J-ACC	3	0.035717594	6
THIGH S-VEL	4	0.035719691	6
HIP P-VEL	5	0.035746144	6
SHANK S-ACC	6	0.036075667	6
WRIST P-ACC	7	0.036825407	6
SHANK S-VEL	8	0.037846491	6
KNEE J-VEL	9	0.03882457	6
WRIST Posit	10	0.044141919	5

Table 9. Top ten minimum values of clustering results

From the Table 9, we can see that the smaller the SA value of 10 attributes has a relatively closer clustering results. In the Equation (28), if using other methods to calculate the distance, such as the Equation (30) and (31), we can compare their 10 minimum value of corresponds to the attributes and found that many of them are same, only individual attribute of exceptions, shown in Table 10. We followed the value of SA from small to large, listed from top to bottom.

$$D_2\left(G_i(j)-C_i\right)=abs(y_{G_i(j)}-y_{c_i}) \tag{30}$$

$$D_3\left(G_i(j)-C_i\right)=\left(y_{G_i(j)}-y_{c_i}\right)^2 \tag{31}$$

Although every time the results of clustering is not exactly the same, but in the course of dozens of experiments, the attributes of the top ten were similar broadly, only slightly changed before and after the order. The values of these attributes are the 10 smallest of SA which value was calculated by three different distance formula D_1, D_2, and D_3. So that you can more clearly see that most of these attributes are overlapped. This indicates that the relationship of that using any distance formula and the selection of attributes was not so great.

Attributes	**SA using D_1**	**Attributes**	**SA using D_2**	**Attributes**	**SA using D_3**
THIGH S-ACC	0.035657274	THIGH S-ACC	0.00017294	THIGH S-ACC	0.000000074
HIP J-ACC	0.035669813	HIP J-ACC	0.000523717	THIGH S-VEL	0.000001067
ANKLE J-ACC	0.035717594	THIGH S-VEL	0.000598035	HIP J-ACC	0.000003165
THIGH S-VEL	0.035719691	ANKLE J-ACC	0.000894828	ANKLE J-ACC	0.000006696
HIP P-VEL	0.035746144	HIP P-VEL	0.001258594	HIP P-VEL	0.000008664
SHANK S-ACC	0.036075667	SHANK S-ACC	0.001953265	SHANK S-ACC	0.000023426
WRIST P-ACC	0.036825407	HIP P-ACC	0.00276713	WRIST Posit	0.000090040
SHANK S-VEL	0.037846491	WRIST P-ACC	0.002879147	ANKLE P-VEL	0.000131324
KNEE J-VEL	0.03882457	WRIST Posit	0.005047818	WRIST P-ACC	0.000172132
WRIST Posit	0.044141919	SHANK S-VEL	0.00685193	HIP Joint	0.000225147

Table 10. Comparison of three distance calculation

We can see Fig. 36 and Fig. 37 are different in shape and the latter are not so beautiful shape. These clusters are very closer to the center of all its members. Perhaps because of the presence of a large offset values, so most of the clusters are compressed in a small range. We can find that clustering results displaying isolated points of the cluster, actually these points show these persons with bad gait symmetry. It is maybe the method to classify asymmetry gait and symmetry gait.

6. Conclusions and discussions

6.1 Main conclusions

In this paper, we have proposed a so-called FL model to analyze the walking stability and symmetry of different age subjects while walking on a normal pace. The most important finding is that human walking stabilities are not strictly monotone decreasing with age. Walking stability of human beings varies with age, but does not reduce in the elderly people always.

1. The variability of footprint increases with age for subjects over 30 years old, and it dramatically increases for the elderly over 60 years old, showing much less footprint stability.
2. The variability of walking cycle declines with age. That is to say, the elderly subjects have more cycle stability.
3. The variability of orbital increases with age for all subjects. In other words, the elderly has weaker orbital stability.
4. Human dynamic stability decreases with age except the twenties, which proves previous assumptions. This data mining technology not only gets the contributing dynamic stability features, but also makes the data acquisition simpler.

6.2 Discussions in clinic

Aging effects on motor control have been implicated as a key factor in adjusting posture during walking. Sensory feedback and muscular strength play important roles in maintaining stability against the presence of unpredictable external perturbations or internal variations of gait.

The footprint stability and walking stability of 20 years old subjects is less than that of over 30 years old. This cannot certify that 20 years old subjects have less quality of neuromuscular control. Nevertheless, they have much strength to control their walking pattern, so it shows a springily walking pattern. The orbital stability is strictly monotone decreasing with age. The orbital stability could express the ability of stability control more appropriately.

As we mentioned above, in most comprehensive opinions, walking stability will decrease with ageing. But the cycle stability increase with age. Why? It seems to be more confused to understand. In fact, in the three kinds of stability, only the cycle stability describes the relative stability of walking, which is the relative relationship among occurrence sequence of cycle events in a walking cycle, while the other two kinds of stability are absolute stability of posture. That indicates that the elderly subjects have a rigid and inflexible walking pattern. The elderly improves his/her walking stability by maintaining cycle stability more carefully, because it needs less strength to control cycle stability than the other two. That is to say, young subjects have more powerful muscles to control walking balance, while elderly subjects improve their walking stability by keeping their fixed walking patterns carefully. This is one of the most important findings of this paper.

One conclusion about gait symmetry is that, according to the attributes that selected out by APCLUSTER algorithm and our calculation analysis, we can classify some test objects in order to better meet the natural age groups. An appropriate grouping method to gait symmetry analysis will make the results of statistical analysis more meaningful.

Another conclusion is that, when the symmetry evaluation of normal walking gait, compared the trunk with the limbs, the latter gave larger contribution. Thus, if we have a device to measure gait symmetry of normal people, it may be wrong to wear it at the waist. It may very appropriate if we paste the device somewhere in the lower extremities (for example, shank or ankle), of course pair-wise and it will be more effective.

The next study is to further deepen the existing clustering classification, including gait symmetry attributes and the relationship between weight and height in order to obtain meaningful results. It is our goal that combining gait symmetry attributes with a number of individual characteristics may construct a simple approach to determine a test object should belong to which group.

Clinical gait analysis is aimed at revealing a key aspect of abnormal gait and impact factors, so as to assist the rehabilitation assessment and treatment, but also help to assist the clinical diagnosis, evaluation. We hope that we can evaluate the symmetry degree of a person gait accurately, not whether symmetry or asymmetry. In other words, it can't use one piece of value, but use a set of indices to evaluate. And then each index may indicate an aspect of gait symmetry.

Further research needs to determine how these gait symmetry is related to actual fall risk. At least to a certain extent, the symmetry between the low-body such as legs seems to codetermine the stability of walking.

7. Acknowledgment

This work is supported in part by the Fukushima Prefectural Foundation for the Advancement of Science and Education (No.F-18-10), Japan, Shanghai, and Shanghai Leading Academic Discipline Project (J50103), China, and Pujiang Program from Science and Technology Commission of Shanghai Municipality, China.

The basic part of this work was implemented in the Biomedical Information Technology Lab, the University of Aizu, Fukushima, Japan.

8. References

Akita, K. (1984). Image Sequence Analysis of Real World Human Motion, *Pattern Recognition*, 17(1),1984, pp. 73-83

Arif, M. Ohtaki, Y. Nagatomi, R. & Inooka, H. (2004). Estimation of the Effect of Cadence on Gait Stability in Young and Elderly People using Approximate Entropy Technique. *Measurement Science Review*, Volume 4, Section 2, 2004, pp.29-40

Cheng, J.C. & Moura, J. M.F.(). Automatic Recognition of Human Walking in Monocular Image Sequences, Journal of VLSI Signal Processing Systems, 20(1-2), 1998, pp. 107–120

Chou, PH.; Chou, YL; Su, FC.; Huang, WK & Lin, TS. (2003). Normal Gait of Children, *Biomedical Engineeringapplications, Basis & Communications,* Vol. 15 No. 4 August 2003, pp. 160-163

Corriveau, H.; Hébert R.; Raîche, M. & Prince, F. (2004). Evaluation of postural stability in the elderly with stroke, *Archives of Physical Medicine and Rehabilitation*, Vol 85, Issue 7, pp.1095-1101

Cunado, D.; Nixon, M.S. & Carter, J.N. (2003). Automatic Extraction and Description of Human Gait Models for Recognition Purposes, *Computer Vision and Image Understanding*, Vol.90, No.1, (April 2003), pp. 1-41, ISSN 1077-3142

Dockstader, S. L.; Bergkessel, K. A. & Tekalp A. M., Feature Extraction for the Analysis of Gait and Human Motion, *Proc. of 16th International Conference on Pattern Recognition,* Canada, 2002,pp.5-8.

Frey, B.J. & Dueck, D. (2007). Clustering by passing messages between data points, *Science*, Vol 315, No 5814, pp 972-976, February 2007

George, F. (2000). Falls in the Elderly, *American Family Physician*, Apr. 2000

Guo, Y.; Xu, G. & Tsuji, S. (1994). Understanding Human Motion Patterns, *Proc. The 12th IAPR International Conference on Pattern Recognition*. Vol.2, 1994, pp. 325-329

Hylton B.M.; Stephen, R. L. and Richard, C. F. (2003). Age-related differences in walking stability. *Age and Ageing* 2003, 32, pp.137-142

Karaharju-Huisnan, T.; Taylor, S.; Begg, R.; Cai, J. & Best, R. (2001). Gait symmetry quantification during treadmill walking, *The Seventh Australian and New Zealand Intelligent Information Systems Conference*, 18-21, Nov. 2001, pp. 203 – 206

Karaulova, I.A.; Hall, P.M. & Marshall, A.D.(2000). A Hierarchical Model of Dynamics for Tracking People with a Single Video Camera, *Proc of the 11th BMVC*, 2000, pp. 262-352

Kavanagh, J. (2006). Dynamic stability of the upper body during walking. *PhD thesis*, School of Physiotherapy and Exercise Science, Griffith Health, Griffith University, 2006.

Lee, L. (2003). Gait Analysis for Classification, *AI Technical Report* 2003-014, Massachusetts Institute of Technology-artificial Intelligence Laboratory, 2003.

Li, Y.; Wen, C.L.; Xie, Z. & Xu, X.H. (2003). Synchronization of batch trajectory based on multi-scale dynamic time warping, *Proceeding of the Second International Conference on Machine Learning and Cybernetics*, 2003.

Marin, L.C.; Kang, H.G. & Dingwell, J.B. (2006). Changes in the Orbital Stability of Walking Across Speeds, *Proceedings of the 30th Annual Meeting of the American Society of Biomechanics*, Blacksburg, VA, September 6-9, 2006.

Menz HB. (2002). Walking Stability in Young, Old and Neuropathic Subjects, *PhD thesis*, School of Physiology and Pharmacology, Faculty of Medicine, University of New South Wales, 2002.

Murray, M.P. (1967). Gait as A Total Pattern of Movement, *American Journal of Physical Medicine*, 46(1), 1967, pp. 290-332.

Nash, J.; Carter, J.N. & Nixon, M.S. (1998). Extraction of Moving Articulated Objects by Evidence Gathering, *Proc. of the 9th British Machine Vision Conference*, ISBN 9781901725049, Southampton, UK, September 14-17, 1998, pp. 609-618

Nichols, D.S. Balance retraining after stroke using force platform biofeedback. Phys Ther. 1997 May; 77(5), pp. 553-8

Rohr, K. (1994). Towards model-based recognition of human movements in image sequences", CVGIP: IU, 74(1), 1994, pp. 94-115

Stirling, J.R. & Zakynthinaki, M.S. (2004). Stability and the maintenance of balance following a perturbation from quiet stance, *Chaos: An Interdisciplinary Journal of Nonlinear Science*, March 2004, Volume 14, Issue 1, pp. 96-105

Sutherland, D.H.; Olshen, R.A.; Cooper, L. & Woo, SLY. (1980). The Development of Mature Walking, *Bone Joint Surg*, 1980,Vol. 62A, No. 3, pp 336-353

Whittle, M. W. (2007). *Gait Analysis: An Introduction*, (4th ed), Elsevier Health Sciences, ISBN 9780750688833, New York

Woollacott, M.H. & Tang, P.F. (1997). Dynamic Balance Control During Walking in the Older Adult: Research and its Implications, *Physical Therapy*, 7(6), 1997, pp. 646-660

Yang N.F. (2001). Coordination Analysis and Parametric Description of Human Movements, *doctoral thesis*, Tsinghua University, 2001

Yoo, J. H.; Nixon, M. S & Harris, C. J. (2002). Extracting Gait Signatures based on Anatomical Knowledge. *Proc. of BMVA Symposium on Advancing Biometric Technologies*, 2002.

Zhang, R.; Vogler, C. & Metaxas, D. (2004). Human Gait Recognition, *Proceedings of the 2004 IEEE Computer Society Conference on Computer Vision and Pattern Recognition Workshops* (CVPRW'04), 2004, pp.1-8

2

Causal Inference in Randomized Trials with Noncompliance

Yasutaka Chiba

Division of Biostatistics, Clinical Research Center, Kinki University School of Medicine, Japan

1. Introduction

In human clinical trials, ethical considerations for study subjects override the scientific requirements of trial design. Noncompliance with an intervention or study procedure for ethical reasons is thus inevitable in practice (Piantadosi, 1997).

The Coronary Drug Project (CDP) trial (CDP Research Group, 1980) was a typical example of trials with noncompliance. The CDP trial was a large, double-blinded, randomized trial testing the effect of the cholesterol-lowering drug, clofibrate, on mortality. Patients were randomly assigned to the clofibrate or placebo groups and were followed for at least 5 years, documenting clinic visits and examinations. During each 4-month follow-up visit, the physician assessed compliance by counting or estimating the number of capsules returned by the patients. In the protocol, good compliers were defined as patients taking more than 80% of the prescribed treatment. Table 1 summarizes the incidence of death during the 5-year follow-up period, based on the treatment assigned and compliance status. Patients who left the trial before the end of the 5-year follow-up period were excluded.

Group	No. of patients	Deaths	Compliance status	No. of patients	Deaths
Clofibrate	1065	194	More than 80%	708	106
			Less than 80%	357	88
Placebo	2695	523	More than 80%	1813	274
			Less than 80%	882	249
Totals	3760	717			

Table 1. The compliance status and incidence of death during a 5-year follow-up period in the CDP trial.

In the clofibrate group, 708 patients were considered good compliers; 106 died during the follow-up period. There were 357 patients considered poor compliers; 88 died. Comparing the compliance status of the proportion of patients that died yields 106/708 – 88/357 = –9.68%. From this result, clofibrate seems to have been beneficial. However, when we make the same comparison for the placebo group, it yields 274/1813 – 249/882 = –13.12%. Surprisingly, we obtain the result that the placebo was more beneficial than clofibrate. However, nobody would interpret the result as being that the placebo had the effect of decreasing death.

Which subgroups to compare to estimate the treatment effect correctly is an important problem. From the viewpoint of treatment compliance, it is considered best to compare the proportion of deaths for the compliers in each group: 106/708 - 274/1813 = -0.14%. This comparison is called the per-protocol (PP) analysis. The PP analysis generally yields biased estimates of treatment effects, because whether patients comply with the assigned treatment is not randomized and several factors may affect it. This problem can be avoided by intention-to-treat (ITT) analysis, in which patients are analyzed according to the assigned treatment regardless of the treatment actually received (Fisher et al., 1990; Lee et al., 1991): 194/1065 - 523/2695 = -1.19%. The ITT estimate may represent the effect of the treatment intended, but generally does not represent the treatment effect itself (Schwartz & Lellouch, 1967; Sheiner & Rubin, 1995).

Noncompliance data may be obtained from actual clinical trials, as in the CDP trial. To estimate the treatment effect correctly from such data, we should consider the expected outcomes if all patients had received the test treatment and the control, and compare them. The effect yielded from such a comparison is called the average causal effect (ACE) (Robins & Tsiatis, 1991; Robins & Greenland, 1994). Several researchers have discussed methodology to estimate ACE (Pearl, 2000; Manski, 2003; Sato, 2006), but as yet, no standard methodology has been developed. Nevertheless, we can derive bounds on ACE using the deterministic causal model (e.g., Pearl, 1995; Cai et al., 2007; Chiba, 2009b). In this chapter, we discuss how estimates from major analyses, such as ITT and PP, are biased and present bounds on ACE under certain assumptions.

To achieve these objectives, this chapter is organized as follows. In Section 2, notation and definitions are provided. Sections 3 and 4 discuss noncompliance by switching the treatment, which, in contrast to the CDP trial, means that non-compliers in a sub-population assigned to treatment A receive treatment B and those assigned to treatment B receive treatment A. We discuss biases from major analyses such as ITT and PP in Section 3, and discuss the bounds on ACE in Section 4. Section 5 discusses noncompliance by receiving no treatment, as in the CDP trial. As in many publications, the instrumental variable (IV) assumption is used in these sections, but this assumption is relaxed in Section 6. Finally, Section 7 offers some concluding remarks. The derivations of equations and inequalities presented in this chapter are outlined in Section 8.

2. Notation and definitions

In the following sections, R is the randomization indicator, where $R = 2$ for subjects randomized to the test treatment and $R = 1$ for subjects randomized to the control. Similarly, X indicates actual (received) treatment that may not be randomized under protocol violations such as noncompliance, where $X = 2$ for subjects who received the test treatment, $X = 1$ for subjects who received the control, and $X = 0$ for subjects who received no treatment. The observed outcome is Y and $Y_{X=x}$ is the counterfactual value (or equally potential outcome) of Y if treatment X was set to x (Rubin, 1974, 1978, 1990). ACE is defined as ACE $\equiv \mathrm{E}(Y_{X=2}) - \mathrm{E}(Y_{X=1})$. Note that ITT and PP estimators are represented by ITT $\equiv \mathrm{E}(Y|R = 2) - \mathrm{E}(Y|R = 1)$ and PP $\equiv \mathrm{E}(Y|X = 2, R = 2) - \mathrm{E}(Y|X = 1, R = 1)$, respectively. Furthermore, we use the notation $E_{xr} = \mathrm{E}(Y|X = x, R = r)$ and $p_{x|r} = \Pr(X = x|R = r)$; then, PP $\equiv E_{22} - E_{11}$.

We require the consistency assumption that $Y_{X=x} = Y$ for all subjects, so that the value of Y that would have been observed if X had been set to what it in fact was is equal to the value of Y that was in fact observed. Thus, this assumption indicates that $\mathrm{E}(Y_{X=x}|X = x) = \mathrm{E}(Y|X = x)$ and furthermore $\mathrm{E}(Y_{X=x}|X = x, R = r) = \mathrm{E}(Y|X = x, R = r)$ (= E_{xr}). We assume that $Y_{X=x}$ is independent from X given R and Z, where Z is a confounder or a set of confounders between X and Y. In Sections 3-5, we also require the instrumental variable (IV) assumption, which states that the potential outcome $Y_{X=x}$ is not affected directly by the treatment assignment R; rather, $Y_{X=x}$ is influenced only by the treatment actually received (Holland, 1986; Angrist et al., 1996). Thus, subjects' potential outcomes are independent of treatment assignment and are constant across the sub-populations of subjects assigned to different treatment arms. The IV assumption is formalized as follows:

ASSUMPTION 1: Instrumental variable (IV)

$$E(Y_{X=x} \mid R = 2) = E(Y_{X=x} \mid R = 1).$$

This assumption may hold in successfully blinded randomized trials, because subjects are not aware of their assigned treatments and so the assigned treatments do not affect the potential outcomes. However, this often may not hold in unblinded trials, in which subjects are aware of the assigned treatment and this knowledge may affect the potential outcomes, and needs to be critically evaluated. Assumption 1 is used in Sections 3-5, but is relaxed in Section 6.

3. Biases of estimates

In this section and the next section, we discuss noncompliance by switching the treatment, which means that non-compliers in a sub-population assigned to treatment A receive treatment B and those assigned to treatment B receive treatment A. In this type of noncompliance, all subjects have the value $X = 1$ or 2 (and not $X = 0$) for both $R = 1$ and 2. Thus, $p_{0|r} = 0$ and $p_{1|r} + p_{2|r} = 1$. The derivations of equations in this section are given in Section 8.1.

In this section, we discuss how estimates from major analyses, such as ITT and PP, are biased. To do so, we introduce the following R-specific bias factors due to confounding between X and Y (Brumback et al, 2004; Chiba et al., 2007):

$$\alpha_r \equiv E(Y_{X=2} \mid X = 2, R = r) - E(Y_{X=2} \mid X = 1, R = r),$$

$$\beta_r \equiv E(Y_{X=1} \mid X = 2, R = r) - E(Y_{X=1} \mid X = 1, R = r),$$

where $r = 1, 2$. α_r and β_r are confounding effects that would arise from R-stratified comparisons of those with $X = 2$ versus those with $X = 1$. When $\alpha_r > 0$ and $\beta_r > 0$, $E(Y_{X=x} \mid X = 2, R = r) > E(Y_{X=x} \mid X = 1, R = r)$, which means that the subjects who received the test treatment tend to have larger outcome values than those who received the control, leading to positive confounding. Conversely, when $\alpha_r < 0$ and $\beta_r < 0$, $E(Y_{X=x} \mid X = 2, R = r) < E(Y_{X=x} \mid X = 1, R = r)$, which means that the subjects who received the test treatment tend to have smaller outcome values than those who received the control, leading to negative confounding. No confounding occurs between X and Y when $\alpha_r = \beta_r = 0$.

Under Assumption 1, using α_r and β_r, $E(Y_{X=2})$ and $E(Y_{X=1})$ are expressed as:

$$E(Y_{X=2}) = E_{2r} - \alpha_r p_{1|r}, \tag{3.1}$$

$$E(Y_{X=1}) = E_{1r} + \beta_r p_{2|r}. \tag{3.2}$$

Using these equations, ITT $\equiv E(Y \mid R = 2) - E(Y \mid R = 1)$ can be expressed by a function of ACE $\equiv E(Y_{X=2}) - E(Y_{X=1})$ and bias factors:

$$\text{ITT} = \text{ACE} + \{\alpha_2 - (E_{22} - E_{12})\}p_{1|2} + \{\beta_1 - (E_{21} - E_{11})\}p_{2|1}. \quad (3.3)$$

Thus, the ITT estimator is generally a biased estimator of ACE, and can be unbiased when $\alpha_2 = E_{22} - E_{12}$ and $\beta_1 = E_{21} - E_{11}$, i.e., $E(Y_{X=2} | X = x, R = r) = E(Y_{X=1} | X = x, R = r)$ for $x \neq r$. This equation implies that the ITT estimate can be unbiased when no treatment effect exists for all subjects (under the sharp null hypothesis: $Y_{X=2} = Y_{X=1}$ for all subjects). Furthermore, equation (3.3) shows that, if we know whether the treatment effect is positive or negative, we can know the sign of bias of the ITT estimate.

Likewise, it can be demonstrated that the PP estimator is generally a biased estimator of ACE, because the difference between equation (3.1) with $r = 2$ and equation (3.2) with $r = 1$ derives:

$$\text{PP} = \text{ACE} + \alpha_2 p_{1|2} + \beta_1 p_{2|1}. \quad (3.4)$$

This equation shows that the PP estimate can be unbiased when $\alpha_2 = 0$ and $\beta_1 = 0$, which imply that whether subjects receive the test treatment or control treatment is randomly determined (no confounder exists between X and Y). Furthermore, if we know the common sign of confounding effects (the common signs of α_r and β_r), we can know the sign of the bias of the PP estimate.

In addition to the ITT and PP estimators, the IV estimator has been developed (Cuzick et al., 1997; Greenland, 2000; Hernán & Robins, 2006). The estimate is calculated by the following formula:

$$\text{IV} \equiv \{E(Y | R = 2) - E(Y | R = 1)\} / (p_{2|2} - p_{2|1})$$

for $p_{2|2} \neq p_{2|1}$. Although the IV estimator may yield a less biased estimate of ACE, it is also generally biased. This is because the IV estimator is expressed using bias factors as follows (Chiba, 2010a):

$$\text{IV} = \text{ACE} - w_1(\alpha_1 - \beta_1) + w_2(\alpha_2 - \beta_2), \quad (3.5)$$

where $w_r = p_{1|r}p_{2|r} / (p_{2|2} - p_{2|1})$ and $p_{2|2} \neq p_{2|1}$. Thus, the IV estimate can be unbiased when $\alpha_r = \beta_r$, i.e., $E(Y_{X=2} - Y_{X=1} | X = 2, R = r) = E(Y_{X=2} - Y_{X=1} | X = 1, R = r)$. Similar to the ITT estimate, the IV estimate can also be unbiased when no treatment effect exists for all subjects (under the sharp null hypothesis: $Y_{X=2} = Y_{X=1}$ for all subjects). Additionally, the IV estimate can be unbiased even when $E(Y_{X=2} - Y_{X=1} | X = x, R = 2) = E(Y_{X=2} - Y_{X=1} | X = x, R = 1)$ (Robins, 1989). Furthermore, as an alternative to the IV estimator, Chiba (2010b) proposed the following estimator of ACE:

$$\text{IV}' \equiv (E_{22}p_{1|1} + E_{12}p_{2|1} - E_{21}p_{1|2} - E_{11}p_{2|2}) / (p_{2|2} - p_{2|1}).$$

This estimator is also generally a biased estimator of ACE, and the estimate can be unbiased under $\alpha_1 = \alpha_2$ and $\beta_1 = \beta_2$, which may be reasonable when the influence of confounding between X and Y is equal in both assigned groups.

4. Bounds on average causal effect

In randomized trials with noncompliance by switching the treatment, we cannot generally estimate ACE in an unbiased manner (Section 3). Thus, in this section, we discuss bounds on ACE. We introduce the bounds under some assumptions in Section 4.1, and illustrate them by using data from a classic randomized trial in Section 4.2. The derivations of inequalities in this section are outlined in Section 8.2.

4.1 Assumptions and bounds

In Section 4.1.1, we introduce bounds on ACE under Assumption 1 only. Because the bounds generally have a broad width, we present the bounds with narrower widths by adding some plausible assumptions in Sections 4.1.2 and 4.1.3.

4.1.1 The instrumental variable

When the outcome Y has a finite range $[K_0, K_1]$, the bounds on ACE under Assumption 1 are as follows (Robins, 1989; Manski, 1990):

$$\max\left\{\begin{matrix} K_0 p_{1|1} + E_{21} p_{2|1} \\ K_0 p_{1|2} + E_{22} p_{2|2} \end{matrix}\right\} - \min\left\{\begin{matrix} E_{11} p_{1|1} + K_1 p_{2|1} \\ E_{12} p_{1|2} + K_1 p_{2|2} \end{matrix}\right\} \leq \text{ACE} \leq \min\left\{\begin{matrix} K_1 p_{1|1} + E_{21} p_{2|1} \\ K_1 p_{1|2} + E_{22} p_{2|2} \end{matrix}\right\} - \max\left\{\begin{matrix} E_{11} p_{1|1} + K_0 p_{2|1} \\ E_{12} p_{1|2} + K_0 p_{2|2} \end{matrix}\right\}. \tag{4.1}$$

Note that $K_0 = 0$ and $K_1 = 1$ in the case of a binary outcome. Furthermore, using a method of linear programming in the case of a binary outcome, Balke and Pearl (1997) presented the following bounds under Assumption 1 only:

$$\max\left\{\begin{matrix} P_{12|2} + P_{01|1} - 1 \\ P_{12|1} + P_{01|2} - 1 \\ P_{12|1} - P_{12|2} - P_{11|2} - P_{02|1} - P_{11|1} \\ P_{12|2} - P_{12|1} - P_{11|1} - P_{02|2} - P_{11|2} \\ -P_{02|2} - P_{11|2} \\ -P_{02|1} - P_{11|1} \\ P_{01|2} - P_{02|2} - P_{11|2} - P_{02|1} - P_{21|1} \\ P_{01|1} - P_{02|1} - P_{11|1} - P_{02|2} - P_{01|2} \end{matrix}\right\} \leq \text{ACE} \leq \min\left\{\begin{matrix} 1 - P_{02|2} + P_{11|1} \\ 1 - P_{02|1} + P_{11|2} \\ P_{02|2} + P_{01|2} + P_{12|1} + P_{01|1} - P_{02|1} \\ P_{12|2} + P_{01|2} + P_{02|1} + P_{01|1} - P_{02|2} \\ P_{12|2} + P_{01|2} \\ P_{12|1} + P_{01|1} \\ P_{12|2} + P_{01|2} + P_{02|1} + P_{12|1} - P_{11|1} \\ P_{12|1} + P_{01|1} + P_{12|2} + P_{11|2} - P_{11|1} \end{matrix}\right\}, \tag{4.2}$$

where $P_{yx|r} = \Pr(Y = y, X = x \mid R = r)$ $(y = 0, 1)$. Inequality (4.2), which is the bounds on ACE having the narrowest width without adding any other assumptions, gives bounds with a narrower width than inequality (4.1) in some situations. However, these bounds generally have broad widths. Thus, in Sections 4.1.2 and 4.1.3, we derive bounds with narrower widths by adding some plausible assumptions.

4.1.2 The monotone treatment response

To derive narrower bounds, Manski (1997) presented the following monotone treatment response (MTR) assumption:

ASSUMPTION 2.1: Monotone treatment response (MTR)

$Y_{X=s} \geq Y_{X=t}$ *for all subjects, where* $s \geq t$.

For $(s, t) = (2, 1)$, the MTR means that a subject takes a larger outcome value if he/she received the test treatment than if he/she received the control. This holds when it is apparent that the test treatment has a positive effect.

Under Assumptions 1 and 2.1, the lower bound on ACE is improved as follows:

$$\text{ACE} \geq \max\{\text{ITT}, -\text{ITT}\}. \tag{4.3}$$

Thus, we can say that ACE is not less than the ITT estimate when the MTR holds. Note that the second and third terms in equation (3.3) are not less than 0 under the MTR, because $E(Y_{X=2} | X = x, R = r) \geq E(Y_{X=1} | X = x, R = r)$, i.e., $\alpha_2 \geq E_{22} - E_{12}$ and $\beta_1 \geq E_{21} - E_{11}$, hold under the MTR.
Using the reverse sign of the inequality in Assumption 2.1, the following reverse MTR (RMTR) assumption can be applied:

ASSUMPTION 2.2: Reverse monotone treatment response (RMTR)
$Y_{X=s} \leq Y_{X=t}$ *for all subjects, where* $s \geq t$.

In contrast to the MTR, for $(s, t) = (2, 1)$, the RMTR means that a subject takes a smaller outcome value if he/she received the test treatment than if he/she received the control. This holds when it is apparent that the test treatment has a negative effect. Under Assumptions 1 and 2.2, the upper bound on ACE is improved as ACE ≤ min{ITT, –ITT}, implying that ACE is not more than the ITT estimate when the RMTR holds.
Assumptions 2.1 and 2.2 are very strict assumptions, because the inequalities must hold for all subjects. In the case of a binary outcome variable, we can use an alternative assumption that is weaker than Assumptions 2.1 and 2.2, but can derive the same bound as those under these assumptions. This is introduced below after the concept of principal stratification (Frangakis & Rubin, 2002).
Based on principal stratification, four types of potential outcomes are defined as follows: doomed $\{Y_{X=2} = 1, Y_{X=1} = 1\}$, which consists of subjects who always experience the event, regardless of the treatment received; preventive $\{Y_{X=2} = 0, Y_{X=1} = 1\}$, which consists of subjects who do not experience the event when they receive the test treatment but do when they receive the control; causative $\{Y_{X=2} = 1, Y_{X=1} = 0\}$, which consists of subjects who experience the event when they receive the test treatment, but not when they receive the control; and immune $\{Y_{X=2} = 0, Y_{X=1} = 0\}$, which consists of subjects who never experience the event, regardless of the treatment received (Greenland & Robins, 1986). Because X and Y are binary, the potential outcomes could be any of these four types. Note that Assumption 2.1 implies that no preventive subject exists: $\Pr(Y_{X=2} = 0, Y_{A=1} = 1) = 0$, because $Y_{X=2} = 0$ and $Y_{X=1} = 1$ cannot hold simultaneously under $Y_{X=2} \geq Y_{X=1}$. Likewise, Assumption 2.2 implies that no causative subject exists.
We can obtain inequality (4.3) even under the following assumption (Chiba, 2011):

ASSUMPTION 3.1
$$\Pr(Y_{X=2} = 1, Y_{X=1} = 0 | X = x, R = r) \geq \Pr(Y_{X=2} = 0, Y_{X=1} = 1 | X = x, R = r).$$

This assumption indicates that the number of causative subjects is not less than the number of preventive subjects within all strata with $X = x$ and $R = r$. Thus, Assumption 3.1 is weaker than Assumption 2.1, because Assumption 2.1 requires that no preventive subject exists but this is not the case for Assumption 3.1.
Likewise, the following assumption, 3.2, can derive the same upper bound as that under Assumption 2.2:

ASSUMPTION 3.2
$$\Pr(Y_{X=2} = 1, Y_{X=1} = 0 | X = x, R = r) \leq \Pr(Y_{X=2} = 0, Y_{X=1} = 1 | X = x, R = r).$$

In contrast to Assumption 3.1, this assumption implies that the number of causative subjects is not more than the number of preventive subjects within all strata with $X = x$ and $R = r$. Again, note that Assumption 2.2 implies that no causative subject exists and thus Assumption 3.2 is a weaker assumption than Assumption 2.2.

4.1.3 The monotone treatment selection

The other assumption to derive narrower bounds is the following monotone treatment selection assumption (Manski & Pepper, 2000; Chiba, 2010c):

ASSUMPTION 4.1: Monotone treatment selection (MTS)
$$E(Y_{X=x} \mid X = s, R = r) \geq E(Y_{X=x} \mid X = t, R = r) \text{ for } s \geq t.$$

For $(s, t) = (2, 1)$, the MTS means that subjects who received the test treatment tend to have larger outcome values than those who received the control within each study treatment-arm subpopulation. For example, when patients with a worse condition prefer to receive the new treatment ($X = 2$), it should be anticipated that the incidence proportion of a bad event ($Y = 1$) such as death will be higher, compared with those who receive the standard treatment ($X = 1$); this indicates that the MTS holds.

Under Assumptions 1 and 4.1, the upper bound on ACE is improved as follows:

$$\text{ACE} \leq \min\{E_{21}, E_{22}\} - \max\{E_{11}, E_{12}\}. \tag{4.4}$$

Specifically, when $\min\{E_{21}, E_{22}\} = E_{22}$ and $\max\{E_{11}, E_{12}\} = E_{11}$, the upper bound is equal to the PP estimator. Thus, ACE is no more than the PP estimate when the MTS holds. Note that this is also verified from equation (3.4) because Assumption 4.1 implies that $\alpha_r \geq 0$ and $\beta_r \geq 0$.

Similar to the RMTR, the following reverse MTS (RMTS) assumption can be applied:

ASSUMPTION 4.2: Reverse monotone treatment selection (RMTS)
$$E(Y_{X=x} \mid X = s, R = r) \leq E(Y_{X=x} \mid X = t, R = r) \text{ for } s \geq t.$$

In contrast to the MTS, for $(s, t) = (2, 1)$, the RMTS means that subjects who received the test treatment tend to have smaller outcome values than those who received the control within each study treatment-arm subpopulation. The lower bound on ACE under the RMTS is ACE $\geq \max\{E_{21}, E_{22}\} - \min\{E_{11}, E_{12}\}$, implying that ACE is not less than the PP estimate when the RMTS holds.

It is obvious that the combination of Assumptions 2.1 and 4.1 improves both the lower and upper bounds:

$$\max\{\text{ITT}, -\text{ITT}\} \leq \text{ACE} \leq \min\{E_{21}, E_{22}\} - \max\{E_{11}, E_{12}\}.$$

Likewise, under the combination of Assumptions 2.2 and 4.2, bounds on ACE are

$$\max\{E_{21}, E_{22}\} - \min\{E_{11}, E_{12}\} \leq \text{ACE} \leq \min\{\text{ITT}, -\text{ITT}\}. \tag{4.5}$$

These inequalities show that ACE exists between ITT and PP estimates under these combinations of assumptions.

By extending a theory developed in the context of observational studies (VanderWeele, 2008a; Chiba, 2009a), Chiba (2009b) presented another assumption that derives the same upper bound as that under the MTS (Assumption 4.1):

ASSUMPTION 5.1: Monotone confounding (MC)
Both $E(Y \mid X = 2, R = r, Z = z)$ *and* $\Pr(X = 2 \mid R = r, Z = z)$ *are non-decreasing or non-increasing in* z *for all* r, *and the components of* Z *are independent of each other.*

For an assumption corresponding to the RMTS (Assumption 4.2), Assumption 5.1 is changed as follows:

ASSUMPTION 5.2: Reverse monotone confounding (RMC)
One of E(Y | X = 2, R = r, Z = z) *and* Pr(X = 2 | R = r, Z = z) *is non-decreasing and the other is non-increasing in z for all r, and the components of Z are independent of each other.*

Although the MTS and MC (RMTS and RMC) give the same upper (lower) bound on ACE, the relationship between them has not been clear. In Section 8.2, we demonstrate that the MC implies the MTS, but it is unclear whether the converse holds.

4.2 Application

For illustration, the assumptions and bounds presented in this section are applied to data from the Multiple Risk Factor Intervention Trial (MRFIT) (MRFIT Research Group, 1982). The MRFIT was a large field trial to test the effect of a multifactorial intervention program on mortality from coronary heart disease (CHD) in middle-aged men with sufficiently high risk levels attributed to cigarette smoking, high serum cholesterol, and high blood pressure. Intervention consisted of dietary advice on ways to reduce blood cholesterol, smoking cessation counseling, and hypertension medication. All subjects were randomly assigned to the intervention program or the control group.

For this illustration, attention is restricted to the effects of cessation of cigarette smoking. This restriction follows other studies (Mark & Robins, 1993; Matsui, 2005; Chiba, 2010a) and was applied due to the paucity of differences achieved for the other risk factors. Table 2 summarizes the incidence of subject mortality due to CHD during the 7-year follow-up period based on the assigned treatment and the actual subject smoking status 1 year after study entry. R represents the assigned group (R = 2 for the test group and R = 1 for the control group), X is the actual smoking status 1 year after entry (X = 2 for smoking cessation and X = 1 for continued smoking), and Y is the incidence of CHD deaths (Y = 1 for dead and Y = 0 for alive). ITT and PP analyses yielded ITT = 69/3833 – 74/3830 = −0.13% and PP = 11/991 – 70/3456 = −0.92%, respectively. IV and IV′ estimates were −0.82% and −0.72%, respectively.

Group	No. of subjects	CHD deaths	Smoking status at 1 year	No. of subjects	CHD deaths
Test	3833	69	Quit	991	11
			Not quit	2842	58
Control	3830	74	Quit	374	4
			Not quit	3456	70
Totals	7663	143			

Table 2. The status of cigarette smoking and the incidence of mortality due to CHD in the MRFIT during a 7-year follow-up period.

To derive the ACE bounds, it is necessary to discuss whether the assumptions in this section hold. It is clear that cessation of cigarette smoking prevents death from CHD. Thus, Assumption 2.2 (RMTR: $Y_{X=2} \le Y_{X=1}$ for all subjects) holds (i.e., no causative subject, who died when they quit smoking but lived when they continued smoking, exists). However, it is possible that such subjects do exist, because the stress of quitting smoking might lead to CHD and this stress would have been lower if the subject had continued smoking (i.e., a causative subject existed). Under this observation, Assumption 2.2 does not hold. However, Assumption 3.2 would still hold, because even if a few causative subjects exist, the number would be the smallest in the four principal strata.

In general, health-conscious individuals may tend not to die from CHD and quit smoking compared with individuals who are not health-conscious. Trial subjects would likely have had similar tendencies, and subjects who quit smoking would logically tend not to have died from CHD. Therefore, it is considered that Assumption 4.2 (RMTS: $E(Y_{X=x} \mid X = 2, R = r) \leq E(Y_{X=x} \mid X = 1, R = r)$ for $x = 1, 2$ and $r = 1, 2$) is valid. Although Assumption 1 may not hold because this trial was an unblinded trial (the details are discussed in Section 6), we here use this assumption for illustrative purposes.

The arguments presented above demonstrate that Assumptions 3.2 and 4.2 can be assumed. Thus, from inequality (4.5), the bounds on ACE become $-0.92\% \leq \text{ACE} \leq -0.13\%$. This result indicates that quitting smoking would prevent death from CHD. Note that the bounds under Assumption 1 only become $-11.31\% \leq \text{ACE} \leq 72.60\%$, where inequalities (4.1) and (4.2) yield the same bounds. While the bounds under Assumption 1 only do not give enough information about ACE, adding Assumptions 3.2 and 4.2 greatly improves the bounds.

5. Noncompliance by receiving no treatment

While noncompliance by switching the treatment was discussed in Sections 3 and 4, this section discusses noncompliance by receiving no treatment, which means that non-compliers receive no treatment. In this type of noncompliance, subjects who are allocated to $R = 2$ take the value of $X = 0$ or 2 (and not $X = 1$) and those who are allocated to $R = 1$ take the value of $X = 0$ or 1 (and not $X = 2$). Thus, $p_{0|2} + p_{2|2} = 1$ and $p_{0|1} + p_{1|1} = 1$. The derivations of equations and inequalities in this section are similar to those in Sections 3 and 4, and can be achieved straightforwardly by replacing $x = 1, 2$ in Sections 3 and 4 to $x = 0, 1$ and $x = 0, 2$. Thus, they are omitted.

5.1 Biases of estimates

By following a similar discussion to Section 3, we show that the ITT and PP estimators generally yield biased estimates of ACE. Unfortunately, the IV estimator cannot be defined in this type of noncompliance.

To express the biases of ITT and PP estimators, we introduce the following bias factors instead of α_r and β_r in Section 3:

$$\gamma \equiv E(Y_{X=2} \mid X = 2, R = 2) - E(Y_{X=2} \mid X = 0, R = 2),$$

$$\delta \equiv E(Y_{X=1} \mid X = 1, R = 1) - E(Y_{X=1} \mid X = 0, R = 1).$$

Similar to α_r and β_r, γ and δ are also confounding effects. γ is interpreted as a confounding effect that would arise from comparisons of those with $X = 2$ versus those with $X = 0$ for the test treatment group. When $\gamma > 0$, $E(Y_{X=2} \mid X = 2, R = 2) > E(Y_{X=2} \mid X = 0, R = 2)$, which means that the subjects who received the test treatment tend to take larger outcome values than those who received no treatment. Conversely, when $\gamma < 0$, $E(Y_{X=2} \mid X = 2, R = 2) < E(Y_{X=2} \mid X = 0, R = 2)$, which means that the subjects who received the test treatment tend to take smaller outcome values than those who received no treatment. Whether subjects in the test treatment group actually receive the treatment is randomly determined when $\gamma = 0$. δ is interpreted using a similar process in the control group.

Biases of ITT and PP estimators can be explained in a similar manner to Section 3, using γ and δ. Because $E(Y_{X=2})$ and $E(Y_{X=1})$ are expressed as $E(Y_{X=2}) = E_{22} - \gamma p_{0|2}$ and $E(Y_{X=1}) = E_{11} - \delta p_{0|1}$, the ITT estimator is given by:

$$ITT = ACE + \{\gamma - (E_{22} - E_{02})\}p_{0|2} - \{\delta - (E_{11} - E_{01})\}p_{0|1}.$$

Therefore, the ITT estimator is generally a biased estimator of ACE, and can be unbiased when $\gamma = E_{22} - E_{02}$ and $\delta = E_{11} - E_{01}$, i.e., $E(Y_{X=r} | X = 0, R = r) = E(Y_{X=0} | X = 0, R = r)$ for $r = 1$, 2. This equation indicates that the ITT estimate can be unbiased when no effect of the treatments exists against no treatment for all subjects (under the sharp null hypothesis: $Y_{X=x} = Y_{X=0}$ for all subjects, where $x = 1, 2$).

The PP estimator is given by:

$$PP = ACE + \gamma p_{0|2} - \delta p_{0|1}.$$

Thus, the PP estimate can be unbiased when $\gamma = 0$ and $\delta = 0$, implying that whether subjects receive the assigned treatment is randomly determined (no confounder exists between X and Y).

In contrast to the case of noncompliance by switching the treatment, it may be difficult to know the signs of biases of ITT and PP estimates.

5.2 Bounds on average causal effect

We extend the bounds concept introduced in Section 4.1 to the case of noncompliance by receiving no treatment.

The bounds under Assumption 1 only are as follows:

$$(E_{22}p_{2|2} + K_0 p_{0|2}) - (E_{11}p_{1|1} + K_1 p_{0|1}) \leq ACE \leq (E_{22}p_{2|2} + K_1 p_{0|2}) - (E_{11}p_{1|1} + K_0 p_{0|1}), \quad (5.1)$$

where $[K_0, K_1]$ is a finite range of outcome Y. In the case of a binary outcome, this inequality is simplified to:

$$P_{12|2} + P_{01|1} - 1 \leq ACE \leq 1 - P_{02|2} - P_{11|1}.$$

As in Section 4.1, the MTR and MTS assumptions and these reverse assumptions can be applied to obtain bounds on ACE with narrower widths. For example, for $(s, t) = (2, 0)$, Assumption 2.1 is $Y_{X=2} \geq Y_{X=0}$, which means that a subject takes a larger outcome value if he/she received the test treatment than if he/she received no treatment. This holds when it is apparent that the test treatment has a positive effect compared with no treatment. The similar interpretation is given for $(s, t) = (1, 0)$ $(Y_{X=1} \geq Y_{X=0})$ in place of the test treatment to the control.

Under Assumptions 1 and 2.1, the lower bound of $E(Y_{X=x})$ becomes $E(Y_{X=x}) \geq E(Y | R = x)$ for $x = 1, 2$, which is derived using $t = 0$ in Assumption 2.1. Likewise, $E(Y_{X=x}) \leq E(Y | R = x)$ under Assumptions 1 and 2.2. Although these bounds of $E(Y_{X=x})$ do not give a bound on ACE in contrast to that in Section 4.1.2, Assumption 2.1 can derive the following bounds by combination with inequality (5.1)[1]:

$$E(Y | R = 2) - (E_{11}p_{1|1} + K_1 p_{0|1}) \leq ACE \leq (E_{22}p_{2|2} + K_1 p_{0|2}) - E(Y | R = 1).$$

Similar to Assumptions 3.1 and 3.2, in the case of a binary outcome variable, we can make weaker assumptions that derive the same bounds as those under Assumptions 2.1 and 2.2, using the principal stratification approach. In the case of noncompliance by receiving no treatment, four types of potential outcomes, based on principal stratification, are re-

[1] If $(s, t) = (2, 1)$ in Assumption 2.1 is used as in Section 4.1, the lower bound on ACE is improved to 0.

defined as follows: doomed $\{Y_{X=x} = 1, Y_{X=0} = 1\}$, which consists of subjects who always experience the event, regardless of whether they receive the assigned treatment; preventive $\{Y_{X=x} = 0, Y_{X=0} = 1\}$, which consists of subjects who do not experience the event when they receive the assigned treatment but do when they receive no treatment; causative $\{Y_{X=x} = 1, Y_{X=0} = 0\}$, which consists of subjects who experience the event when they receive the assigned treatment, but not when they receive no treatment; and immune $\{Y_{X=x} = 0, Y_{X=0} = 0\}$, which consists of subjects who never experience the event, regardless of whether they receive the assigned treatment. In the definition, $x = 2$ for the test treatment group ($R = 2$) and $x = 1$ for the control group ($R = 1$). Similar to Section 4.1.2, Assumption 2.1 implies that no preventive subject exists, and Assumption 2.2 implies that no causative subject exists.

Under this definition of principal strata, alternative assumptions of Assumptions 2.1 and 2.2 are as follows:

ASSUMPTION 3.3

$$\Pr(Y_{X=x} = 1, Y_{X=0} = 0 \mid X = R = x) \geq \Pr(Y_{X=x} = 0, Y_{X=0} = 1 \mid X = R = x) \textit{ for } x = 1, 2.$$

ASSUMPTION 3.4

$$\Pr(Y_{X=x} = 1, Y_{X=0} = 0 \mid X = R = x) \leq \Pr(Y_{X=x} = 0, Y_{X=0} = 1 \mid X = R = x) \textit{ for } x = 1, 2.$$

Assumption 3.3 implies that the number of causative subjects is not less than the number of preventive subjects, and Assumption 3.4 implies that the number of causative subjects is not more than the number of preventive subjects, within both assigned groups. Thus, these Assumptions are weaker than assumptions 2.1 and 2.2. Nevertheless, they can give the same bounds as those under Assumptions 2.1 and 2.2.

The MTS and RMTS (Assumptions 4.1 and 4.2) can also be applied to the case of noncompliance by receiving no treatment. For example, for $(s, t) = (2, 0)$ and $r = 2$, Assumption 4.1 is $E(Y_{X=x} \mid X = 2, R = 2) \geq E(Y_{X=x} \mid X = 0, R = 2)$, which means that subjects who received the assigned test treatment (i.e., compliers) tend to have larger outcome values than those who received no treatment (i.e., non-compliers) for the test treatment group. Under Assumptions 1 and 4.1, the upper bound of $E(Y_{X=x})$ becomes $E(Y_{X=x}) \geq E_{xx}$ ($E(Y_{X=x}) \leq E_{xx}$ under Assumptions 1 and 4.2) for $x = 1, 2$. Thus, the combination with inequality (5.1) derives bounds on ACE of:

$$(E_{22}p_{2|2} + K_0 p_{0|2}) - E_{11} \leq \text{ACE} \leq E_{22} - (E_{11}p_{1|1} + K_0 p_{0|1}).$$

When both MTR and MTS hold, the bounds on ACE are:

$$E(Y \mid R = 2) - E_{11} \leq \text{ACE} \leq E_{22} - E(Y \mid R = 1),$$

because $E(Y \mid R = x) \leq E(Y_{X=x}) \leq E_{xx}$ for $x = 1, 2$. When both RMTR and RMTS hold, these signs of inequalities for $E(Y_{X=x})$ are reversed.

Finally, we note that the MC and RMC (Assumptions 5.1 and 5.2), which derive the same bounds as those under the MTS and RMTS (Assumptions 4.1 and 4.2), are changed as follows for the case of noncompliance by receiving no treatment:

ASSUMPTION 5.3: Monotone confounding (MC)

Both $E(Y \mid X = R = x, Z = z)$ *and* $\Pr(X = x \mid R = x, Z = z)$ *are non-decreasing or non-increasing in* z *for* $x = 1, 2$ *and all* r*, and the components of* Z *are independent of each other.*

ASSUMPTION 5.4: Reverse monotone confounding (RMC)

One of E(Y | X = R = x, Z = z) *and* Pr(X = x | R = x, Z = z) *is non-decreasing and the other is non-increasing in z for x* = 1, 2 *and all r, and the components of Z are independent of each other.*

In some actual situations, assumptions presented in this section may hold for one of the test treatment and control groups but not for the other. In such cases, the assumptions can be applied only to one group. This example is introduced in the next sub-section.

5.3 Application

We apply the assumptions and bounds presented in Section 5.2 to the CDP trial introduced in Section 1 (Table 1). R represents the assigned group (R = 2 for the clofibrate group and R = 1 for the placebo group), and X is the compliance status (X = 2 for compliers in the clofibrate group, X = 1 for compliers in the placebo group, and X = 0 for non-compliers). Here, compliers and non-compliers are patients receiving more or less than 80% of the assigned treatment, respectively. Y is the incidence of deaths (Y = 1 for dead and Y = 0 for alive). Again, we note that ITT and PP analyses yielded ITT = 194/1065 – 523/2695 = –1.19% and PP = 106/708 – 274/1813 = –0.14%, respectively.

As in Section 4.3, it is necessary to discuss whether the assumptions hold. There may be a placebo effect, but it is not thought that the proportion of deaths will increase by receiving the placebo. Thus, Assumptions 2.2 (RMTR) and 3.4 can be assumed for (s, t) = (1, 0) and x = 1. However, a preventive effect of clofibrate may not be present (i.e., these assumptions may not be assumed for (s, t) = (2, 0) and x = 2) because of side-effects. The World Health Organization (WHO) has reported that in a large randomized trial, there were 25% more deaths in the clofibrate group than in the comparable high serum cholesterol control group (WHO, 1980). Because it is not clear whether the clofibrate has a positive or negative effect, we cannot assume the MTR or RMTR (and Assumption 3.3 or 3.4) for the clofibrate group.

Relating to the patients in this trial, health-oriented subjects might tend not to die and be more likely to comply with the assigned treatment, compared with subjects not concerned about their health. Under this observation, the RMTS (Assumption 4.4) would hold for both assigned groups. However, we note that some researchers may criticize this because some patients might not receive the treatment due to side-effects. In such a case, the RMTS may not hold for the clofibrate group. Nevertheless, we assume the RMTS for both assigned groups for illustrative purposes. Assumption 1 would hold because this trial was a double-blinded trial.

The arguments presented above demonstrate that the RMTR and RMTS can be assumed for the placebo group. Therefore, the bounds of E($Y_{X=1}$) are E_{11} ≤ E($Y_{X=1}$) ≤ E(Y | R = 1), which yield 15.11% ≤ E($Y_{X=1}$) ≤ 19.41%. For the clofibrate group, the RMTS is assumed and then the bounds of E($Y_{X=2}$) are E_{22} ≤ E($Y_{X=2}$) ≤ $E_{22}p_{2|2} + K_1 p_{0|2}$ for K_1 = 1, which yields 14.97% ≤ E($Y_{X=2}$) ≤ 43.47%. In conclusion, the bounds on ACE are −4.43% ≤ ACE ≤ 28.36%. Unfortunately, we cannot conclude whether clofibrate is effective. However, the bounds improve those under Assumption 1 only: −32.94% ≤ ACE ≤ 33.31%, especially the lower bound.

6. Monotone instrumental variable

Sections 3-5 assumed the IV assumption (Assumption 1). As mentioned in Section 2, however, this assumption often may not hold in unblinded trials, in which subjects are aware of the assigned treatment and this knowledge may affect the potential outcomes. In the MRFIT (Section 4.3), subjects would have been aware of their assigned group because it was an unblinded trial, and thus the intervention itself might have evoked a psychological response. Furthermore, in addition to smoking cessation counseling, the intervention consisted of dietary advice to reduction blood cholesterol and hypertension medication. These interventions might also have influenced the incidence of CHD independent of smoking status. Thus, in this section, we relax the IV assumption to the following monotone instrumental variable (MIV) assumption (Manski & Pepper, 2000, 2009):

ASSUMPTION 6.1: Monotone instrumental variable (MIV)

$$E(Y_{X=x} \mid R = 2) \geq E(Y_{X=x} \mid R = 1).$$

The MIV assumption is only the replacement of equality in the IV assumption with inequality, and means that the values of potential outcomes for subjects assigned to $R = 2$ are overall larger than those assigned to $R = 1$. For example, consider an unblinded trial to compare a new treatment with a standard treatment, where the outcome is a measure such that a larger value is better for the subject's health. In such a trial, subjects may think that the new treatment is more effective than the standard treatment, and this thinking may give rise to better results for subjects assigned to the new treatment than those assigned to the standard treatment; this indicates that the MIV holds.

We can also consider the following reverse MIV (RMIV) assumption:

ASSUMPTION 6.2: Reverse monotone instrumental variable (RMIV)

$$E(Y_{X=x} \mid R = 2) \leq E(Y_{X=x} \mid R = 1).$$

We discuss the bounds on ACE under Assumptions 6.1 and 6.2 instead of Assumption 1. Noncompliance by switching the treatment (as in Sections 4) is discussed in Section 6.1, and noncompliance by receiving no treatment (as in Section 5) is discussed in Section 6.2. The derivations of inequalities in this section are outlined in Section 8.3.

6.1 Noncompliance by switching the treatment

The bounds introduced in Section 4 are extended to those under the MIV and RMIV (Assumptions 6.1 and 6.2). Under the MIV and RMIV, the bounds on ACE are:

$$(E_{21}p_{2|1} + K_0p_{1|1}) - (E_{12}p_{1|2} + K_1p_{2|2}) \leq \text{ACE} \leq (E_{22}p_{2|2} + K_1p_{1|2}) - (E_{11}p_{1|1} + K_0p_{2|1}), \quad (6.1)$$

$$(E_{22}p_{2|2} + K_0p_{1|2}) - (E_{11}p_{1|1} + K_1p_{2|1}) \leq \text{ACE} \leq (E_{21}p_{2|1} + K_1p_{1|1}) - (E_{12}p_{1|2} + K_0p_{2|2}). \quad (6.2)$$

These inequalities correspond to inequalities when a or b in $\max\{a, b\}$ and $\min\{a, b\}$ in inequality (4.1) are used. Therefore, the MIV and RMIV assumptions yield bounds on ACE with the same or broader width in comparison with the bounds under the IV assumption.

Even under the MIV (or RMIV) assumption, but not IV assumption, we can derive bounds on ACE with narower widths by applying assumptions in Section 4.2 (Chiba, 2010c). Each combination of the MIV or RMIV and the MTR or RMTR derives the improved lower or upper bounds on ACE in Table 3. Likewise, each combination of the MIV or RMIV and the MTS or RMTS derives the improved lower or upper bounds on ACE in Table 4.

Assumptions	Improved bound on ACE
MIV + MTR	ACE ≥ max{−ITT, 0}
RMIV + MTR	ACE ≥ max{ITT, 0}
MIV + RMTR	ACE ≤ min{ITT, 0}
RMIV + RMTR	ACE ≤ min{−ITT, 0}

Table 3. Improved bound on ACE under the MIV or RMIV and the MTR or RMTR, where $\text{ITT} \equiv E(Y \mid R = 2) - E(Y \mid R = 1)$.

Assumptions	Improved bound on ACE
MIV + MTS	ACE ≤ E_{22} − E_{11}
RMIV + MTS	ACE ≤ E_{21} − E_{12}
MIV + RMTS	ACE ≥ E_{21} − E_{12}
RMIV + RMTS	ACE ≥ E_{22} − E_{11}

Table 4. Improved bound on ACE under the MIV or RMIV and the MTS or RMTS.

Eight lower or upper bounds in Tables 3 and 4 yield the same or broader bounds as those under the IV assumption. Note that we can use Assumptions 3.1 and 3.2 instead of the MTR and RMTR (Assumptions 2.1 and 2.2), respectively, and Assumptions 5.1 and 5.2 instead of the MTS and RMTS (Assumptions 4.1 and 4.2), respectively. Further combinations of the above bounds can derive further improved bounds; for example, max{−ITT, 0} ≤ ACE ≤ PP under the MIV, MTR and MTS assumptions.

For illustration, we apply the bounds presented here to the MRFIT (Table 2), in which the IV assumption may not hold, as discussed above. Because the intervention consisted of dietary advice and hypertension medication as well as the therapy itself that might have evoked a psychological response, the potential incidence of CHD for subjects assigned to the test group might have been reduced, compared with subjects assigned to the control group. This observation shows that Assumption 6.2 (RMIV: $E(Y_{X=x} \mid R = 2) \le E(Y_{X=x} \mid R = 1)$) is reasonable. Additionally, as discussed in Section 4.3, the RMTR (or Assumption 3.2) and RMTS are reasonable assumptions in this trial. In conclusion, the RMIV, RMTR and RMTS can be assumed, and then bounds on ACE become PP ≤ ACE ≤ min{−ITT, 0}, which yield −0.92% ≤ ACE ≤ 0%. In comparison with the IV (plus RMTR and RMTS) in Section 4.2 (−0.92% ≤ ACE ≤ −0.13%), the lower bound is the same but the upper bound is larger.

6.2 Noncompliance by receiving no treatment

The bounds introduced in Section 5 are extended to those under the MIV and RMIV (Assumptions 6.1 and 6.2). Under these assumptions, the bounds on ACE are:

$$K_0 - K_1 \le \text{ACE} \le (E_{22}p_{2|2} + K_1 p_{0|2}) - (E_{11}p_{1|1} + K_0 p_{0|1}), \quad (6.3)$$

$$(E_{22}p_{2|2} + K_0 p_{0|2}) - (E_{11}p_{1|1} + K_1 p_{0|1}) \le \text{ACE} \le K_1 - K_0, \quad (6.4)$$

respectively. The upper bound in inequality (6.3) is equal to that in inequality (5.1) and the lower bound in inequality (6.4) is equal to that in inequality (5.1). Unfortunately, the respective lower and upper bounds in inequalities (6.3) and (6.4) do not give any information.

As discussed in the above sub-section, by combining the MTR (or RMTR) and MTS (or RMTS), the bounds on ACE can be improved. Table 5 summarizes the bounds under the MIV or RMIV and the MTR and RMTR, and Table 6 summarizes those under the MIV or RMIV and the MTS and RMTS. The bounds in Tables 5 and 6 include K_0 or K_1, which is the finite range of Y. Specifically, in Table 6, the lower or upper bounds are not improved even when the MTS or RMTS is added. Thus, the bounds may not be greatly improved. However, further combinations of these assumptions can remove K_0 and K_1 from one of the lower and upper bounds. Such bounds are summarized in Table 7.

Assumptions	Bounds on ACE
MIV + MTR	$E(Y \mid R=1) - (E_{22}p_{2\mid 2} + K_1 p_{0\mid 2}) \le \text{ACE} \le (E_{22}p_{2\mid 2} + K_1 p_{0\mid 2}) - E(Y \mid R=1)$
RMIV + MTR	$E(Y \mid R=2) - (E_{11}p_{1\mid 1} + K_1 p_{0\mid 1}) \le \text{ACE} \le K_1 - (E_{02}p_{0\mid 2} + K_0 p_{2\mid 2})$
MIV + RMTR	$K_0 - (E_{02}p_{0\mid 2} + K_1 p_{2\mid 2}) \le \text{ACE} \le E(Y \mid R=2) - (E_{11}p_{1\mid 1} + K_0 p_{0\mid 1})$
RMIV + RMTR	$(E_{22}p_{2\mid 2} + K_0 p_{0\mid 2}) - E(Y \mid R=1) \le \text{ACE} \le E(Y \mid R=1) - (E_{22}p_{2\mid 2} + K_0 p_{0\mid 2})$

Table 5. Bounds on ACE under the MIV or RMIV and the MTR or RMTR[2].

Assumptions	Bounds on ACE
MIV + MTS	$K_0 - K_1 \le \text{ACE} \le E_{22} - (E_{11}p_{1\mid 1} + K_0 p_{0\mid 1})$
RMIV + MTS	$(E_{22}p_{2\mid 2} + K_0 p_{0\mid 2}) - E_{11} \le \text{ACE} \le K_1 - K_0$
MIV + RMTS	$K_0 - K_1 \le \text{ACE} \le (E_{22}p_{2\mid 2} + K_1 p_{0\mid 2}) - E_{11}$
RMIV + RMTS	$E_{22} - (E_{11}p_{1\mid 1} + K_1 p_{0\mid 1}) \le \text{ACE} \le K_1 - K_0$

Table 6. Bounds on ACE under the MIV or RMIV and the MTS or RMTS.

Assumptions	Bounds on ACE
MIV + MTR + MTS	$E(Y \mid R=1) - (E_{22}p_{2\mid 2} + K_1 p_{0\mid 2}) \le \text{ACE} \le E_{22} - E(Y \mid R=1)$
RMIV + MTR + MTS	$E(Y \mid R=2) - E_{11} \le \text{ACE} \le K_1 - (E_{02}p_{0\mid 2} + K_0 p_{2\mid 2})$
MIV + RMTR + RMTS	$K_0 - (E_{02}p_{0\mid 2} + K_1 p_{2\mid 2}) \le \text{ACE} \le E(Y \mid R=2) - E_{11}$
RMIV + RMTR + RMTS	$E_{22} - E(Y \mid R=1) \le \text{ACE} \le E(Y \mid R=1) - (E_{22}p_{2\mid 2} + K_0 p_{0\mid 2})$

Table 7. Bounds on ACE under some combinations of assumptions[3].

For illustration, we apply the bounds presented here to the CDP trial (Table 1). Although the IV (Assumption 1) would hold in this trial because it was a double-blinded trial, we here relax this assumption to the MIV and RMIV (Assumptions 6.1 and 6.2), and yield bounds on ACE under both assumptions. As discussed in Section 5.3, we assume the RMTS for the clofibrate group and the RMTR and RMTS for the placebo group. Then, under the MIV, the bounds of $E(Y_{X=2})$ and $E(Y_{X=1})$ are $K_0 \le E(Y_{X=2}) \le E_{22}p_{2\mid 2} + K_1 p_{0\mid 2}$ and $E_{11} \le E(Y_{X=1}) \le E_{02}p_{0\mid 2} + K_1 p_{2\mid 2}$, respectively, where $K_0 = 0$ and $K_1 = 1$ because Y is binary. These bounds yield bounds on ACE of $-74.74\% \le \text{ACE} \le 28.36\%$. Likewise, under the RMIV, the bounds on ACE become $-4.43\% \le \text{ACE} \le 90.05\%$, because $E_{22} \le E(Y_{X=2}) \le K_1$ and $E_{22}p_{2\mid 2} + K_0 p_{0\mid 2} \le E(Y_{X=1}) \le E(Y \mid R = 1)$. Unfortunately, these bounds have a very broad width, and thus they do not provide enough information about treatment effects of clofibrate.

7. Conclusion

This chapter has presented bounds on ACE in randomized trials with noncompliance. Although the results presented here are relevant to the causal differences, they can also be readily applied to the causal risk ratio when the outcome is binary.

---

[2] If $(s, t) = (2, 1)$ in the MTR and RMTR (Assumptions 2.1 and 2.2) is used, the lower bound is 0 under the MTR and the upper bound is 0 under the RMTR.

[3] If $(s, t) = (2, 1)$ in the MTR and RMTR (Assumptions 2.1 and 2.2) is additionally used, a candidate of the lower bound is 0 under the MTR and that of the upper bound is 0 under the RMTR.

It is generally thought that the ITT analysis is likely to yield a downwardly biased estimate of causal effects (Sheiner & Rubin, 1995), whereas the PP analysis is likely to yield an upwardly biased estimate (Lewis & Machine, 1993). Thus, the ACE probably exists between the results of the ITT and PP analyses. As shown in Section 4.1, this is true under IV + MTR + MTS or under IV + RMTR + RMTS for noncompliance by switching the treatment. However, as shown in Sections 5 and 6, we cannot be certain that this is true when noncompliance is due to receiving no treatment and/or the IV assumption does not hold. Thus, investigators should not simply conclude that the ACE exists between the results of the ITT and PP analyses. Unfortunately, no standard method currently exists for estimating the ACE in randomized trials with noncompliance issues. Investigators should consider whether the assumptions presented in this chapter are valid and then yield bounds on ACE using the methodology described herein.

The needs from further methodologies in this field are three-fold. The first is to find weaker assumptions than those given here, which nevertheless can derive the same bounds. The second is to make assumptions that can derive the bounds with a narrower width, which are still reasonable in some situations. The ideal is to make a reasonable assumption that can give a point estimator. The third and final need is to extend the discussions in this chapter to more complex situations: for example, two types of noncompliance in this chapter may occur simultaneously, and more than two arms may be compared (Cheng & Small, 2006).

The other recent interest in causal inference is statistical analysis concerning the role of an intermediate variable between a particular treatment and outcome (Rubin, 2004; Joffe et al., 2007; VanderWeele, 2008b). Investigators are often interested in understanding how the effect of a treatment on an outcome may be mediated through an intermediate variable. For example, in the MRFIT, this implies that investigators are interested in how the effect of a multifactor intervention program on CHD mortality may be mediated through the smoking status 1 year after entry, rather than the effect of the smoking status 1 year after entry on CHD mortality. Such statistical analyses are closely related to issues of inference with a surrogate marker and issues of post-randomization selection bias and truncation-by-death (Zhang & Rubin, 2003; Chiba & VanderWeele, 2011). Further methodological research is needed to answer these issues.

8. Appendix: Derivations of equations and inequalities

This section outlines the derivations of the equations and inequalities presented in Sections 3, 4 and 6, which are outlined in Sections 8.1, 8.2 and 8.3, respectively.

8.1 Derivations of equations in Section 3

Equation (3.1) can be derived as follows:

$$\begin{aligned}
\mathrm{E}(Y_{X=2}) &= \mathrm{E}(Y_{X=2} \mid R=r) \\
&= \sum_{x=1,2} \mathrm{E}(Y_{X=2} \mid X=x, R=r)\Pr(X=x \mid R=r) \\
&= (E_{2r} - \alpha_r)p_{1|r} + E_{2r}p_{2|r} \\
&= E_{2r} - \alpha_r p_{1|r}.
\end{aligned}$$

The first equation holds by Assumption 1, and the third equation is derived by substituting $\mathrm{E}(Y_{X=2} \mid X = 1, R = r) = \mathrm{E}(Y_{X=2} \mid X = 2, R = r) - \alpha_r$ and applying the consistency assumption: $\mathrm{E}(Y_{X=2} \mid X = 2, R = r) = \mathrm{E}(Y \mid X = 2, R = r)$ (= E_{2r}). A similar calculation derives equation (3.2).

To derive equation (3.3), we consider the difference between $E(Y|R = 2)$ and $E(Y_{X=2})$ and between $E(Y|R = 1)$ and $E(Y_{X=1})$. The former difference derives:

$$\begin{aligned} E(Y \mid R=2)-E(Y_{X=2}) &= \sum_{x=1,2} E_{x2} p_{x|2} - (E_{22} - \alpha_2 p_{1|2}) \\ &= (E_{12} + \alpha_2) p_{1|2} - E_{22}(1 - p_{2|2}) \\ &= \{\alpha_2 - (E_{22} - E_{22})\} p_{1|2}. \end{aligned}$$

By a similar calculation, the latter difference becomes $E(Y|R = 1) - E(Y_{X=1}) = \{\beta_1 - (E_{21} - E_{11})\}p_{2|1}$. The difference between these equations derives equation (3.3).
The derivation of equation (3.5) is as follows. Simple algebra, $p_{2|r} \times$ equation (3.1) plus $p_{1|r} \times$ equation (3.2), yields $p_{2|r}\mathrm{ACE} + E(Y_{X=1}) = E(Y|R = r) - (a_r - \beta_r)p_{1|r}p_{2|r}$. The difference between this equation with $r = 2$ and that with $r = 1$ is:

$$(p_{2|2} - p_{2|1})\mathrm{ACE} = E(Y|R = 2) - E(Y|R = 1) - (a_2 - \beta_2)p_{1|2}p_{2|2} + (a_1 - \beta_1)p_{1|1}p_{2|1}.$$

This equation implies equation (3.5) for $p_{2|2} \neq p_{2|1}$.

8.2 Derivations of inequalities in Section 4

Inequality (4.1) can be derived as presented below. By substituting $K_0 \leq E(Y_{X=x}|X = x^*, R = r) \leq K_1$ for $x \neq x^*$ and $E(Y_{X=x}|X = x^*, R = r) = E(Y|X = x, R = r)$ $(= E_{xr})$ for $x = x^*$ (consistency assumption) into:

$$E(Y_{X=x} \mid R=r) = \sum_{x^*=1,2} E(Y_{X=x} \mid X = x^*, R=r)\Pr(X = x^* \mid R = r), \tag{8.1}$$

we obtain:

$$E_{xr}p_{x|r} + K_0 p_{x^*|r} \leq E(Y_{X=x} \mid R = r) \leq E_{xr}p_{x|r} + K_1 p_{x^*|r} \tag{8.2}$$

for $x \neq x^*$. Because $E(Y_{X=x}) = E(Y_{X=x}|R = r)$ by Assumption 1, the bounds of $E(Y_{X=x})$ become:

$$\max\begin{Bmatrix} E_{x1}p_{x|1} + K_0 p_{x^*|1} \\ E_{x2}p_{x|2} K_0 p_{x^*|2} \end{Bmatrix} \leq E(Y_{X=x}) \leq \min\begin{Bmatrix} E_{x1}p_{x|1} + K_1 p_{x^*|1} \\ E_{x2}p_{x|2} + K_1 p_{x^*|2} \end{Bmatrix}$$

for $x \neq x^*$. The difference between the lower and upper bounds of this inequality for $x = 1, 2$ is inequality (4.1).
Inequality (4.3) can be also derived using equation (8.1). Assumption 2.1 implies that $E(Y_{X=2}|X = x, R = r) \geq E(Y_{X=1}|X = x, R = r)$. Thus, by substituting this inequality with $x = 1$ into equation (8.1), we obtain:

$$\begin{aligned} E(Y_{X=2}) &= E(Y_{X=2} \mid R=r) \\ &\geq \sum_{x=1,2} E(Y_{X=x} \mid X = x, R = r)\Pr(X = x \mid R = r) \\ &= \sum_{x=1,2} E(Y \mid X = x, R = r)\Pr(X = x \mid R = r) \\ &= E(Y \mid R = r), \end{aligned} \tag{8.3}$$

and thus $E(Y_{X=2}) \geq \max\{E(Y|R = 1), E(Y|R = 2)\}$. Similarly, $E(Y_{X=1}) \leq \min\{E(Y|R = 1), E(Y|R = 2)\}$ by substituting $E(Y_{X=2}|X = 2, R = r) \geq E(Y_{X=1}|X = 2, R = r)$ into equation (8.1). The difference between them is inequality (4.3).

In the case of a binary outcome variable, inequality (4.3) can also be derived under Assumption 3.1. By adding $\Pr(Y_{X=2} = 1, Y_{X=1} = 1 | X = x, R = r)$ on both sides of the inequality in Assumption 3.1: $\Pr(Y_{X=2} = 1, Y_{X=1} = 0 | X = x, R = r) \geq \Pr(Y_{X=2} = 0, Y_{X=1} = 1 | X = x, R = r)$, we obtain $\Pr(Y_{X=2} = 1 | X = x, R = r) \geq \Pr(Y_{X=1} = 1 | X = x, R = r)$. Because this inequality is a binary outcome version of $E(Y_{X=2} | X = x, R = r) \geq E(Y_{X=1} | X = x, R = r)$, inequality (4.3) is derived.

Inequality (4.4) can be derived as follows. Substituting $E(Y_{X=2} | X = 2, R = r) \geq E(Y_{X=2} | X = 1, R = r)$ ($x = 2$ and $(s, t) = (2, 1)$ in Assumption 4.1) into equation (8.1) yields:

$$\begin{aligned} E(Y_{X=2}) &= E(Y_{X=2} \mid R = r) \\ &\leq \sum_{x=1,2} E(Y_{X=2} \mid X = 2, R = r)\Pr(X = x \mid R = r) \\ &= E(Y \mid X = 2, R = r)(= E_{2r}), \end{aligned} \tag{8.4}$$

and thus $E(Y_{X=2}) \leq \min\{E_{21}, E_{22}\}$. Similarly, $E(Y_{X=1}) \geq \max\{E_{11}, E_{12}\}$ by substituting $E(Y_{X=1} | X = 2, R = r) \geq E(Y_{X=1} | X = 1, R = r)$ ($x = 1$ and $(s, t) = (2, 1)$ in Assumption 4.1) into equation (8.1). The difference between them is inequality (4.4).

Inequality (4.4) can also be derived under Assumption 5.1. To prove this, we need the following lemma (Esary et al., 1967):

LEMMA 1

Let f and g be functions with n real-valued arguments such that both f and g are non-decreasing or non-increasing in each of their arguments. If $Z = (Z_1, \ldots, Z_n)$ is a multivariate random variable with n components such that each component is independent of the other components, then $\mathrm{Cov}\{f(Z), g(Z)\} \geq 0$.

Let $f_r(Z) = E(Y | X = 2, R = r, Z = z)$, $g_r(Z) = \Pr(X = 2 | R = r, Z = z)$ and $F_{Z|R=r}$ denote the cumulative distribution function of Z conditional on $R = r$. Then, by Lemma 1, we obtain:

$$E_{F_{Z|R=r}}\{f_r(Z)g_r(Z)\} - E_{F_{Z|R=r}}\{f_r(Z)\}E_{F_{Z|R=r}}\{g_r(Z)\} = \mathrm{Cov}_{F_{Z|R=r}}\{f_r(Z), g_r(Z)\} \geq 0,$$

if both $f_r(Z)$ and $g_r(Z)$ are non-decreasing or non-increasing in z and the components of Z are independent. Thus, using the assumption that $Y_{X=x}$ is independent from X given R and Z, the following inequality is derived:

$$\begin{aligned} E(Y_{X=2} \mid X = 1, R = r) &= \sum_z E(Y_{X=2} \mid X = 1, R = r, Z = z)\Pr(Z = z \mid X = 1, R = r) \\ &= \sum_z \frac{E(Y \mid X = 2, R = r, Z = z)\Pr(X = 1 \mid R = r, Z = z)\Pr(Z = z \mid R = r)}{\Pr(X = 1 \mid R = r)} \\ &= E_{F_{Z|R=r}}[f_r(Z)\{1 - g_r(Z)\}]/\Pr(X = 1 \mid R = r) \\ &\leq E_{F_{Z|R=r}}\{f_r(Z)\}E_{F_{Z|R=r}}\{1 - g_r(Z)\}/\Pr(X = 1 \mid R = r) \\ &= E_{F_{Z|R=r}}\{f_r(Z)\} \\ &= E_{F_{Z|R=r}}\{f_r(Z)\}E_{F_{Z|R=r}}\{g_r(Z)\}/\Pr(X = 2 \mid R = r) \\ &\leq E_{F_{Z|R=r}}\{f_r(Z)g_r(Z)\}/\Pr(X = 2 \mid R = r) \\ &= \sum_z \frac{E(Y \mid X = 2, R = r, Z = z)\Pr(X = 2 \mid R = r, Z = z)\Pr(Z = z \mid R = r)}{\Pr(X = 2 \mid R = r)} \\ &= E(Y \mid X = 2, R = r). \end{aligned}$$

The second equation holds because $E(Y_{X=2} \mid X = 1, R = r, Z = z) = E(Y_{X=2} \mid X = 2, R = r, Z = z) = E(Y \mid X = 2, R = r, Z = z)$ by the independency and consistency assumptions. The fourth inequality holds because $1 - g_r(Z)$ is non-increasing when $g_r(Z)$ is non-decreasing. The fifth and sixth equations hold because:

$$E_{F_{Z|R=r}}\{g_r(Z)\} = \sum_z \Pr(X = 2 \mid R = r, Z = z)\Pr(Z = z \mid R = r) = \Pr(X = 2 \mid R = r).$$

A similar calculation derives $E(Y_{X=1} \mid X = 2, R = r) \geq E(Y \mid X = 1, R = r)$. The inequalities derived here are the same as those in Assumption 4.1. Therefore, inequality (4.4) can be derived under Assumption 5.1.

8.3 Derivations of inequalities in Section 6

$E(Y_{X=x})$ can be expressed as $E(Y_{X=x}) = E(Y_{X=x} \mid R = 1)\Pr(R = 1) + E(Y_{X=x} \mid R = 2)\Pr(R = 2)$. Therefore,

$$E(Y_{X=x} \mid R = 1) \leq E(Y_{X=x}) \leq E(Y_{X=x} \mid R = 2) \tag{8.5}$$

under Assumption 6.1 (MIV: $E(Y_{X=x} \mid R = 1) \geq E(Y_{X=x} \mid R = 0)$). All bounds under the MIV are derived based on inequality (8.5), while those under the IV (Assumption 1) are based on $E(Y_{X=x}) = E(Y_{X=x} \mid R = r)$. This is why inequality (6.1) corresponds to it when a or b in $\max\{a, b\}$ and $\min\{a, b\}$ in inequality (4.1) is used. This is also similar under the RMIV (Assumption 6.2), and then inequality (6.2) and the bounds in Tables 3 and 4 also correspond to those when a or b in $\max\{a, b\}$ and $\min\{a, b\}$ in the bounds presented in Section 4.1 are used. Therefore, the derivations of bounds in Section 6.1 are simple. Inequality (6.1) is derived by the combination of inequalities (8.2) and (8.5).

In Table 3, $ACE \geq \max\{-ITT, 0\}$ under the MIV and MTR is derived as follows. Because $E(Y_{X=2}) \geq E(Y_{X=2} \mid R = 1)$ from inequality (8.5), $E(Y_{X=2}) \geq E(Y \mid R = 1)$ from inequality (8.3) with $r = 1$. Likewise, $E(Y_{X=1}) \leq E(Y \mid R = 2)$ by $E(Y_{X=1}) \leq E(Y_{X=1} \mid R = 2)$ and the MTR (Assumption 2.1). The difference between these inequalities derives $ACE \geq -ITT$. Additionally, the MTR derives $ACE = E(Y_{X=1}) - E(Y_{X=0}) \geq 0$ directly. The other bounds in Table 3 can be derived in a similar way.

In Table 4, $ACE \leq E_{22} - E_{11}$ under the MIV and MTS is derived as follows. Because $E(Y_{X=2}) \leq E(Y_{X=2} \mid R = 2)$ from inequality (8.5), $E(Y_{X=2}) \leq E_{22}$ from inequality (8.4) with $r = 2$. Likewise, $E(Y_{X=1}) \geq E_{11}$ by $E(Y_{X=1}) \geq E(Y_{X=1} \mid R = 1)$ and the MTS (Assumption 4.1). The difference between these inequalities derives $ACE \leq E_{22} - E_{11}$. The other bounds in Table 4 can be derived in a similar way.

The inequalities in Section 6.2 can be derived in straightforward manner as the derivations of those in Section 6.1 by replacing $x = 1, 2$ in Section 6.1 to $x = 0, 1$ and $x = 0, 2$, although they may be somewhat complex.

9. Acknowledgment

This work was supported partially by Grant-in-Aid for Scientific Research (No. 23700344) from the Ministry of Education, Culture, Sports, Science, and Technology of Japan.

10. References

Angrist, J.D.; Imbens, G.W. & Rubin, D.B. (1996). Identification of causal effects using instrumental variables (with discussions). *Journal of the American Statistical Association*, Vol.91, No.434, (June 1996), pp.444-472, ISSN 0162-1459

Balke, A. & Pearl, J. (1997). Bounds on treatment effects from studies with imperfect compliance. *Journal of the American Statistical Association*, Vol.92, No.439, (September 1997), pp.1171-1176, ISSN 0162-1459

Brumback, B.A.; Hernán, M.A.; Haneuse, S.J.P.A. & Robins, J.M. (2004). Sensitivity analyses for unmeasured confounding assuming a marginal structural model for repeated measures. *Statistics in Medicine*, Vol.23, No.5, (March 2004), pp.749–767, ISSN 1097-0258

Cai, Z.; Kuroki, M. & Sato, T. (2007). Non-parametric bounds on treatment effects with non-compliance by covariate adjustment. *Statistics in Medicine*, Vol.26, No.16, (July 2007), pp.3188-3204, ISSN 1097-0258

Cheng, J. & Small, D.S. (2006). Bounds on causal effects in three-arm trials with non-compliance. *Journal of the Royal Statistical Society, Series B*, Vol.68, No.5, (November 2006), pp.815-836, ISSN 0964-1998

Chiba, Y. (2009a). The sign of the unmeasured confounding bias under various standard populations. *Biometrical Journal*, Vol.51, No.4, (August 2009), pp. 670-676, ISSN 0323-3847

Chiba, Y. (2009b). Bounds on causal effects in randomized trials with noncompliance under monotonicity assumptions about covariates. *Statistics in Medicine*, Vol.28, No.26, (November 2009), pp.3249-3259, ISSN 1097-0258

Chiba, Y. (2010a). Bias analysis of the instrumental variable estimator as an estimator of the average causal effect. *Contemporary Clinical Trials*, Vol.31, No.1, (January 2010), pp.12-17, ISSN 1551-7144

Chiba, Y. (2010b). An approach for estimating causal effects in randomized trials with noncompliance. *Communications in Statistics – Theory and Methods*, Vol.39, No.12, (January 2010), pp.2146-2156, ISSN 0361-0926

Chiba, Y. (2010c). The monotone instrumental variable in randomized trials with noncompliance. *Japanese Journal of Biometrics*, Vol.31, No.2, (December 2010), pp.93-106, ISSN 0918-4430

Chiba, Y. (2011). An alternative assumption for assessing the sign of causal effects. *Oriental Journal of Statistical Methods, Theory and Applications*, in press, ISSN Awaited

Chiba, Y.; Sato, T. & Greenland, S. (2007). Bounds on potential risks and causal risk differences under assumptions about confounding parameters. *Statistics in Medicine*, Vol.26, No.28, (December 2007), pp. 5125-5135, ISSN 1097-0258

Chiba, Y. & VanderWeele, T.J. (2011). A simple method for principal strata effects when the outcome has been truncated due to death. *American Journal of Epidemiology*, Vol.173, No.7, (April 2011), pp.745-751, ISSN 0002-9262

Coronary Drug Project Research Group (1980). Influence of adherence to treatment and response of cholesterol on mortality in the coronary drug project. *New England Journal of Medicine*, Vol.303, No.18, (October 1980), pp.1038-1041, ISSN 0028-4793

Cuzick, J.; Edwards, R. & Segnan, N. (1997). Adjustment for non-compliance and contamination in randomized clinical trials. *Statistics in Medicine*, Vol.16, No.9, (May 1997), pp.1017-1029, ISSN 1097-0258

Esary, J.D.; Proschan, F. & Walkup, D.W. (1967). Association of random variables, with applications. *Annals of Mathematical Statistics*, Vol.38, No.5, (October 1967), pp.1466-1474, ISSN 0003-4851

Fisher, L.D.; Dixon, D.O.; Herson, J.; Frankowski, R.; Hearron, M. & Peace, K.E. (1990). Intention to treat in clinical trials, In: *Statistical Issues in Drug Research and Development*, K.E. Peace (Ed.), 331-350, Marcel Dekker, ISBN 0-8247-8290-9, New York, USA

Frangakis, C.E. & Rubin, D.B. (2002). Principal stratification in causal inference. *Biometrics* Vol.58, No.1, (March 2002), pp.21-29, ISSN 0006-341X

Greenland, S. (2000). An introduction to instrumental variables for epidemiologists. *International Journal of Epidemiology*, Vol.29, No.4, (August 2000), pp.722-729, ISSN 0300-5771

Greenland, S. & Robins, J.M. (1986). Identifiability, exchangeability and epidemiologic confounding. *International Journal of Epidemiology*, Vol.15, No.3, (June 1986), pp.413-419, ISSN 0300-5771

Hernán, M.A. & Robins, J.M. (2006). Instruments for causal inference: An epidemiologist's dream? *Epidemiology*, Vol.17, No.4, (July 2006), pp.360–372, ISSN 1044-3983

Holland, P.W. (1986). Statistics and causal inference (with discussions). *Journal of the American Statistical Association*, Vol.81, No.396, (December 1986), pp.945-970, ISSN 0162-1459

Joffe, M.; Small, D. & Hsu, C.-Y. (2007). Defining and estimating intervention effects for groups that will develop an auxiliary outcome. *Statistical Science*, Vol.22, No.1, (February 2007), pp.74-97, ISSN 0883-4237

Lee, Y.; Ellenberg, J.; Hirtz, D. & Nelson, K. (1991). Analysis of clinical trials by treatment actually received: Is it really an option? *Statistics in Medicine*, Vol.10, No.10, (October 1991), pp.1595-1605, ISSN 1097-0258

Lewis, J.A. & Machine, D. (1993). Intention to treat - who should use ITT? *British Journal of Cancer*, Vol.68, No.4, (October 1993), pp.647-650, ISSN 0007-0920

Manski, C. F. (1990). Nonparametric bounds on treatment effects. *American Economic Review*, Vol.80, No.2, (May 1990), pp.319-323, ISSN 0002-8282

Manski, C.F. (1997). Monotone treatment response. *Econometrica*, Vol.65, No.6, (November 1997), pp.1311-1334, ISSN 0012-9682

Manski, C.F. (2003). *Partial identification of probability distributions*, Springer-Verlag, ISBN 0-387-00454-8, New York, USA

Manski, C.F. & Pepper, J.V. (2000). Monotone instrumental variables: With an application to the returns to schooling. *Econometrica*, Vol.68, No.4, (July 2000), pp.997-1010, ISSN 0012-9682

Manski, C.F. & Pepper, J.V. (2009). More on monotone instrumental variables. *Econometrics Journal*, Vol.12, No.S1, (January 2009), pp.S200-S216, ISSN 1368-4221

Mark, S.D. & Robins, J.M. (1993). A method for the analysis of randomized trials with noncompliance information: An application to the multiple risk factor intervention trial. *Controlled Clinical Trials*, Vol.14, No.2, (April 1993), pp.79-97, ISSN 1551-7144

Matsui, S. (2005). Stratified analysis in randomized trials with noncompliance. *Biometrics*, Vol.61, No.3, (September 2005), pp.816-823, ISSN 0006-341X

Multiple Risk Factor Intervention Trial Research Group (1982). Multiple risk factor intervention trial: Risk factor changes and mortality results. *Journal of the American Medical Association*, Vol.248, No.12, (September 1982), pp.1465-1477, ISSN 0098-7484

Piantadosi, S. (1997). *Clinical Trials: A Methodologic Perspective*, Wiley, ISBN 0-471-16393-7, New York, USA

Pearl, J. (1995). Causal inference from indirect experiments. *Artificial Intelligence in Medicine,* Vol.7, No.6, (December 1995), pp.561-582, ISSN 0933-3657

Pearl, J. (2000). *Causality: Models, Reasoning, and Inference,* Cambridge University Press, ISBN 0-521-77362-8, Cambridge, USA

Robins, J.M. (1989). The analysis of randomized and non-randomized AIDS treatment trials using a new approach to causal inference in longitudinal studies, In: *Health Service Research Methodology: A Focus on AIDS,* L. Sechrest, H. Freeman & A. Mulley (Eds), 113-159, DHHS Publication No.(PHS)89-3439, U.S. Public Health Service, Washington DC, USA

Robins, J.M. & Greenland, S. (1994). Adjusting for differential rates of PCP prophylaxis in high- versus low-dose AZT treatment arms in an AIDS randomized trial. *Journal of the American Statistical Association,* Vol.89, No.427, (September 1994), pp.737-749, ISSN 0162-1459

Robins, J.M. & Tsiatis, A.A. (1991). Correcting for non-compliance in randomized trials using rank preserving structural failure time models. *Communications in Statistics – Theory and Methods,* Vol.20, No.8, (January 1991), pp.2609-2631, ISSN 0361-0926

Rubin, D.B. (1974). Estimating causal effects of treatments in randomized and nonrandomized studies. *Journal of Educational Psychology,* Vol.66, No.5, (October 1974), pp.688-701, ISSN 0022-0663

Rubin, D.B. (1978). Bayesian inference for causal effects: The role of randomization. *Annals of Statistics,* Vol.6, No.1, (January 1978), pp.34-58, ISSN 0090-5364

Rubin, D. B. (1990). Formal models of statistical inference for causal effects. *Journal of Statistical Planning and Inference,* Vol.25, No.3, (July 1990), pp.279-292, ISSN 0378-3758

Rubin, D.B. (2004). Direct and indirect effects via potential outcomes. *Scandinavian Journal of Statistics,* Vol.31, No.2, (June 2004), pp.161-170, ISSN 1467-9469

Sato, T. (2006). Randomization-based analysis of causal effects, In: *Handbook of Clinical Trials: Design and Analysis,* T. Tango & H. Uesaka (Eds.), 535-556, Asakura Publishing, ISBN 978-4-254-32214-9, Tokyo, Japan (in Japanese)

Schwartz, D. & Lellouch, J. (1967). Explanatory and pragmatic attitudes in therapeutic trials. *Journal of Chronic Diseases,* Vol.20, No.8, (August 1967), pp.637-648, ISSN 0021-9681

Sheiner, L. & Rubin, D.B. (1995). Intention-to-treat analysis and the goals of clinical trials. *Clinical Pharmacology and Therapeutics,* Vol.57, No.1, (January 1995), pp.6-15, ISSN 0009-9236

VanderWeele, T.J. (2008a). The sign of the bias of unmeasured confounding. *Biometrics,* Vol.64, No.3, (September 2008), pp.702-706, ISSN 0006-341X

VanderWeele, T.J. (2008b). Simple relations between principal stratification and direct and indirect effects. *Statistics and Probability Letters,* Vol.78, No.17, (December 2008), pp.2957-2962, ISSN 0167-7152

World Health Organization (1980). W.H.O. cooperative trial on primary prevention of ischaemic heart disease using clofibrate to lower serum cholesterol: Mortality follow-up: Report of the committee of principal investigators. *Lancet,* Vol.316, No.8191, (August 1980), pp.379-385, ISSN 0140-6736

Zhang, J.L. & Rubin, D.B. (2003). Estimation of causal effects via principal stratification when some outcomes are truncated by "death." *Journal of Educational and Behavioral Statistics,* Vol.28, No.4, (December 2003), pp.353-368, ISSN 1076-9986

3

Design of Scoring Models for Trustworthy Risk Prediction in Critical Patients

Paolo Barbini and Gabriele Cevenini
Department of Surgery and Bioengineering, University of Siena
Italy

1. Introduction

Prediction of an adverse health event (AHE) from objective data is of great importance in clinical practice. A health event is inherently dichotomous as it either happens or does not happen, and in the latter case, it is a favourable health event (FHE).

In many clinical applications, it is relevant not only to predict AHEs happening (diagnostic ability) but also to estimate in advance their individual risk of occurrence using ordered multinomial or quantitative scales (prognostic ability) such as probability. An estimated probability of a patient's outcome is usually preferred to a simpler binary decision rule. However, models cannot be designed by optimising their fit to true individual risk probabilities because the latter are not intrinsically known, nor can they be easily and accurately associated with an individual's data. Classification models are therefore usually trained on binary outcomes to provide an orderable or quantitative output, which can be dichotomised using a suitable cut-off value.

Model discrimination refers to accurate identification of actual outcomes. Model calibration, or goodness of fit, is related to the agreement between predicted probabilities and observed proportions and it is an important aspect to consider in evaluating the prognostic capacity of a risk model (Cook, 2008). Model calibration is independent of discrimination, since there are risk models with good discrimination but poor calibration. A well-calibrated model gives probability values that can be reliably associated with the true individual risk of outcomes.

Many models have recently been proposed for diagnostic purposes in a wide range of medical applications and they also provide reliable estimates of individual risk probabilities. Two different approaches have been used to predict patient risk. The first approach is based on estimation of risk probability by sophisticated mathematical and statistical methods, such as logistic regression, the Bayesian rule and artificial neural networks (Dreiseitl & Ohno-Machado, 2002; Fukunaga, 1990; Marshall et al., 1994). Despite their great accuracy, these models are unfortunately not widely used because they are hard to design and call for difficult calculations, often requiring dedicated software and computing knowledge that doctors do not welcome, besides being difficult to incorporate in clinical practice. The second approach creates scoring systems, in which the predictor variables are usually selected and scored subjectively by expert consensus or objectively using statistical methods (den Boer et al., 2005; Higgins et al., 1997; Vincent & Moreno, 2010).

Despite their lower accuracy, scoring models are usually preferred to probability models by clinicians and health operators because they allow immediate calculation of individual patient scores as a simple sum of integer values associated with binary risk factors, without the need for any data processing system. It has also been demonstrated that in most cases, where a considerable amount of clinical information is available, their diagnostic accuracy is similar to that of probability models (Cevenini & P. Barbini, 2010, as cited in Cevenini et al., 2007). Computation facility of score models should be carefully evaluated in conjunction with their predictive performance. Too many simple models can lead to misleading estimates of a patient's clinical risk, which can be useless, counterproductive or even dangerous.

Any risk model, even if sophisticated and accurate in the local specific condition in which it was designed, loses much of its predictive power when exported to different clinical scenarios. Locally customized scoring models generally provide better performances than exported probability models. This reinforces the clinical success and effectiveness of scoring systems, the design and customisation to local conditions and/or institutions of which are usually much easier.

A limit of many scoring systems is their complex, involuted and even arbitrary design procedure that often involves contrivances to round off parameters of more sophisticated probability models to integer values. This can make their design even more complicated than that of probability models. Scoring often involves dichotomisation of continuous clinical variables to binary risk factors by identifying cut-off values from subjective clinical criteria not based on suitable optimisation techniques. However, whatever the design procedure, the main weakness of scoring models regards the interpretation of individual scores in terms of prognostic probabilities (model calibration), the reliability of which depends on the availability of a sufficient proportion of adverse outcomes and of a design procedure that provides precise individual risk estimation (Cevenini & P. Barbini, 2010). The Hosmer-Lemeshow test is commonly used to assess the calibration of probability models and therefore to manage their learning, but its results are unreliable when applied to models with discrete outputs, such as scoring systems (Finazzi et al., 2011).

This chapter provides an initial brief overview of general issues for the correct design of predictive models with binary outcomes. It broadly describes the main modelling approaches, then illustrates in more detail a method for creating score models for predicting the risk of an AHE. The method tackles and overcomes many of the above-mentioned limits. It uses a well-founded numerical bootstrap technique for appropriate statistical interpretation of simple scoring systems, and provides useful and reliable diagnostic and prognostic information (Carpenter & Bithell, 2000; DiCiccio & Efron, 1996). The whole design procedure is set out and validated by a simulation approach that mimics realistic clinical conditions. Finally, the method is applied to an actual clinical example, to predict the risk of morbidity of heart surgery patients in intensive care.

2. Model issues

Various pattern recognition approaches can be used to design models for separating and classifying patients into the two independent classes of adverse or favourable health outcome, AHE and FHE. The approaches fall into two main categories.

1. Probability models estimate a class-conditional probability, $P(AHE|x)$, of developing the adverse outcome AHE, given a set of chosen predictor variables or features x

(Bishop, 1995; Dreiseitl & Ohno-Machado, 2002; Fukunaga, 1990; Lee, 2004). A probability threshold value, P_t, is identified for classification, over which AHE is recognized to occur, that is when $P(AHE \mid x) > P_t$; the choice of P_t depends on the clinical cost of a wrong decision and influences model classification performance (E. Barbini et al., 2007).

2. Score models evaluate risk by a discrete scale of n positive integer values s_i ($i = 0, 1, 2, ..., n$) which includes zero to represent null risk, but rarely provides a threshold value for classification purposes (Cevenini & P. Barbini, 2010; Vincent & Moreno, 2010).

2.1 Discrimination and calibration

Whatever the risk model, its prediction power is generally expressed by discrimination and calibration (Cook, 2008; Diamond, 1992).

Discrimination is the capacity of a classification model to correctly distinguish patients who will develop an adverse outcome from patients who will not. It must be optimized during model design by ascertaining that the model learns all the discrimination properties valid for the population, correctly from the training sample and therefore shows similar performance in different samples (generalisation ability) (Dreiseitl & Ohno-Machado, 2002; Vapnik, 1999). Though many criteria exist for evaluating model discrimination capacity (Fukunaga, 1990), sensitivity (SE) and specificity (SP), which measure the fractions of correctly classified sick and healthy patients, respectively, are commonly used for statistical evaluations of binary diagnostic test performance. SE end SP are combined in the receiver operating characteristic (ROC) curve which is a graphic representation of the relationship between the true-positive fraction (TPF = SE) and false-positive fraction (FPF = 1-SP) obtained for all possible choices of P_t. The area under the ROC curve (AUC) is the most widely used index of total discrimination capacity in medical applications (Lasko et al., 2005).

Calibration, or goodness of fit, represents the agreement between model-predicted and true probabilities of developing the adverse outcome (Hosmer & Lemeshow, 2000). Retrospective training data only provides dichotomous responses, that is presence or absence of the AHE, so true individual risk probabilities cannot intrinsically be known. The only way to derive them directly from sample data is to calculate the proportion of AHEs in groups of patients, but this obviously becomes less accurate as group size decreases. Nevertheless, from a health or clinical point of view, it is often useful to have an estimation of the level at which each event happens, using a continuous scale, such as probability. For probability models with dichotomous outcomes, calibration capacity can be evaluated by the Hosmer-Lemeshow (HL) goodness-of-fit test, based on two alternative chi-squared statistics, $\hat{H}$ and $\hat{C}$ (Hosmer & Lemeshow, 2000). The first formulation compares model-predicted and observed outcome frequencies of fixed deciles of predicted risk probability; the second compares by partitioning observations into ten groups of the same size (the last group can have a slightly different number of cases) and calculating model-predicted frequencies from average group probabilities. The $\hat{C}$-statistic is generally preferred because it avoids empty groups, although it depends heavily on sample size and grouping criterion (den Boer et al., 2005). The HL test cannot really be applied to models with discrete outputs, such as score systems, because group sizes should themselves be adjusted on the basis of discrete values (Finazzi et al., 2011).

Calibration can be improved, without changing discrimination capacity, by suitable monotonic mathematical transformations of model predicted probabilities (Harrell et al., 1996). The mean squared error between model predicted probability and observed binary outcomes is sometimes calculated as a global index of model accuracy, and has been demonstrated to incorporate both discrimination and calibration capacities (Murphy, 1973).

2.2 Generalisation, cross-validation and variable selection

Generalisation is defined as the capacity of the model to maintain the same predictive performance on data not used for training, but belonging to the same population. A high generalisation power is of primary importance for predictive models designed on a sample data set of correctly classified cases (training set). Many different procedures, which involve different correctly classified data sets for testing model performance (testing sets), have been used to control model generalisation (Bishop, 1995; Fukunaga, 1990; Vapnik, 1999). A model generalises when differences between errors of testing and training sets are not statistically significant.

Theoretically, the optimal model is the simplest possible model designed on training data and has the highest possible performance on any other equally representative set of testing data. Excessively complex models tend to overfit, i.e. give significantly lower errors on the training data than on the testing data. Overfitting produces data storage rather than learning of prediction rules. Models must be designed to avoid overfitting and improve generalisation through efficient control of the training process. This control often includes suitable techniques for the selection of predictor variables (Guyon & Elisseeff, 2003).

Computer algorithms for properly controlling overfitting are known as cross-validation or rotation techniques and make efficient use of all available data to train and test the model (Vapnik, 1999). The most common type of cross-validation procedure is k-fold, where the original sample is randomly partitioned into k subsamples, one of which is used as testing set and the other k–1 as training set. The process is then repeated k times, changing the testing set each time so that all subsamples are used for testing. A convenient variant, more appropriate in dichotomous classification, selects each subsample to contain approximately the same proportion of cases in the two classes. When k is equal to sample size, n, the procedure is called leave-one-out. One case is tested at a time at each of the n training sessions using n–1 training cases. Resampling methods also exist, and include bootstrap methods that produce different data samples by randomly extracting cases with replacement from the original dataset (Chernick, 2007).

Cross-validation can be used to compare the performance of different predictive modelling procedures and, specifically, to select different sets of predictor variables with the same model. In fact, it is convenient to select the best minimum subset of predictor variables to control generalisation and to avoid information overlap due to correlation between variables. Computer-aided stepwise techniques are usually used to obtain optimal nested subsets of variables for this purpose. To train the model, a variable is entered or removed from the predictor subset on the basis of its contribution to a significant increase in discrimination performance (typically the AUC for dichotomous classification) at each step of the process. The stepwise process stops when no variable satisfies the statistical criterion for inclusion or removal (Guyon & Elisseeff, 2003).

3. Probability models

We now provide an overview of four approaches for estimating AHE risk probability: the Bayesian classification rule (Lee, 2004), k-nearest neighbour discrimination (Beyer et al., 1999), logistic regression (Dreiseitl & Ohno-Machado, 2002; Hosmer & Lemeshow, 2000), and artificial neural networks (Bishop, 1995; Dreiseitl & Ohno-Machado, 2002). Linear and quadratic discriminant analyses and related Fisher discriminant functions were not considered because they are strictly classification methods, and although they also enable easy derivation of prediction probabilities, they have been demonstrated to be equivalent to Bayesian methods (Fukunaga, 1990).

3.1 Bayesian classifiers

Bayes's rule allows the posterior conditional probability of AHEs to be predicted as follows (Lee, 2004):

$$P(AHE\,|\,x)=\frac{P(AHE)\,p(x\,|\,AHE)}{P(AHE)\,p(x\,|\,AHE)+P(FHE)\,p(x\,|\,FHE)} \tag{1}$$

where P(AHE) and P(FHE) = 1-P(AHE) are the prior probabilities of the adverse and favourable health events, respectively, p(x | AHE), and p(x | FHE) are the corresponding class-conditional probability density functions (CPDFs) of selected features x. Posterior probability of class FHE is simply P(FHE | x) = 1-P(AHE | x).

Setting the posterior class-conditional probability threshold P_t at 0.5, the Bayes decision rule gives minimum error. It amounts to assigning patients to the class with the largest posterior probability. A higher/lower value of P_t gives rise to a smaller/larger number of patients classified at risk.

Lack of knowledge about prior probability P(AHE), i.e. the prevalence of AHE, does not affect the discrimination performance of the Bayesian classifier since it can be counterbalanced by different choices of P_t. On the contrary, a reliable estimate of prognostic probability P(AHE | x) can be obtained only if all prior probabilities and CPDFs are correctly known.

Statistical assumptions are usually made about whether CPDFs have parametric or non parametric structure. In many cases they are assumed to be of the parametric Gaussian type, because this has been proven to provide good discrimination performance, especially if a subset of predictors can be optimally selected from a large set of clinically available variables (E. Barbini et al., 2007; Fukunaga, 1990).

3.2 K-nearest neighbour algorithms

The k-nearest neighbour algorithm is among the simplest non parametric methods for assigning patients based on closest training examples in the space of features x (Beyer et al., 1999). Euclidean distance is usually used to measure between-point nearness but other metrics must be introduced if non continuous variables are considered.

In our binary classification scheme, the training phase simply consists in partitioning feature space into the two regions or classes, AHE and FHE, based on the positions of training cases. Each new patient is assigned to the region in which the greatest number of its k neighbours occurs, where k is of course a positive integer.

With two classes, it is convenient to choose an odd k to avoid situations of equality. Typically, the choice of neighbourhood size depends on the type and size of the training set;

larger values of k generally reduce the effect of noise on classification at the expense of distinction between classes.

Heuristic techniques are used to obtain the optimal value of k. A common choice is to take k equal to the square root of the total number of training cases, but cross-validation methods, such as bootstrap, are often preferred.

Although k-nearest neighbour is not strictly a probability method, it has been demonstrated that the fraction of k neighbourhood training cases falling in the AHE region is a good estimate of class-conditional risk probability (Beyer et al., 1999).

3.3 Logistic regression

Logistic regression is perhaps the most popular method for estimating risk probabilities in the medical field (Hosmer & Lemeshow, 2000). Logistic regression is a variation of ordinary regression: it belongs to the family of methods called generalized linear models, which include a linear part followed by some associated function. It can be considered a predictive model to use when the dependent response variable is dichotomous and the independent predictor variables are of any type, i.e. continuous, categorical, or both. In d-dimensional feature space, the form of the model is:

$$\log\frac{P(AHE\,|\,x)}{1-P(AHE\,|\,x)}=c_0+c_1x_1+c_2x_2+\ldots+c_dx_d \tag{2}$$

where "log" is the natural logarithm function, x_k (k = 1, 2, …, d) the observation data set and c_k (k = 0, 1, 2, ..., d) regression coefficients estimated from training data using maximum likelihood criteria.

The inverse of eq. 2 allows the posterior probability of AHE risk, P(AHE | x), to be modelled by a continuous S-shaped curve, even if all predictor variables are categorical. The argument of the logarithm of eq. 2 defines the probability of the outcome event occurring divided by the probability of the event not occurring and is known as the odds ratio. When it is specifically associated with dichotomous predictor variables (risk factors), it is a useful measure of the relative risk due to single risk factors. The reliability of logistic regression results is affected by linear correlations and interaction effects between predictor variables, dependence between error terms, and especially outliers.

3.4 Artificial neural networks

Artificial neural networks (or simply neural networks) are mathematical models miming the physiological learning functions of the human brain. They can be designed and trained to create optimal input-output maps of any physical or statistical phenomenon, the relationships of which may even be complex or unknown. They do not require sophisticated statistical hypotheses and account for all possible interrelations between predictor variables in a natural way. In this sense, neural networks can be considered universal approximators (Bishop, 1995).

A preliminary definition of network architecture is needed and should include number of neurons, number of layers, number and type of connections among neurons, type of neuronal activation functions and so on. Learning is the trickiest phase of neural networks: it consists of estimating network parameters (connection weights and activation thresholds) iteratively from training data, to minimize error between actual and model-estimated outputs. Feed-forward neural networks can be designed to directly estimate class-conditional posterior probabilities from predictor variables, without requiring sophisticated statistical hypotheses. Their architecture can be variably complex, but should provide one output neuron with a logistic sigmoid activation function, generating an output between 0 and 1. Neural networks have been demonstrated to provide reliable estimates of class-conditional posterior probabilities, such as the AHE risk probability, P(AHE|x), that is (Bishop, 1995):

$$P(AHE|x)=\frac{1}{1+\exp(-f)} \quad (3)$$
$$f=b+w_1u_1+w_2u_2+...+w_nu_n$$

where f is a linear function of n neuron inputs u_k (k = 0, 1, 2, ..., n), originating from the outputs of n preceding connected neurons, the parameters of which are connection weights, w_k, and neuron activation bias, b.

Under-learning can lead to high prediction errors, whereas over-learning can cause overfitting which produces loss of generalisation. Artificial neural network design is therefore anything but simple. Experience is necessary to manipulate heuristic procedures for suitable definition of network architecture and to correctly use iterative numerical training techniques that stop learning when the network begins to overfit.

4. Direct score model

A scoring model is a formula that assigns points based on known information, in order to predict an unknown future outcome. Many integer score systems have been designed for clinical application to critical patients. The most popular were derived from simplification of any of the above probability models by rounding their parameters to integer values. In particular, many approximate the coefficients of logistic regression models to the nearest integer values (Higgins et al., 1997). We do not dwell on the methodology of these score models here, directing readers to the specialised literature (Vincent & Moreno, 2010). Our main interest is to identify score values that give reliable probabilities of individual risk for prognostic purposes. We discuss on the design of a very simple score system that we call a "direct score model". We also provide a correct and useful statistical interpretation of model prognostic capacity, which can easily be extended to any other score model, even more sophisticated ones (Cevenini & P. Barbini, 2010).

4.1 Model design

Only binary predictor variables (risk factors) are used in this score model. The automatic computer procedure and model training is described by the following steps:

- All quantitative predictor variables are dichotomised by ROC curve analysis, identifying cut-off values giving equal sensitivity and specificity in relation to adverse outcomes.
- Risk factors over or under the cut-off value are coded 0 or 1, depending on whether the risk of AHE decreases or increases, respectively.
- The odds ratio of each binary variable is evaluated on the basis of the corresponding confidence interval (CI) (Agresti, 1999): variables with odds ratios not significantly greater than 1 are discarded.

- A forward iterative procedure is applied to a data sample (training set) which sums selected binary variables stepwise.
- All binary factors are reconsidered at each step, so that multiple selection of one factor gives rise to a multiple integer contribution to the score.
- At each step the risk factor providing the highest increment to AUC is included.
- Training is stopped when the cumulative increment in AUC obtained in five consecutive steps is less than 1%. This rather soft stopping criterion is used instead of well-established statistical methods (Zhou et al., 2008) to avoid selecting too few predictors, which reduces the possibility of associating an effective probability of AHE with each integer score.
- A testing dataset of the same size as the training set is used to evaluate model generalisation and to guide conclusive selection of the optimal predictor set.

Backward sessions and cross-validation trials cannot be applied because the model is non-parametric. Optimal model selection is carried out by a step-by-step analysis of model prognostic and diagnostic power. At each step w, the conditional probability of the adverse outcome (prognostic risk probability), $P_w(AHE|S_k)$, associated with each kth integer score value S_k, is estimated from sample data as the ratio of adverse events to the total number of events determining a model score S_k.

The bias-corrected and accelerated bootstrap method is applied to estimate 95% CIs of $P_w(AHE|S_k)$ using 2000 bootstrapped samples. This method makes it possible to infer complex statistics that are difficult or even impossible to represent mathematically and have proven to be theoretically and practically more accurate than other bootstrap methods (Cevenini & P. Barbini, 2010; DiCiccio & Efron, 1996). By graphic inspection of results, the convenience of grouping close scores having large 95% CI because of excessively low data frequencies is considered. The model is chosen to correspond to the iteration providing the largest number of score values or classes having sufficiently narrow and separate 95% CIs with respect to the training data, and at the same time giving testing-data probabilities falling within their 95% CIs.

Once the model is created, the score, S, associated with a generic patient is simply given by:

$$S=\sum_{i=1}^{d} p_i s_i \tag{4}$$

where d is the number of predictors in the model, p_i the binary value of the ith predictor, and s_i, its model-identified associated score. Finally, model discrimination and calibration performance are compared with a logistic regression model designed on the same training data.

All statistical procedures are evaluated at a significance level of 95%.

4.2 Simulation

Many realistic simulation experiments are carried out to validate and optimise model design. Predictor variables are all taken in binary form, skipping the dichotomisation of continuous variables. In particular, we consider d dichotomised binary predictors, obtaining $n = 2^d$ different combinations of these predictors. Each combination identifies one value of a discrete variable $x_j = j/n$ ($j = 0, 1, 2, ..., n-1$) ranging from 0 to 1. In this way two different beta probability density functions can be associated with adverse and favourable outcomes.

Beta distribution is particularly suitable for representing multinomial phenomena, such as that described by the above n discrete values. In detail, we refer to the discrete probability distribution of a multinomial variable x, the probability values of which are calculated using a beta probability density function.

Figure 1 shows an example with two different choices of the beta probability density function shape parameters, α and β, to simulate healthy and sick subjects. When the class-conditional probability density functions of a two-class classification problem are known, the highest achievable discrimination level is related to the areas of overlap. The lowest error probability of classification, ε, is given by:

$$\varepsilon=\int_{-\infty}^{+\infty}\min\{P(C_1)p(x\,|\,C_1),P(C_2)p(x\,|\,C_2)\}dx \tag{5}$$

where $P(C_h)$ and $p(x\,|\,C_h)$ are the prior probability and the class-conditional probability density function for class C_h ($h = 1, 2$), respectively. Prior probability of an adverse outcome, P(AHE), is also known as prevalence, π, and prior probability of favourable outcome, P(FHE), is $1-\pi$. Because of the discrete nature of variable x, in our simulation study, eq. 5 can be approximated as:

$$\begin{aligned}&\varepsilon=\frac{1}{n}\sum_{j=0}^{n-1}\min\left[\pi\times p(x_j|\,AHE),(1-\pi)\times p(x_j|\,FHE)\right]\\&p(x_j|\,AHE)=B(x_j,\alpha_{AHE},\beta_{AHE})\\&p(x_j|\,FHE)=B(x_j,\alpha_{FHE},\beta_{FHE})\end{aligned} \tag{6}$$

where α_{AHE}, β_{AHE}, α_{FHE} and β_{FHE} are the corresponding shape parameters of beta functions, $B_{AHE}= B(x_j,\alpha_{AHE},\beta_{AHE})$ and $B_{FHE}= B(x_j,\alpha_{FHE},\beta_{FHE})$, related to adverse and favourable outcomes, respectively.

Eq. 6 shows that ε depends on prevalence and beta parameters. At any iteration w of the above-mentioned stepwise procedure, for any k^{th} integer value of score S_k, the simulated "true" conditional risk probability, $P_w^t(AHE|S_k)$, can be calculated using the Bayes theorem, considering AHE prevalence, π, and the class-conditional score probabilities, $P_w^t(S_k\,|AHE)$ and $P_w^t(S_k\,|FHE)$, of adverse and favourable outcomes, respectively:

$$P_w^t(AHE\,|\,S_k)=\frac{\pi\, P_w^t(S_k|\,AHE)}{\pi\, P_w^t(S_k|\,AHE)+(1-\pi)\, P_w^t(S_k|\,FHE)} \tag{7}$$

By assuming mutually exclusive x_j events, the true class-conditional probabilities are simply obtained from the two simulated beta distributions as the sum of all the discrete probabilities corresponding to the x_j values giving the score S_k, that is:

$$\begin{aligned}&P_w^t(S_k|\,AHE)=\frac{1}{n}\sum_{x_j\in S_k}B(x_j,\alpha_{AHE},\beta_{AHE})\\&P_w^t(S_k|\,FHE)=\frac{1}{n}\sum_{x_j\in S_k}B(x_j,\alpha_{FHE},\beta_{FHE})\end{aligned} \tag{8}$$

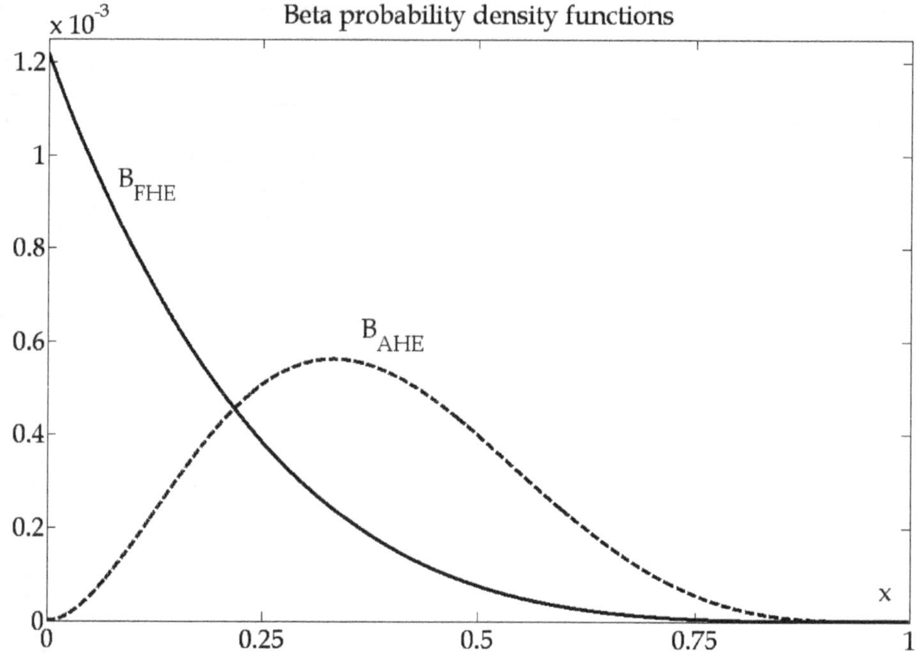

Fig. 1. Simulated probability density functions, B_{FHE} and B_{AHE}, for favourable and adverse outcomes, respectively: example with beta parameters $\alpha_{FHE} = 1$, $\alpha_{AHE} = 3$, $\beta_{AHE} = \beta_{FHE} = 5$

4.2.1 Simulation experiments

Simulation experiments are performed by randomly extracting $N = N_{AHE} + N_{FHE}$ data items from beta distributions of adverse and favourable outcomes, B_{AHE} and B_{FHE}, respectively, to form two samples of size $N_{AHE} = \pi \cdot N$ and $N_{FHE} = (1-\pi) \cdot N$. Each extracted item x_j ($j = 1, 2, ..., N$) is represented as a d-dimensional point in the discrete space of binary variables.

We use $d = 12$ binary variables and simulate nine different conditions corresponding to the combinations of three prevalence values and three levels of separation between event classes, obtained by changing the parameters of beta distributions. Low, medium and high separation between AHEs and FHEs are reproduced by increasing only the values of parameter α_{AHE}, specifically equal to 2, 3 and 5, respectively. The other three beta parameters are kept constant at $\alpha_{FHE} = 1$, $\beta_{AHE} = \beta_{FHE} = 5$. Prevalence values of 5%, 20% and 40% are tried. For each condition, six samples with progressively doubled sizes, namely $N = 250, 500, 1000, 2000, 4000$ and 8000, are extracted for a total of 54 simulation experiments covering a wide range of actual clinical situations (see also Table 1). Training data is not used because the simulation process enables the true probabilities, described above, to be evaluated exactly.

All computations are performed using MATLAB code.

4.2.2 Simulation results

The method is illustrated in detail by describing the results of a simulation of the 54 experiments performed. The experiment corresponding to N = 1000, π = 20% and α_{AHE} = 3 is illustrated, because it is similar to an actual clinical condition that will be shown below.

Figure 2 shows the AUC values obtained using the forward selection of model features from simulated training data described above. The stopping criterion arrested the stepwise algorithm at the eleventh step, after 5 out of 12 predictor variables had been selected. In fact, the cumulative increment in AUC was about 0.8% in the last five steps (nos. 7-11). The variables are numbered in order of decreasing discrimination power. The most discriminating variable, no. 1, was entered five times (s_1 = 5) in the model, variable no. 2 three times (s_2 = 3) and variables nos. 3-5 only once each ($s_{3\text{-}5}$ = 1).

Figure 3 shows the 95% confidence interval of score-associated risk probabilities identified by the bias-corrected and accelerated bootstrap method applied to simulated sample data, from step no. 2 to step no. 9. For each integer score value, the estimated 95% CI is plotted together with the corresponding true probability of AHE (calculated from the beta distribution) and the percentage of cases. The discrimination capacity of the model can be detected at every step by observing the growth of estimated AHE probability with the score, whereas calibration is demonstrated by true risk probabilities (stars), which fall in the corresponding 95% confidence interval of the training data, with the sole exception of certain high scores, where there may be too few cases.

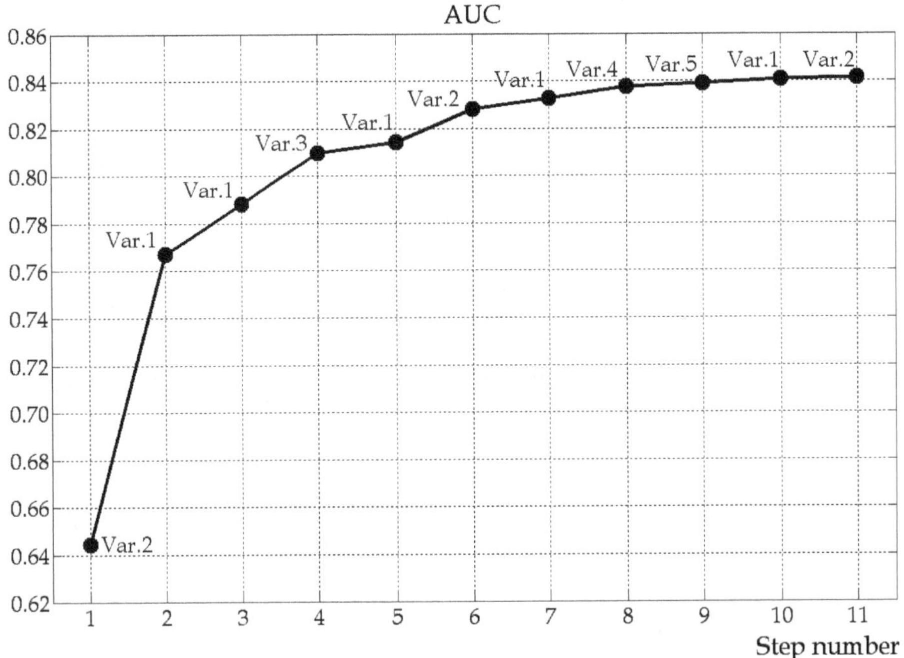

Fig. 2. Area under the ROC curve (AUC) during stepwise selection of model features from simulated data. The predictor variables entered are also indicated

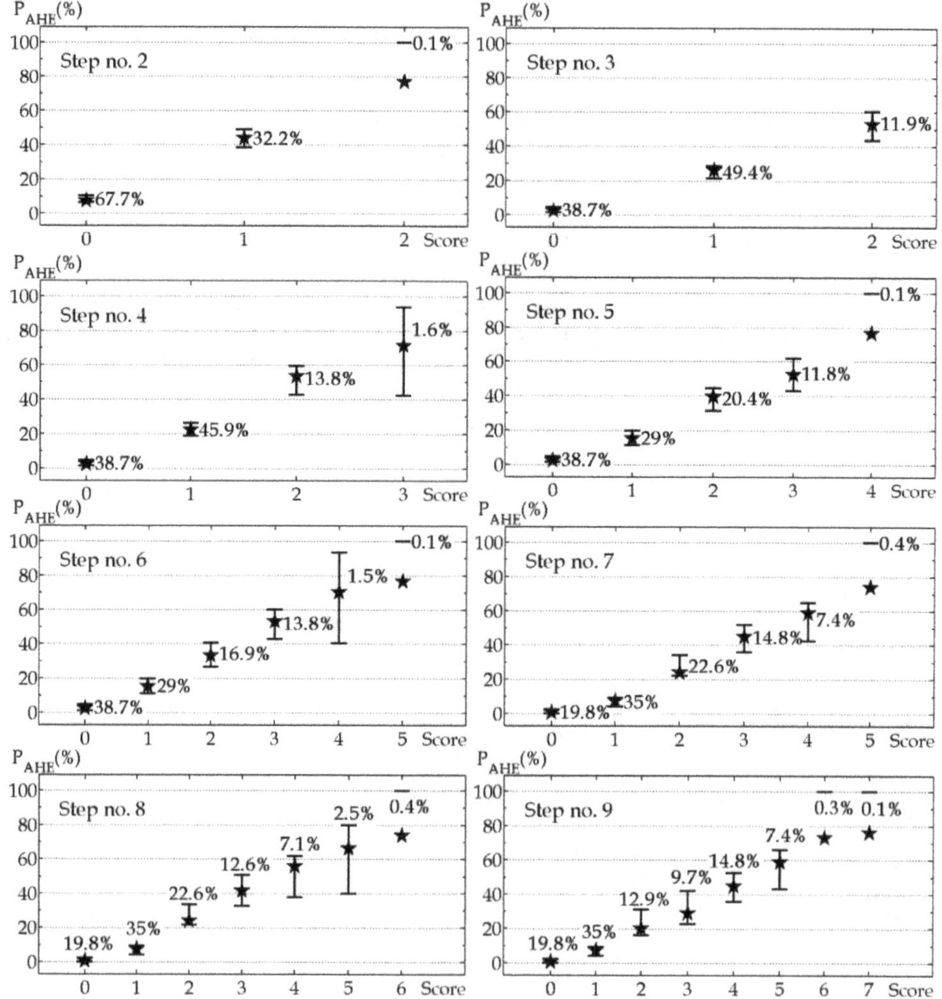

Fig. 3. 95% confidence intervals of AHE score probability, estimated from simulated training data, percentages of score cases and true probabilities (stars)

Now it is necessary to identify a model that reconciles calibration and discrimination. Excessively simple score models (few steps) have low discrimination power (low AUC) and give inopportunely separated 95% CIs. This can be observed at steps nos. 2 and 3 of Fig. 3 where only three score values (0, 1 and 2) are obtained: CIs between scores have very large gaps, suggesting that finer partitioning of the score axis can be achieved with a larger number of steps. Figure 2 indicates poor discrimination capacity of the scoring system at these initial steps.

On the contrary, if too many scores are used, as in steps nos. 7-9, the CIs are either too wide or overlap, worsening calibration accuracy. The width of score CIs increases significantly with decreasing observed frequency. For example, at step no. 4, score of 3 has only 16 cases (1.6%) and the corresponding 95% CI is so large that it completely overlaps with the previous score of 2. When the number of cases is even lower, as in step no. 9, where the highest scores of 6 and 7 have four and one cases, respectively, the bootstrap method fails to correctly estimate the CIs and the corresponding scores are totally unreliable in prognostic terms. Hence the need to combine neighbouring scores with too few cases. It is particularly convenient to pool the highest scores, which often have few cases, into a single class having a sufficient data frequency to significantly narrow the 95% CIs. For example, at step no. 6 it is useful to pool the last two scores of 4 and 5 into a single class. The pooling of adjacent scores with small data frequency enhances model prognostic reliability, usually with an insignificant reduction in discrimination capacity.

From the simulated experiment of Fig. 3, five score classes were identified as a suitable compromise between calibration and discrimination. At any step from no. 6 to no. 9, it is worthwhile combining scores greater than or equal to 4 and leaving the lower scores of 0-3 ungrouped, so as to form five score classes: 0, 1, 2, 3 and ≥ 4.

Figure 4 shows the results of pooling the three highest scores of step no. 8, which is preferred to the previous steps no. 6 and no. 7, because besides having higher discrimination capacity, the pooled class contains a greater number of cases, which narrows the related 95% CI to a greater extent. Just a small gap and a slight overlap can be observed in Fig. 4 between scores of 1 and 2, and between scores of 3 and the class of scores ≥ 4, respectively. Step no. 9 and subsequent steps not reported in Fig. 3 are discarded because no improvement can be obtained with respect to step no. 8 and CI overlap increases. Indeed, to improve the accuracy of estimates of individual probability of AHE, it could be worthwhile increasing the number of classes, tolerating a greater CI overlap. This can be done by analysing and selecting a step beyond the eighth, where the observed frequency in each class is of course significantly reduced, especially for high scores.

Comparison of the results of the three-step model with those of the eight-step pooled model shown in Fig. 4 indicates that the scoring system with five classes effectively fills the gaps between adjacent CIs of the simpler score model. At step no. 8, pooling of the highest scores does not significantly influence the discrimination capacity of the scoring system: the estimated AUC decreases slightly from 0.838 (95% CI, 0.781-0.885) to 0.827 (95% CI, 0.777-0.869).

Stepwise logistic regression applied to the training data used for the simulation example, set at statistical significance levels of 95% and 90% to enter and remove variables, respectively, selected the first five binary variables. Figure 5 compares ROC curves of the logistic model and the score model of Fig. 4. The ROC curve of true probability values, calculated from training data using beta distributions and the Bayes theorem, is also plotted (dashed line). AUCs of true data and the logistic model were 0.845 and 0.849, respectively.

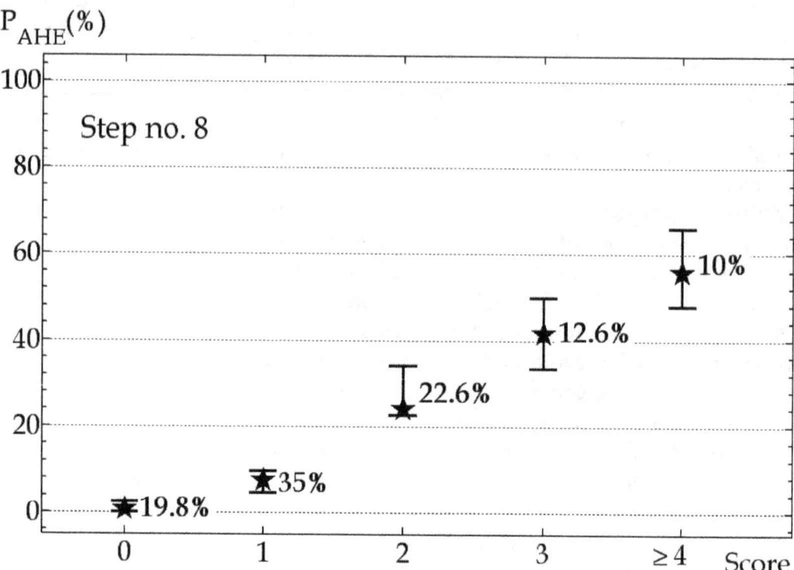

Fig. 4. 95% confidence intervals of AHE score probabilities estimated from simulated training data, percentages of score cases and true probabilities (stars) for the model identified at step no. 8

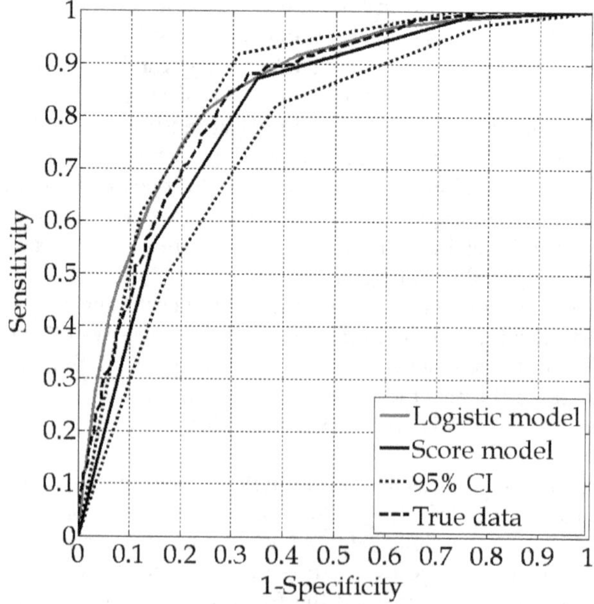

Fig. 5. ROC curves from simulated sample data. 95% CI refers to score model

When comparing model discrimination power by AUC, we have to consider that the ROC curve of the score model (continuous line) is drawn by connecting only 5 discrete points (score classes), whereas the logistic model curve (gray line) is based on more probability values. Figure 5 shows that the score model is close enough to the logistic and true ROC curves. Clearly, discretisation leads to a lower AUC, resulting in underestimation of score-model discrimination capacity. In addition, the true and logistic curves are to a large extent within the 95% CI of the score curve. Finally, in real clinical applications, logistic regression often includes continuous variables that may improve discrimination performance.

The HL goodness-of-fit test (Hosmer & Lemeshow, 2000) showed good calibration performance of the logistic model ($p = 0.751$). However, 95% of the training-data errors between model-estimated and true percentage risk probabilities were from about -10.5% (underestimation) and +12.0% (overestimation), revealing similar uncertainty to that of the score model.

Table 1 gives the number of score values or classes identified by the same procedure, for each of the 54 simulation experiments. It shows that the number of score classes increases with increasing sample size, prevalence and separation between event classes (decreasing error ε). The importance of estimating uncertainty suggests to keep 95% CIs of between-class probabilities separate, or slightly overlapping. This limits the identifiable number of score classes and provides reliable probability estimates. Enlargement and overlapping of 95% CIs and consequent loss of prognostic probability information depends heavily on the data frequency of score values or classes and their rate of AHEs influenced by prevalence. Small samples and/or low prevalence make it necessary to pool neighbouring scores to form classes with a sufficient number of cases to ensure a reliable estimate (narrow CI) of class probabilities.

	Low separation $\alpha_{AHE} = 2$			Medium separation $\alpha_{AHE} = 3$			High separation $\alpha_{AHE} = 5$		
Π%	5	20	40	5	20	40	5	20	40
ε% / N	5.0	20.0	32.9	5.0	17.7	23.9	4.6	11.4	13.7
250	2	3	3	3	4	4	3	4	4
500	3	4	4	4	5	5	4	5	5
1000	4	4	4	4	5	5	4	5	6
2000	4	5	5	5	5	6	5	6	6
4000	5	5	5	5	6	6	5	6	6
8000	5	6	6	6	6	7	6	7	7

Table 1. Simulation experiments: largest number of score classes having sufficiently narrow and separate 95% confidence intervals of prognostic probability. αAHE = shape parameter of AHE beta distribution; Π = prevalence; ε = lowest error probability of classification; N = sample size

Simulation experiments suggests grouping scores into classes when frequencies are less than about 3% and 10% of the whole sample for N = 8000 and N = 250, respectively. Only two classes are recognised in the worst condition of minimum sample size (N = 250), minimum prevalence ($\Pi = 5\%$) and low separation between health events ($\alpha_{AHE} = 2$). A maximum of seven score-classes is identified in conditions of large sample size (N = 8000), high prevalence and high separation between event classes. Although more score classes could be achieved with greater CI overlap, the cost would be unreliable estimates.

The discrimination of the different simulation experiments is assessed by AUC of true simulated probability calculated using beta functions. Conditions of large overlap between areas of beta functions ($\alpha_{AHE} = 2$) lead to values of true AUC ranging from 0.72 to 0.75; medium overlap ($\alpha_{AHE} = 3$) gives AUC values in the range 0.82-0.85 and the conditions of greatest separation ($\alpha_{AHE} = 5$) produce AUCs between 0.92 and 0.95.

4.3 Clinical example

The approach was applied to actual clinical data of critical patients in the intensive care unit to evaluate their risk of morbidity after heart surgery.

We used a sample of 1040 adult patients younger than 80 years, who underwent coronary artery bypass grafting and were admitted to the intensive care unit of the Department of Surgery and Bioengineering of Siena University. 212 patients developed at least one serious postoperative complication (cardiovascular, respiratory, neurological, renal, infectious or hemorrhagic), corresponding to a morbidity of 20.4% (Cevenini & P. Barbini, 2010, as cited in Cevenini et al., 2007). The data was split randomly into a training and a testing set of the same size (520 cases), with the same number of patients with morbid conditions in each set (106 cases) to avoid misleading bias in the results.

Table 2 describes the 15 clinical variables used for score model design, six of which were binary in origin. The other nine continuous variables were dichotomised using cut-off values associated with the point of equal sensitivity and specificity on the respective ROC curves. Three of the resulting 15 binary variables were discarded because their odds ratios of morbidity were not significantly greater than 1. This left a total of 12 variables for training the score model, as in the simulation experiments.

This real clinical situation was similar to the simulation experiment with N = 500 and $\Pi = 20\%$ (see Table 1). Consulting Table 1, we expected to develop a score model with 4 or 5 classes, depending on the level of data separation between normal and morbid patients.

Figure 6 shows the stepwise procedure used to select the model variables. After step no. 8, AUC values of testing data (dashed line with stars) decreased and diverged from training data AUCs (continuous line with dots). This indicated overfitting that was possible because the criterion used to stop the training procedure was deliberately soft, to allow inclusion of more steps than needed for generalisation. In fact, as previously illustrated in the simulation results, investigation of extra steps can be useful to optimise model prognostic power through score pooling. Steps nos. 6, 7 and 8 gave similar prognostic performance, so we chose step no. 8, thus obtaining higher discrimination (greater AUC). A convenient class was formed by pooling scores greater than 3, as shown in Fig. 7. All 95% CIs of adjacent scores or classes were well-separated and all testing score probabilities (stars) fell within their corresponding CIs, thereby ensuring high prognostic reliability of the model. The pooling of the highest scores of the eight-step model led to a slight but not statistically significant reduction in discrimination performance: the estimated training and testing AUCs decreased from 0.851 (95% CI, 0.781-0.909) to 0.835 (95% CI, 0.764-0.895) and from 0.841 (95% CI, 0.775-0.900) to 0.816 (95% CI, 0.743-0.879), respectively.

Variable description	**Acronym**	**Type**	**Cut-off**	**Steps**	
Inotropic heart drugs	IHD	Binary		1,4,10	(LR)
O_2 delivery index	DO_2I	Continuous	< 280 ml/min/m^2	2	(LR)
Peripheral vascular disease	PVD	Binary		3,9	(LR)
O_2 extraction ratio	O_2ER	Continuous	≥ 38%	5	(LR)
Emergency	EM	Binary		6	
CO_2 production	VCO_2	Continuous	< 180 ml/min	7	
Pulmonary artery hypertension	PAH	Binary		8	(LR)
Cardio-pulmonary bypass time	CPB	Continuous	≥ 2 hours	11	(LR)
Intra aortic balloon pump	IABP	Binary		12	(LR)
Creatinine	Cr	Continuous	≥ 1 mg/l	NE	(LR)
Potassium	K	Continuous	≥ 4.1 mEq/l	NE	(LR)
Haemoglobin	Hb	Continuous	< 9.6 g/dl	NE	
Cardiac index	CI	Continuous	< 2.4 l/min/m^2	NS	(LR)
Mean arterial pressure	MAP	Continuous	> 95 mmHg	NS	
Previous heart surgery	Re-do	Binary		NS	

Table 2. Clinical variables, cut-off values for the dichotomisation of continuous variables and score-model entry steps. NE = not entered; NS = not statistically significant; LR = variable selected by stepwise logistic regression

Two logistic regression models were designed to compare the score model results on the same training data with the 15 clinical variables of Table 2. The first model, named LogCV, used the original continuous variables and the second (LogBV) dichotomised them (see Table 2). The stepwise regression procedure selected ten clinical variables (see Table 2) and provided training-data AUC values of 0.906 (HL test, p = 0.135) and 0.871 (HL test, p = 0.557) for LogCV and LogBV, respectively. Figure 8 compares the ROC curves. The LogCV ROC curve (continuous gray line) showed the greatest discrimination performance, mainly because the model selected many continuous variables (6 out of 10). Except for the highest specificity values, where the discretisation effect of scoring was more evident, the score model ROC curve (continuous black line) did not differ significantly from that of LogBV (dashed gray line), which was inside the respective 95% CI and close enough to the score-model points. Model scores computed using the testing data gave a ROC curve (dashed black line) not significantly different from the training data curve. Finally, it should be noted that the discrimination performance of logistic models decreased considerably when applied to testing data (ROC curves not reported in Fig. 8): AUCs of logCV and logBV were reduced to 0.879 and 0.826, respectively, thus suggesting a possible overfitting.

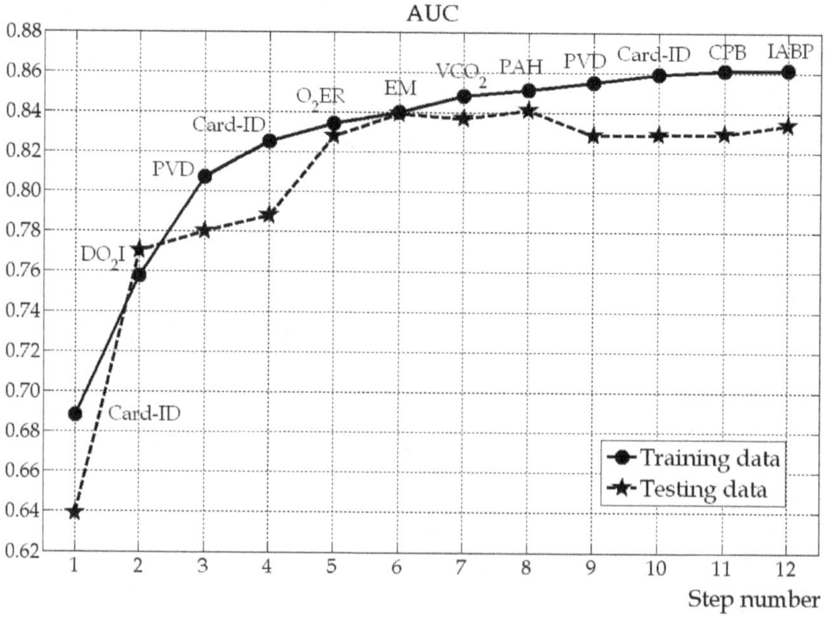

Fig. 6. Area under the ROC curve (AUC) during the stepwise selection of model features from clinical data. The predictor variables entered are also indicated

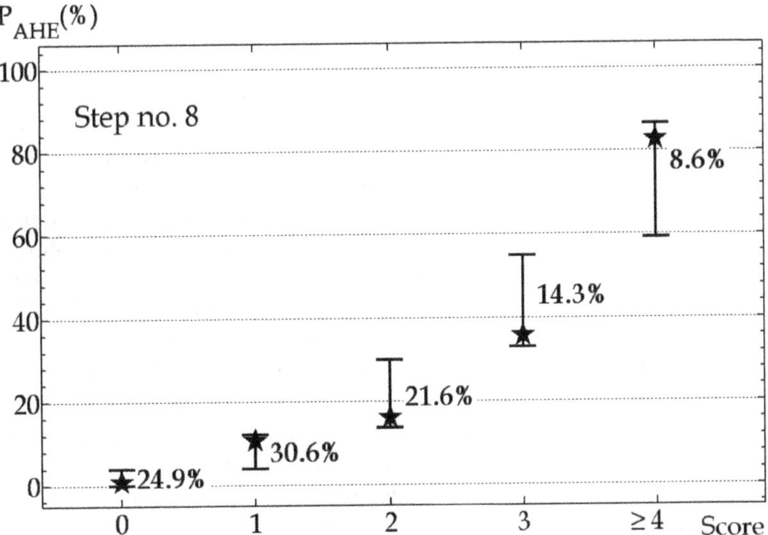

Fig. 7. Estimated 95% confidence intervals of AHE score probabilities from clinical training data, percentages of score cases and testing-data probabilities (stars) for the eight-step model chosen

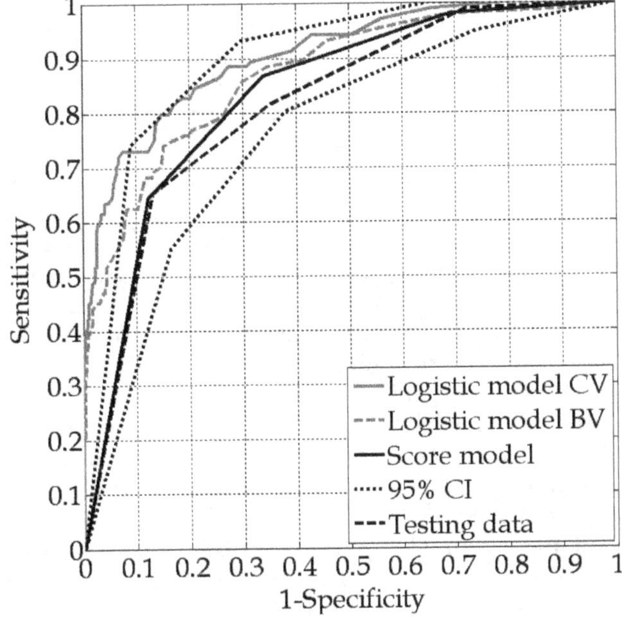

Fig. 8. ROC curves from clinical data. 95% CI refers to the score model. CV = also with continuous variables; BV = with binary variables only

5. Discussion

Many quantitative methods for assessing the health risk of critical patients have been developed in past and recent literature (E. Barbini et al., 2007; den Boer et al., 2005; Vincent & Moreno, 2010). They aim to provide objective and accurate information about patient diagnosis and prognosis. Experience has shown that simplicity of use and effectiveness of implementation are the most important requirements for their success in routine clinical practice. Scoring systems respond well to these requirements because their outcomes are accessible in real time without the use of advanced computational tools, thus allowing decisions to be made quickly and effectively. Many clinical applications can profit from their simplicity. For example, they are often used to suggest alternative treatments and organize intensive care resources, where surveillance of vital functions is the primary goal.

Other important benefits of score models are their easy updating and customisation to local institutions. In fact, because the standardisation of local practices is difficult and patient populations may differ, it is now accepted that predictive models must be locally validated, tuned and periodically updated to provide correct risk-adjusted outcomes. All models suffer from the limitation of foreseeing better future treatments and improving prognosis (den Boer et al., 2005). Even very accurate predictive models, when exported to clinical contexts different from those in which they were designed, have often proved unreliable (Murphy-Filkins et al., 1996). Appropriate design and local customisation of excessively sophisticated models is often easier said than done, especially in health centres where there is little technical expertise in developing models that can generalise, i.e. preserve their predictive performance on future data. On the contrary, simple score models can easily and frequently be updated to learn from new correctly-classified cases and are quite tolerant to missing data. This is very useful in clinical practice where data is usually scarce and training on as much available data as possible is of fundamental importance (Cevenini & P. Barbini, 2010, as cited in P. Barbini et al., 2007).

A major problem with score models is that they are difficult to calibrate, i.e. associate reliable estimates of prognostic risk probability with each score. Nevertheless, correct estimation of individual probability of adverse outcome for hospitalized critical patients is useful for prevention, treatment and quantification of health problems and costs. It can help experienced physicians to improve clinical management by optimizing the monitoring of patient status and enhancing the quality of care, and allow new generations of doctors to be better trained during postgraduate specialization and internship. Moreover, reliable knowledge of risk factors and their impact on clinical course and future quality of life can encourage public health policy for risk reduction (Hodgman, 2008).

The proposed method offers a simple risk-assessment system that associates a reliable estimate of the individual probability of developing an adverse event with predicted scores. The model is a very simple score of risk factors chosen, one or more times, by a stepwise procedure based on maximising discrimination through ROC analysis. No hypotheses or statistical models are involved. Since conventional methods for evaluating calibration, such as the Hosmer-Lemeshow test (Hosmer & Lemeshow, 2000), are unreliable for scoring systems, we analysed the 95% confidence interval of sample-estimated risk probabilities associated with each score step by step. The experimental score probability is easily evaluated by calculating the sampling rate of adverse outcomes having that score.

Unfortunately, the statistics of the sampling error are not simple to derive. We therefore preferred to use bootstrap resampling, a method commonly used in statistical inference to estimate confidence intervals (Carpenter & Bithell, 2000; DiCiccio & Efron, 1996). The bootstrap method is simpler and more general than conventional approaches; it requires no great expertise in mathematics or probability theory and is based on assumptions that are less restrictive and easier to control. The method can be used to evaluate statistics that are difficult or impossible to determine by conventional methods. We used an elaboration of the simplest bootstrap method of percentile intervals, known as bias-corrected and accelerated intervals, which avoids estimate bias and offers substantial advantages over other bootstrap methods, both in theory and practice (Chernick, 2007). Our simulation experiments confirmed the method's accuracy in estimating 95% CI of prognostic probabilities: when true probabilities were related to score values, or classes, with a sufficient number of sampled training data, they always fell within bootstrap-estimated 95% CIs (see Fig. 3). Bootstrap techniques are not too complex in a clinical environment, since nowadays many available packages for data processing include them for calculating confidence intervals. In any case, they are used exclusively during model design.

As shown in Fig. 3, step by step graphical inspection of probability CIs made it possible to choose the best model to compromise between calibration and discrimination, also suggesting convenient pooling of adjacent scores that gave large and overlapping CIs due to an insufficient number of cases or adverse events. The controlled simulation experiments showed that good calibration was achieved with a limited number of score classes, up to a maximum of seven in experiments with the biggest sample size, and high prevalence and separation between event classes (see Table 1). More classes could be identified if greater overlap of close scores were allowed, but when the number of classes became excessive, there were problems of overfitting. We also saw that a logistic model designed on the same training data provided nearly continuous probability estimates, the uncertainty of which was similar to that achieved by the score model. Significant improvement of discrimination performance could only be appreciated when continuous variables were also included in the logistic model, as in the clinical example described. This analysis can enable medical staff to select the best scoring system for any specific clinical context.

6. Conclusion

In critical care medicine, scoring systems are often designed exclusively on the basis of discrimination and generalisation characteristics (diagnostic capacity), at the expense of reliable individual probabilities (prognostic capacity). Our proposed approach that weighs both these capacities is validated by suitable simulation experiments, which also allow design conditions and application limits of scoring systems to be investigated for correct prediction of critical patient risk in a real clinical context.

The bias-corrected and accelerated bootstrap method for evaluating the 95% confidence interval, CI, of individual prognostic probabilities provides reliable estimates of true simulated probabilities. CIs are calculated for each score and at each step of scoring-system design. By increasing the number of steps, model discrimination power (greater AUC) and prognostic information (greater number of different score values) increases but widening and overlap of 95% CIs soon occurs, so that it becomes convenient to pool adjacent scores into score classes. The maximum number of different score classes giving distinct prognostic information, that is having narrow and less overlapping 95% CIs, increases with increasing sample size and prevalence of adverse outcome and decreasing error probability of classification. It is strongly limited by reduced frequency of score cases and the respective rate of adverse events: in our simulated experiments, which covered a wide range of real conditions, it varied from 2 to 7.

Application of the method to a real clinical situation demonstrated that the technique can be a simple practical tool, providing useful additional prognostic information to associate with classes of scores, and enabling doctors to choose the best risk score model to use in their specific clinical context.

7. Acknowledgment

This work was partly financed by the University of Siena, Italy.

8. References

Agresti, A. (1999). On Logit Confidence Intervals for the Odds Ratio with Small Samples. *Biometrics,* Vol.55, pp. 597-602, ISSN 0006-341X

Barbini, E.; Cevenini, G.; Scolletta, S.; Biagioli, B.; Giomarelli, P. & Barbini, P. (2007). A Comparative Analysis of Predictive Models of Morbidity in Intensive Care Unit after Cardiac Surgery - Part I: Model Planning. *BMC Medical Informatics and Decision Making,* Vol.7, No.35, (22 November 2007), pp. 1-16, ISSN 1472-6947, Available from http://www.biomedcentral.com/1472-6947/7/35

Beyer, K.; Goldstein, J.; Ramakrishnan, R. & Shaft, U. (1999). When is Nearest Neighbor Meaningful?, *Proceedings of the 7th International Conference on Database Theory,* pp. 217-235, ISBN 3-540-65452-6, Jerusalem, Israel, January 10-12, 1999

Bishop, C.M. (1995). *Neural Networks for Pattern Recognition,* Oxford University Press, ISBN 0-19-853864-2, Oxford, UK

Carpenter, J. & Bithell, J. (2000). Bootstrap Confidence Intervals: When, Which, What? A Practical Guide for Medical Statisticians. *Statistics in Medicine,* Vol.19, No.9, pp. 1141-1164, ISSN 0277-6715

Chernick, M.R. (2007). *Bootstrap Methods: A Guide for Practitioners and Researchers,* Wiley, ISBN 978-0-471-75621-7, New York, USA

Cevenini, G. & Barbini, P. (2010). A Bootstrap Approach for Assessing the Uncertainty of Outcome Probabilities when Using a Scoring System. *BMC Medical Informatics and Decision Making,* Vol.10, No.45, (26 August 2010), pp. 1-9, ISSN 1472-6947, Available from http://www.biomedcentral.com/1472-6947/10/45

Cook, N.R. (2008). Statistical Evaluation of Prognostic versus Diagnostic Models: Beyond the ROC Curve. *Clinical Chemistry,* Vol.54, pp. 17-23, ISSN 1339-1348, Available from http://www.clinchem.org/cgi/content/full/54/1/17

den Boer, S.; de Keizer, N.F. & de Jonge, E. (2005). Performance of Prognostic Models in Critically Ill Cancer Patients - A Review. *Critical Care,* Vol.9, pp. R458-R463, (8 July 2005), ISSN 1364-8535, Available from http://ccforum.com/content/9/4/R458

Diamond, G.A. (1992). What Price Perfection? Calibration and Discrimination of Clinical Prediction Models. *Journal of Clinical Epidemiology,* Vol.45, No.1, pp. 85-89, ISSN 0895-4356

DiCiccio, T.J. & Efron, B. (1996). Bootstrap Confidence Intervals. *Statistical Science,* Vol.11, pp. 189-228, ISSN 0883-4237

Dreiseitl, S. & Ohno-Machado, L. (2002). Logistic Regression and Artificial Neural Network Classification Models: A Methodology Review. *Journal of Biomedical Informatics,* Vol.35, no.5-6, pp. 352-359, ISSN 1532-0464

Finazzi, S.; Poole, D.; Luciani, D.; Cogo, P.E. & Bertolini, G. (2011). Calibration Belt for Quality-of-Care Assessment Based on Dichotomous Outcomes. *PLoS One,* Vol.6, No.2, (23 February 2011), e16110, ISSN 1932-6203, Available from http://www.plosone.org/article/info%3Adoi%2F10.1371%2Fjournal.pone.0016110

Fukunaga, K. (1990). *Introduction to Statistical Pattern Recognition,* Academic Press, ISBN 978-0-12-269851-4, Boston, USA

Guyon, I. & Elisseeff, A. (2003). An Introduction to Variable and Feature Selection. *Journal of Machine Learning Research,* Vol.3, No.7-8, pp. 1157-1182, ISSN 1532-4435

Harrell, F.E. Jr; Lee, K.L. & Mark, D.B. (1996), Multivariable Prognostic Models: Issues in Developing Models, Evaluating Assumptions and Adequacy, and Measuring and Reducing Errors. *Statistics in Medicine,* Vol.15, No.4, pp. 361-387, ISSN 0277-6715

Higgins, T.L.; Estafanous, F.G.; Loop, F.D.; Beck, G.J.; Lee, J.C.; Starr, N.J.; Knaus, W.A. & Cosgrove III, D.M. (1997). ICU Admission Score for Predicting Morbidity and Mortality Risk after Coronary Artery Bypass Grafting. *The Annals of Thoracic Surgery,* Vol.64, No.4, pp. 1050-1058, ISSN 0003-4975

Hodgman, S.B. (2008). Predictive Modeling & Outcomes. *Professional Case Management,* Vol.13, pp. 19-23, ISSN 1932-8087

Hosmer, D.W. & Lemeshow, S. (2000). *Applied Logistic Regression,* Wiley, ISBN 0-4716-1553-6, New York, USA

Lasko, T.A.; Bhagwat, J.G.; Zou, K.H. & Ohno-Machado, L. (2005). The Use of Receiver Operating Characteristic Curves in Biomedical Informatics. *Journal of Biomedical Informatics,* Vol.38, No.5, pp. 404-415, ISSN 1532-0464

Lee, P.M. (2004). *Bayesian Statistics - An Introduction,* Arnold, ISBN 0-340-81405-5, London, UK

Marshall, G.; Shroyer, A.L.W.; Grover, F.L. & Hammermeister K.E. (1994). Bayesian-Logit Model for Risk Assessment in Coronary Artery Bypass Grafting. *The Annals of Thoracic Surgery,* Vol.57, No.6, pp. 1492-1500, ISSN 0003-4975

Murphy, A.H. (1973). A New Vector Partition of the Probability Score. *Journal of Applied Meteorology,* Vol.12, No.4, pp. 595-600, ISSN 0021-8952, Available from http://journals. ametsoc.org/toc/jam/12/4

Murphy-Filkins, R.; Teres, D.; Lemeshow, S. & Hosmer, D.W. (1996). Effect of Changing Patient Mix on the Performance of an Intensive Care Unit Severity-of-Illness Model: How to Distinguish a General from a Specialty Intensive Care Unit. *Critical Care Medicine,* Vol.24, No.12, pp. 1968-1973, ISSN 0090-3493

Vapnik, V.N. (1999). *The Nature of Statistical Learning Theory,* Springer-Verlag, ISBN 0-387-98780-0, New York, USA

Vincent, J.L. & Moreno, R. (2010). Clinical Review: Scoring Systems in the Critically Ill. *Critical Care,* Vol.14, No.2 (207), pp. 1-9, ISSN 1364-8535

Zhou, X.H.; Li, S.M. & Gatsonis, C.A. (2008). Wilcoxon-Based Group Sequential Designs for Comparison of Areas Under Two Correlated ROC Curves. *Statistics in Medicine,* Vol.27, No.2, pp. 213-223, ISSN 0277-6715

4

The Role of Mass Media Communication in Public Health

Daniel Catalán-Matamoros
University of Almería
Spain

1. Introduction

The mass media are intensively employed in public health. Vast sums are spent annually for materials and salaries that have gone into the production and distribution of booklets, pamphlets, exhibits, newspaper articles, and radio and television programs. These media are employed at all levels of public health in the hope that three effects might occur: the learning of correct health information and knowledge, the changing of health attitudes and values and the establishment of new health behavior.

Mass media campaigns have long been a tool for promoting public health (Noar, 2006) being widely used to expose high proportions of large populations to messages through routine uses of existing media, such as television, radio, and newspapers. Communication campaigns involving diverse topics and target audiences have been conducted for decades. Some reasons why information campaigns fail' is an early landmark in the literature. Exposure to such messages is, therefore, generally passive (Wakefield, 2010). Such campaigns are frequently competing with factors, such as pervasive product marketing, powerful social norms, and behaviours driven by addiction or habit.

Mass media campaigns have generally aimed primarily to change knowledge, awareness and attitudes, contributing to the goal of changing behaviour. There has not normally been a high expectation that such campaigns on their own would change people's behaviour. Theory suggests that, as with other preventive health efforts, mass media campaigns are most likely to reduce unhealthy attitudes if their messages are reinforced by other efforts. Reinforcing factors may include law enforcement efforts, grassroots activities, and other media messages.

There is a vast literature relating to public health information campaigns. Much theoretical literature is devoted to the topic of effectiveness of health communication strategies. Mass media campaigns have usually been one element of broader health promotion programmes with mutually reinforcing components:

1. Mobilising and supporting local agencies and professionals who have direct access to individuals within the target population.
2. Bringing together partnerships of public, voluntary and private sector bodies and professional organisations.
3. Informing and educating the public, but also setting the agenda for public debate about the health topic, thereby modifying the climate of opinion surrounding it.

4. Encouraging local and national policy changes so as to create a supportive environment within which people are more able to change their behaviour.

This book chapter will first focus on some key concepts such as communication campaigns *vs* mass media campaigns, advertising *vs* communication campaigns, the concept of risk and risk communication campaigns. Later on, the chapter will focus on the effectiveness of public health campaigns using mass media communication.

2. Communication campaigns *vs* mass media campaigns

There is often confusion between the labels campaign, communication campaign or program, media or mass media campaign, and intervention. No particular definition adequately covers current practice, and there are many local variations of what is meant by these labels. Indeed, a variety of definitions exists in the literature but the following elements of a *communication* campaign are essential (Rogers and Storey 1987).

Firstly, a campaign is purposive. The specific outcomes can be extremely diverse ranging from individual level cognitive effects to societal or structural change.

Secondly, a communication campaign is aimed at a large audience. Rogers and Storey (1987) note that 'large' is used to distinguish campaigns from interpersonal persuasive communications by one individual (or a few people) aiming to seek to influence only a few others.

Thirdly, communication campaigns have a specified time limit. This is not to state that all campaigns are short lived. For example, the initial Stanford Heart Disease Prevention Program ran for three years, however follow-up investigations were conducted over decades.

The fourth point is that a communication campaign comprises a designed set of organised activities. This is most evident in message design and distribution. Messages are organised in terms of both form and content, and responsibility is taken for selecting appropriate communication channels and media. As Rogers and Storey (1987) point out, even those campaigns whose nature or goal is emancipation or participation involve organised message production and distribution.

In summary, the term communication campaign implies that:

- it is planned to generate specific outcomes;
- in a relatively large number of individuals;
- within a specified time period; and
- uses an organised set of communication activities.

Rogers and Storey (1987) observe that in the modern communication campaign, modest changes in audience behaviour are frequently achievable, and it is important for the campaign planner to set modest and realistic expectations about what can be achieved. They argue that a health promotion campaign might be considered successful or effective if about five percent of the target (or segmented) audience does adopt measurable changes in health behaviour over the longer-term.

In this context, it is important to define a communication campaign. It should be noted that the word communication is used to highlight the fact that not all campaigns necessarily involve mass media messages, or mass media messages in isolation, and that communication campaigns may be small-scale in scope and audience reach.

3. Advertising and communication campaigns

Elliott (1987), one of Australia's leading communication practitioners, offers a particularly informative look at the differences between advertising and communication campaigns. His literature review and analyses of campaigns are especially relevant because they are based largely on experience. He defines a set of parameters for considering and planning for a campaign's realistic outcomes.

Elliott's (1987) basic premise is that the objectives and processes that are appropriate for commercial advertising are usually inappropriate for health promotion. The essential differences between advertising and health campaigns lie in the nature of the product, the processes involved in promotion and, of course, in the nature of audiences. Elliott argues that advertising by itself will not result in fundamental changes in behaviour: "Commercial products are regarded by many as trivial and superficial, not as central and ego-involving to the individual as ill health. They are positive and attractive and can be relatively easily obtained. By contrast, health publicity is largely negative: it preaches the avoidance of something negative (which is enjoyable), often involving short-term unpleasantness, for the sake of benefits that are long-term, probabilistic and not guaranteed".

Elliott (1987) draws on previous research to demonstrate once again that advertising does not have massive effects on potential consumers, as many might believe. However, he notes that small changes in market share for a particular product that are achieved as a consequence of advertising may result in greatly increased sales and profits. In this regard, it is useful to recall Rogers and Storey's (1987) assertion that a health promotion campaign might be considered successful if five percent of the target audience make long-term changes in overt health behaviour.

Commercial advertising techniques are but one element of a communication campaign using mass media. The following table is comparing communication campaigns and advertising.

Typical Communication Campaign	Typical Advertising Campaign
Persuasive focus involving response shaping, reinforcement attitude change; behavioural change.	Focus on feelings and perceptions toward product. Not attitude change.
Difficult to specify individual desires and wants.	Based on the idea of satisfying desires and wants.
Designed to meet societal or individual needs in face of risk.	May be designed to create desire and need.
May not be in line with prevailing attitudes and opinions.	Plays on prevailing attitudes and opinions.
Usually against the tide of public opinion.	Tries to stay with the tide of public opinion.
Not usually seen as a personal benefit as such and may be designed to create a social benefit.	Usually, if not exclusively, a personal benefit.

Typical Communication Campaign	Typical Advertising Campaign
Involves personal cost, sometimes even discomfort.	Cost is one of choice among competing brands.
Message is that all people should adopt or comply.	Products/services that are not accepted fail.
Often difficult to see short-term outcomes.	Easy to see, and outcomes can usually be quantified.
Reward difficult to see.	Reward easy to see.
People may express support for socially desirable behaviour but not adopt the behaviour.	
Experience is the best way to change attitudes – not mass media.	
Tries to define communication objectives as changes in individuals: • Increased salience; • Strengthening or attitude change; • More positive disposition to behave in a desired direction; • Adoption of behaviour either in the short or long term; • Awareness of unintended consequences.	Market objectives often confused with communication objectives. Focus on behavioural outcomes with intermediary objectives such as reinforcing loyal buyers' beliefs, creating consumer satisfaction, maintaining brand salience.
May be very sensitive, obtrusive, and emotional.	May not involve great emotional or affective attachment.
Many times involves an organisational bias – in the 'public service/interest'. Educational campaigns favoured even when evidence shows previous similar campaigns failed.	Campaigns that fail or result in loss lead to immediate action.
Sometimes, objectives confused with education or mere dissemination of information.	
Organisation may constrain budget, processes and structure of the campaign.	All about excitement, sexuality, self-indulgence, and even power.
Government equated to what ought to be done, what should be done, etc. It is the 'parental' mode.	Talks to the child in us.

Typical Communication Campaign	Typical Advertising Campaign
Information often perceived to be unreliable because: •Most groups perceive others as the problem or cause. •Many see themselves compliant with the attitudes or behaviour, when they are not •People seek justification for non-compliance and may give misleading information in any evaluation.	Easy to get information about products and services. Yet, advertising does not work in the way that most people believe. Advertising does not have massive effects on people.
Some people have pre-existing beliefs or ideas about 'communication'. Unrealistic expectations about what can be achieved.	Can be targeted to specific audiences or segments and expectations adjusted.
Often difficult to identify target audience. Audience could be everyone. Expectations should be low.	
Secondary audiences may be critical in facilitating change.	Secondary audiences rarely critical in mass advertising.
Usually a major objective related to a social concern.	Usually aiming at slight modifications.
Tends to be strategy based on modifications/change or slow down of undesirable attitudes/behaviours.	Tends to be strategy based on start or stop.
Slow processes involved over time.	May see instant results.
Television's commercial 'values' may be inappropriate to the campaign's message.	Commercial television is commercial television advertising; the program is designed to deliver an audience to an advertiser.

Table 1. Comparison of communication and advertising campaigns

4. The concept of risk

Most health communication campaigns involve risk, i.e. risks to people and societal risks. The concept of risk has been at the focus of contemporary thinking in recent years because of the salience and threat of environmental issues, which have received extensive public and media attention.

Giddens (1999) observes that most traditional cultures did not have a concept of risk and argues that it is a concept associated with modern industrialised civilisation, embodying ideas about controlling or conquering the future. People are forced to negotiate their lives around risks, and to rely increasingly on their own judgments about risks. Experts can assess the likelihood and magnitude of a given risk, however the public understanding of a given risk takes on meaning through our cultural practices.

One important cultural site for the production of meanings about risk is media content, including communication campaigns. The meaning of a particular health risk to various groups in society, for example, develops through the continuing and often changing representations of that risk in media content, and in scientific and medical discourses, as well as through other social and cultural practices. It is against this background of changing technical, media and public discourses that communication campaigns are planned.

Wynne (1996) argues that, just as expert opinion is central to ideas about risk, so too is lay criticism and comment. He observes that, while risks may be debated within scientific or 'public accountability' discourses, they are dealt with by most people as individuals in very specific situations, at the level of the local, the private, the mundane, the everyday, and intimate experiences. Wynne argues that it is essential to examine how perceptions of risks are constructed by local, or as he terms it 'situated', knowledge, as well as by expert knowledge. For example, there are profound differences across class, gender, race, ethnicity, age and other variables in the ways people understand, interpret and respond to health risks. Individualism might suggest a degree of choice in negotiating risk, but it is recognised that, within the power structures of our society, some people have more authority over the ways risks are identified, defined as public, and managed, than do other people. Anecdotally, it has been noted that a teenage boy will ask for the cigarette packet with the warning label 'Smoking is dangerous to pregnant women' because 'it doesn't apply to him'.

This risk perspective offers invaluable insights for communication campaign planners. This section of communication literature has one point of origin in the environmental sciences, and is particularly important to review because of its parallels to more general communication campaigns.

4.1 Risk communication campaigns

Risk communication campaigns offer the promise of resolving public conflict and diminishing fear about new large-scale technologies, such as nuclear power, as well as promoting safety campaigns concerned with science, technology and health. The concept of communication being 'in the public interest' was viewed as essential in fulfilling the public's need for information and education, or for promoting behavioural change and protective action, in the face of an anticipated disaster or hazard.

Brown and Campbell (1991) note that many western societies recognised the need for public information about science and technological risks. They link heightened interest in risk communication to the emergence of environmental impact legislation and the requirement to inform the public. The early risk communication campaign model involved 'experts'attempting to persuade the public of the validity of their scientific and technical risk assessments of a particular hazard. It is perhaps unsurprising that many such campaigns met with limited success, as the reviews outlined above would predict.

A fundamental change in campaign planning occurred with the recognition that public perceptions of various risks differed widely. This change is viewed historically as a turning point for risk communication research. As Hadden (1989) observes, old risk communication models, such as those involving scientific experts attempting to persuade lay people of the validity of their risk assessments and decisions, are impeded by lay risk perceptions, by lay people's difficulties in understanding mathematical probabilities, and by technical and scientific difficulty.

Leiss (1998) argues that the changed research direction is a shift in emphasis from 'risk' to 'communication' in the concept of risk communication. In other words, it involves 're-framing the issue of risk communication as a problem in communication theory and practice, rather than in the concept of risk'. Risks perceived as familiar, controlled, voluntary, beneficial, and fair are more likely to be acceptable to most people than risks perceived in opposite ways (Slovic, 1994). For example, the perceived health risks of chemical pollution from a local industrial factory are different from the perceived risks from exceeding the speed limit on a country road: the first is involuntary and unfamiliar, while the latter may be considered voluntary and familiar.

Risk perception research adds to the body of knowledge in this area by accounting for seemingly irrational responses by various publics to identified and potential hazards. It should be noted that the same risk might in fact produce very different perceptions in differing groups of people, depending upon the context in which the risk is understood and interpreted. These varied perceptions may produce differing policy or strategic decisions about risk 'management' and responses by 'experts'. Rowan (1996) puts forward the following argument about generalised perception factors: [The factors] are expressions of various types of power: informational, decisional and distributional. People who feel deprived of facts, unable to control their own lives, and forced to bear the costs but not the benefits are likely to be outraged by news of some new risk. To be effective risk communication must involve power sharing. Therefore, risk communication may not reduce conflict and smooth risk management. Empowerment can be destabilising in the short term, but it leads to more broadly based policy decisions, which can hold up over the long term.

As a consequence, contemporary risk communication campaigns attempt to be more individually reflexive and, as Hadden (1989) argued, the key to this approach lies in establishing dialogue or conversations with the public. The notion of one-way, top-down, expert-to-public campaigns is replaced with a more interactive process designed to empower various publics. Campaigns recognise that understanding the complexities of health issues, including technical knowledge, are not necessarily beyond ordinary people. They also highlight the potential importance of the interplay between scientific forms of knowledge and those that may be considered are more cultural. In other words, lay knowledge about health issues cannot be ignored in communication campaigns.

Hadden (1989) notes that campaigns that emphasise dialogue among parties and active participation in assessing and managing risk, are 'impeded by the lack of, or difficulty in establishing, participatory institutions'. Similarly, in a health context, Needleman (1987) notes that the goal of empowering those at risk to make an informed choice is laudable, however the risk communication intervention needs to be more than merely the dissemination of information:

The intervention must, somewhere along the line, stimulate individual and/or collective behavioural changes that reduce health risks. Otherwise, the risk communication becomes a kind of *ritualistic activity*, an end in itself in which the formal aspects of conveying risk information take precedence over their actual health impact.

The emergence of a participatory or dialogue model, which attempts to explore the disparity between expert information and a diverse public knowledge, has challenged both the 'scientific' approach to the problem of risk communication, and indeed the later perception research.

Brown and Campbell (1991) have placed risk communication models within a two by two matrix that categorises the underlying approach in terms of low and high power devolvement, and low and high community interaction. Older models of risk communication are low in terms of both power sharing and community interaction, in contrast to newer dialogue models that are high in power sharing and high in community interaction (see Table 2).

		Community Interaction	
Power sharing	Low	Low "Information" Leaflets Displays	High "Consultation" Public meetings Planning Inquiries
	High	"Canvassing" Surveys Groups Interviews	Conversation Searching focus Planning cells

Table 2. Risk Communication "Conversation Models"

The key message from Brown and Campbell's (1991) table to communication planners is to take full account of the day-to-day experiences, perceptions and cultural values of various audiences in the formative stages of any campaign. Formative research should go beyond simple quantitative measures to include more reflexive, cultural understandings of campaign messages and audiences. Of equal importance is the need to understand what various audiences bring to the reception process in their use of mass media, and their use of mass media in terms of understanding health issues.

British researcher Jenny Kitzinger, who has completed many studies on health issues, says (1994): We are none of us self-contained, isolated, static entities; we are part of complex and overlapping, social, familial and collegiate networks. Our personal behaviour is not cut off from public discourses and our actions do not happen in a 'cultural vacuum'. We make sense of things through talking with and observing other people, through conversations at home or at work; and we act (or fail to act) on that knowledge in a social context. When researchers want to explore people's understandings, or to influence them, it makes sense to employ methods, which actively encourage the examination of these social processes in action.

The notion of an active dialogue model may appear idealistic or impractical, however it should be contrasted with the failures of the dominant 'top-down' campaign strategies, which comprised the older risk communication approach. An active dialogue model examining expert and lay knowledge should not be viewed as ignoring technical health knowledge. The approach explicitly acknowledges the legitimacy of all sources of knowledge central to risk dialogue, including technical knowledge (Handmer 1995). It acknowledges the importance of investigating the interplay between various discourses, including scientific, medical, health, media, and lay discourses, in planning any communication campaign.

The key message from Brown and Campbell's (1991) table to communication planners is to take full account of the day-to-day experiences, perceptions and cultural values of various audiences in the formative stages of any campaign. Formative research should go beyond simple quantitative measures to include more reflexive, cultural understandings of campaign messages and audiences. Of equal importance is the need to understand what various audiences bring to the reception process in their use of mass media, and their use of mass media in terms of understanding health issues.

British researcher Jenny Kitzinger, who has completed many studies on health issues, says (1999): We are none of us self-contained, isolated, static entities; we are part of complex and overlapping, social, familial and collegiate networks. Our personal behaviour is not cut off from public discourses and our actions do not happen in a 'cultural vacuum'. We make sense of things through talking with and observing other people, through conversations at home or at work; and we act (or fail to act) on that knowledge in a social context. When researchers want to explore people's understandings, or to influence them, it makes sense to employ methods, which actively encourage the examination of these social processes in action. The notion of an active dialogue model may appear idealistic or impractical, however it should be contrasted with the failures of the dominant 'top-down' campaign strategies, which comprised the older risk communication approach. An active dialogue model examining expert and lay knowledge should not be viewed as ignoring technical health knowledge. The approach explicitly acknowledges the legitimacy of all sources of knowledge central to risk dialogue, including technical knowledge. It acknowledges the importance of investigating the interplay between various discourses, including scientific, medical, health, media, and lay discourses, in planning any communication campaign.

5. Content and delivery of mass media campaigns

Several aspects of mass media campaigns may influence their effectiveness. These can be categorized into variables related to message content and to message delivery.

5.1 Message content

One important aspect of message content involves the themes used to motivate the desired behavior change. Some common motivational themes in mass media campaigns to prevent unhealthy behabiours include:

- fear of legal consequences
- promotion of positive social norms
- fear of harm to self, others, or property
- and stigmatizing unhealthy behabiours as irresponsible and dangerous

The actions promoted by the campaigns also vary, ranging from messages related to abstinence or moderation to more specific behavioural recommendations. Decisions related to message content are generally made based on the opinions expressed by experts or focus groups rather than on evidence of effectiveness in changing behaviour (Randy et al., 2004).

Another aspect of message content relates to the optimal amount of anxiety produced (Witte & Allen, 2000; Tay, 2002). The effectiveness of "fear-based" campaigns is the subject of a long-standing controversy. Some level of anxiety arousal is generally seen as a desirable motivator. However, several authors have cautioned that generating intense anxiety by emphasizing the severity of a problem and the audience's susceptibility to it can cause some people to ignore or discount the campaign messages. Although this caution appears to be justified, increasing the strength of a fear appeal also increases the probability that the audience will change their attitudes, intentions, and behaviours. These changes are maximized, and defensive avoidance minimized, when the anxiety-arousing message is accompanied by specific information about actions that people can take to protect themselves. The degree of persuasion versus defensive avoidance produced may be influenced by interactions between the message content and characteristics of the recipient. For instance, strong fear appeals may be more effective for motivating a response among segments of the audience that initially do not view the problem addressed as being important or relevant to them. They may also be more persuasive to people who are already engaging in the desired behaviour.

5.2 Message delivery

A mass media campaign cannot be effective unless the target audience is exposed to, attends to, and comprehends its message. Two important aspects of message delivery are control over message placement and production quality. Control over message placement helps to ensure that the intended audience is exposed to the messages with sufficient frequency to exceed some threshold for effectiveness.

It also allows for the optimal timing and placement of those messages. This control can only be assured with paid campaigns. Those that rely solely on donated public service time may attain adequate exposure, but message placement and frequency are ultimately left to media schedulers and station management; paid advertising time always gets preferential placement. Assuming that the target audience is adequately exposed, high production quality of the campaign messages may maximize the probability that the audience will pay attention to them. High production quality may also improve the chances of eliciting the intended emotional impact.

5.3 Message pretesting

Pretesting of campaign themes and messages is also thought to be important for a successful outcome (Hornik & Woolf, 1999). Pretesting can help to assess which themes or concepts are most relevant to the target audience. It can also help to ensure that the target audience will attend to and comprehend the specific messages presented. The importance of pretesting is highlighted by an evaluation of a mass media campaign designed to prevent alcohol-related problems by encouraging drinking in moderation. No pretesting of ads was done for this campaign, and a survey conducted at midcampaign found that over a third of respondents thought that the ads were promoting alcohol consumption. Many mistook them for beer ads.

6. Effectiveness of the mass media campaigns

An Australian review of mass media health promotion campaigns in two areas, cardiovascular risk behavior and safety restraints (Redman, Spencer, and Sanson-Fisher, 1990) illustrates these moderate effects. The authors began with 24 studies but determined that only nine met their criteria for adequate evaluation methodologies. These nine were further divided into two models of media effects: media only and media as agenda-setting plus community programming. Not surprisingly, they concluded that media only campaigns had discouraging results but that most studies of media plus intensive community interventions reported significant changes in behavior. The authors, however, challenged these positive results by questioning how important the media component was to the success of such combined programs.

It is probably time to consider a fourth era and that one is characterized by the use of the internet and by paid media rather than relying on public service time. It is too early to have much data from this fourth era but the White Houses' Office of the Drug Czar's anti-drug campaign shows some promising results as do many of the state anti-smoking campaigns.

What has been missing from these previous reviews is a systematic analysis of the size of effects achieved for different types of objectives, e.g., awareness, knowledge, attitudes, and behaviors. It was addressed this gap by identifying and reviewing the extant empirical data from evaluations of mass mediated health campaigns.

Campaign Objective	Average Size of Change %
Awareness (N=16)	56
Knowledge change (N=15)	22
Attitude change (N-21)	8
Behavior change (N=29)	13

Table 3. Average changes achieved after mass-mediated health campaigns

6.1 Changing knowledge and awareness

Changing behaviour is the highest priority in any public health campaign, however, most of the mass media will change knowledge and awareness more easily than behaviour.

Theoretically, the mass media are supposed to be most effective in achieving awareness. This review supports that expectation. When measuring awareness as simple recognition of the message, up to 83% levels of awareness have been reported, with a median of 48%. Although, without a pre message measure, some of this (perhaps up to 9%) may be measurement error, e.g., a desire to please the interviewer.

Ceiling effects must also be considered. If awareness is moderately high before the campaign, there are ceilings on the increases possible and probably these increases are harder to achieve. If both pre and post levels of awareness are available, increases can be calculated based on the percent of audience possible to change. For example, if awareness of the seriousness of colon cancer was 11% prior to a campaign and 40% after it, the increase, instead of being 29% would be 29% of the possible change of 89% which is 33%.

Knowledge gain is clearly achievable using mass mediated health campaigns. When exposure is guaranteed, dramatic increases in knowledge (as large as 60%) have been observed. When exposure is not guaranteed but the campaign can saturate a community, knowledge gains around 25% seem feasible. The size of these knowledge gains decrease when the campaigns are national in scope and must compete with numerous other stimuli. Still, most of the campaigns were successful in achieving some knowledge gain, although around 10% appears to be a more achievable increase. Multi—channel campaigns appear to be much more successful than single channel, especially print only campaigns.

Below there is some evidence about changes in levels of knowledge and awareness during mass media public health campaigns:

Alcohol

- Awareness of 'sensible drinking message' unit - up from 39 to 76%, 1989–94
- Knowledge of units in popular drinks - up 300%, 1989–94
- People's accurate assessment of their own drinking - up 5%, 1990–94.

HIV/AIDS

- Changes in levels of tolerance: those in the general public who say that homosexual relations are always or mostly wrong - 74% in 1987; 44% in 1997

- Attitudes to people with HIV infection: those who think people with AIDS have only themselves to blame - 57% in 1987; 36% in 1996
- Belief that a condom protects against HIV: 66% in 1986; 95% in 1997
- Women aged 18–19 whose partners used condoms: 6% in 1986; 22% in 1993.

Folic acid

- Spontaneous awareness of folic acid - 9% in 1995; 39% in 1997
- Sales of folic acid supplements and prescription rates - up 50% in an eight-month period.

Immunisation - the Hib vaccine

- Awareness of the Hib vaccine: 5% in 1992; 89% in 1993.

Skin cancer

- Proportion of the public who thought a suntan was important -28% in 1995; 25% in 1996
- Proportion of people who say they use a sunscreen when sunbathing in this country - 34% in 1995; 41% in 1996.

Note

With complex interventions that are intended to work synergistically it is difficult to attribute impacts to particular intervention components. Also, factors external to interventions - particularly if they are about sensitive subjects - may add to or subtract from their impact.

6.2 Changing attitudes and behaviours

All but four of the 21 evaluations of these health communication campaigns showed significant attitude change. The actual amount of change varied considerably. These results suggest that if exposure is insured, considerable attitude change is possible. The greatest amount of change (+38% for an AIDS video shown in waiting rooms of STD clinics (Solomon & DeJong, 1986) a case of forced exposure. The ARTA campaign (Woods, Davis, & Stover, 1991) also demonstrated considerable attitude change, an average of 20% across five attitude items, however, it must be remembered that the ARTA camp has received unusually high exposure for a PSA campaign, and was only part of extensive media coverage of HIV/AIDS. Therefore, it is impossible to know how much of that change is attributable to the campaign itself. Some of the evaluations clearly suffered from ceiling effects and the results are difficult to interpret. The surveys measuring outcomes of one of the Cancer Prevention Awareness campaigns, for example, found pre—campaign levels of 90+% on some of the items leaving little room to measure change. In spite of more control over airing than the typical PSA, the single channel campaigns did not achieve as much attitude change.

Although behaviour is normally considered one of the most difficult objectives to achieve in mediated health campaigns, the campaigns reviewed here were quite successful. Only six of the 29 behavioral change campaigns identified failed to achieve some level of change. The average change reported was 13% should be noted that these results may be biased by the tendency toward not publishing non—significant findings.

The literature is beginning to amass evidence that targeted, well-executed health mass media campaigns can have small-to-moderate effects not only on health knowledge, beliefs, and attitudes, but on behaviours as well, which can translate into major public health impact given the wide reach of mass media. Such impact can only be achieved, however, if principles of effective campaign design are carefully followed.

There is renewed interest in the possibility of achieving policy goals through behaviour change. For example, a recent report commissioned for the Cabinet Office (Halpern and Bates, 2004) states that: 'Behaviourally based interventions can be significantly more cost-effective than traditional service delivery.' Interventions to change health-related behaviour may range from a simple, face-to-face consultation between professional and patient to a complex programme, often involving the use of mass media. This briefing looks first at the evidence on the effectiveness of interventions in changing behaviour generally; and second at the evidence concerning mass media campaigns.

A range of types of intervention aim to change 'risky' behaviours:

- Increasing knowledge and awareness of risks (through information and awareness-raising), or knowledge and awareness of services to help prevent risks
- Changing attitudes and motivations, eg through messages aimed at young people about the harm smoking does to skin and appearance
- Increasing physical or interpersonal skills, eg in using condoms, or deploying assertiveness skills to suggest that condoms be used
- Changing beliefs and perceptions, eg through interventions aimed at increasing testicular self-examination in men by raising their awareness of risk and 'normalising' self-examination
- Influencing social norms, eg by changing public perceptions of secondary smoking, or public acceptance of breastfeeding
- Changing structural factors and influencing the wider determinants of health, eg by implementing clean-air policies to decrease pollution and improve health
- Influencing the availability and accessibility of health services.

The evidence suggests that the following characteristics are the key elements for success in changing behaviour:

- Using theoretical models in developing interventions
- Intervening at multiple levels when appropriate
- Targeted and tailored (in terms of age, gender, culture, etc), making use of needs assessment or formative research
- Providing basic, accurate information through clear, unambiguous messages
- Using behavioural skills training, including self-efficacy
- Joining up services with other community provisions, eg providing transport links from community centres to clinics, or situating health services in accessible community settings
- Working with community members as advocates of appropriate services
- Providing alternative choices and risk reduction (eg promoting condom use), rather than simply telling people not to do something (eg don't take drugs, don't have sex)
- Addressing peer norms and social pressures.

Even though mass media health campaigns are used extensively, considerable debate continues over their effectiveness. This review differed from previous ones in that it included only those campaign evaluations that collected quantitative evidence of impact and it organized these data according to campaign objectives. In general, the results confirm Rogers and Storey's (1987) description of the era of moderate effects. As McGuire's (1989) hierarchy of effects model would predict, the size of the effects were greater at the earlier steps, i.e., awareness, and knowledge than the later stages of attitude change, and behavior change.

7. Lessons about implementing mass media campaigns

A report published by the National Health Services in UK (2004) on anti-smoking campaigns in the 1990s high-lighted lessons, some of which may be of general value:

- Campaigns need to contain a variety of messages – 'threatening' and 'supportive' styles of delivery can complement each other
- Anti-smoking advertising has to compete in a crowded media marketplace – a hook is needed to engage the emotions of the target audience
- Emotions can be engaged using humour, fear, sympathy or aspiration
- TV advertising, in particular, is better at jolting smokers than delivering encouraging or supportive messages
- Smokers want help and encouragement to quit
- Advertising should not tell people what they should do
- Smokers are motivated by knowing that they are not alone, and that support and help are available – they need reminding of the benefits of not smoking
- Content and style of delivery are of equal importance – smokers can accept unpalatable messages if the context is encouraging and supportive.

8. Conclusion

Mass media health campaigns clearly can be an effective tool for health promotion whether the effort is on a national or local scale. We should stop arguing whether they are more or less effective than other strategies or whether one channel is better than another. Instead we should carefully formulate our conceptual model of how we expect an intervention to work and then evaluate it accordingly. Health promotion interventions are not like pills – they are much more complex and indirect in the way they work. Therefore our evaluation designs may be very different allowing us to track a social influence process and document its effects on social and political institutions as well as on individuals.

8.1 When to use the media

It is apparent from the evidence that the media can be an effective tool in health promotion, given the appropriate circumstances and conditions. Some of the situations in which media have been found to be most appropriate are as follows.

1. When wide exposure is desired. Mass media offer the widest possible exposure, although this may be at some cost. Cost–benefit considerations are at the core of media selection.
2. When the timeframe is urgent. Mass media offer the best opportunity for reaching either large numbers of people or specific target groups within a short timeframe.
3. When public discussion is likely to facilitate the educational process. Media messages can be emotional and thought provoking. Because of the possible breadth of coverage, they can be targeted at many different levels, stimulating discussion and thereby expanding the impact of a message.
4. When awareness is a main goal. By their very nature, the media are awareness-creating tools. Where awareness of a health issue is important to its resolution, the mass media can increase awareness quickly and effectively.
5. When media authorities are 'on-side'. Where journalists, editors and programmers are on-side with a particular health issue, this often guarantees greater support in terms of space and editorial content.

6. When accompanying back-up can be provided on the ground. Regardless of whether media alone are sufficient to influence health behaviour, it is clear that the success of media will be improved with the support of back-up programmes and services.
7. When long-term follow-up is possible. Most changes in health behaviour require constant reinforcement. Media programmes are most effective where the opportunity exists for long-term follow-up. This can take the form of short bursts of media activity over an extended period, or follow-up activities unrelated to media.
8. When a generous budget exists. Paid advertising, especially on television, can be very expensive. Even media with limited reach, such as pamphlets and posters, can be expensive depending on the quality and quantity. For media to be considered as a strategy in health promotion, careful consideration of costs and benefits needs to be undertaken.
9. When the behavioural goal is simple. Although complex behaviour change such as smoking cessation or exercise adoption may be initiated through media programmes, the nature of media is such that simple behaviour changes such as immunisation or cholesterol testing are more easily stimulated through the media. In general, the more complex the behaviour change, the more back-up is required to supplement a media health programme.
10. When the agenda includes public relations. Many, if not most, health promotion programmes have an agenda which is not always explicit - maybe to gain public support or acknowledgement, to solicit political favour, or to raise funds for further programmes. Where public relations are either an explicit or implicit goal of a programme, mass media are effective because of their wide-ranging exposure.

8.2 Further research questions

1. *Evaluating message content effects:* What is the relative effectiveness and cost-effectiveness of various campaign themes (e.g., law enforcement, legal penalties, social stigma, guilt, injury to self and others) for reducing unhealthy behaviours? For influencing public support for stronger prevention activities?
2. *Evaluating message delivery effects:* What is the dose–response curve for varying levels of advertising exposure (e.g., none, light, moderate, and heavy)? Does the shape of this curve vary according to message content and the outcome evaluated? What is the relative effectiveness and cost-effectiveness of different media types (TV, radio, etc.)? Paid advertising and public service announcements? What is the optimal exposure schedule for public health mass media campaigns (e.g., intermittent waves of messages vs a steady flow)? How should mass media campaigns be adapted to the changing media environment (e.g., market segmentation, Internet, message filtering devices)?
3. *Evaluating message/recipient interactions:* To what extent are certain population groups more or less likely to be influenced by mass media campaigns? Are some themes more likely than others to influence "hard-to-reach" target groups (e.g., enforcement themes for "hard-core" drinking drivers)?
4. *Improving research design:* What measurement issues need to be addressed to improve assessment of media and message exposure? What research designs can best address problems in measuring exposure?

9. References

Brown, J. & Campbell, E. (1991). Risk communication: Some underlying principles. *Journal of Environmental Studies*, Vol. 38, 1991, 297-303.

Elliott, B.J. (1987). *Effective Mass Communication Campaigns: A Source Book of Guidelines*. Elliott & Shanahan Research, North Sydney.

Giddens, A. (1999). Risk and Responsibility. *Modern Law Review*, Vol. 62, No. 1, 1999, 1-10.

Hadden, S.G. (1989). Institutional Barriers to Risk Communication. *Risk Analysis*, Vol. 9, 1989, 301–308.

Halpern, D. and Bates, C. (2004) Personal responsibility and changing behaviour: the state of knowledge and its implications for public policy. London: Cabinet Office, Prime Minister's Strategy Unit. www.strategy.gov.uk/files/pdf/pr.pdf

Hornik, R., Woolf, K.D. (1999). Using cross-sectional surveys to plan message strategies. *Soc Marketing Q*, Vol. 5, 1999; 34–41.

Kitzinger, J. (1999). Researching risk and the media. *Health, risk & Society*, Vol. 1, No. 1, 1999, 55-69.

Leiss, W. (1998). Risk Communication and public knowledge. In: *Communication Theory Today*, Crowley, D. &. Mitchell, D. (Eds.), Polity Press, Oxford.

McGuire, W.J. (1989). Theoretical Foundations of Campaigns. In: *Public Communication Campaigns*, Rice, R.E. & Atkin, C. (Eds.), 43-65, Newbury Park, Sage Publications, CA.

Needleman, C. (1987). Ritualism in communicating risk information. *Sci Tech Hum Values*, Vol. 12, 1987, 20-25.

Noar, S.M. (2006). A 10-Year Retrospective of Research in Health Mass Media Campaigns: Where Do We Go From Here?. *Journal of Health Communication: International Perspectives*, Vol. 11, No. 1, 2006, 21 - 42, 1087-0415.

Randy, W.E., Shults, A., Sleet, D., Faahb, J.L., Thompson, R.S. & Rajab, W. (2004). Effectiveness of Mass Media Campaigns for reducing drinking and driving and alcohol-involved crashes. Am J Prev Med, Vol. 27, No. 1, 2004, 57-65.

Redman, S., Spencer, E.A., & Sanson-Fisher, R.W. (1990). The role of mass media in changing health-related behavior: a critical appraisal of two models. *Journal of Health Promotion of Australia*, Vol. 7, No. 2, 1990, 91-99.

Rogers, E.M. & Storey, J.D. (1987). Communication campaigns. In: *Handbook of communication science*, C. Berger & S. Chaffee (Eds.), 817-846, Newbury Park, Sage, CA.

Rowan, F. (1996). The high stakes of risk communication. *Preventive Medicine*, Vol. 25, 1996, 26-29.

Slovic, P. (1994). Perceptions of risk: Challenge and paradox. In: *Future and risk management*, Brehmer, B. & Sahlin, N.E. (Eds.), 63-78, Kluwer Academic Publishers, NY.

Solomon, D.S. (1982). Health campaigns on television. In: *Television and behavior*. Pearl, D., Bouthilet, L. & Lazar, J. (Eds.). NIMH Technical Reviews, Washington, DC.

Szerzynski, B., & Wynne, B. (1996). *Risk, Environment and Modernity. Towards a new Ecology*, SAGE Publications, London.

Tay, R. (2002). Exploring the effects of a road safety advertising campaign on the perceptions and intentions of the target and nontarget audiences to drink and drive. *Traffic Inj Prev*, Vol. 3, 2002, 195–200.

Wakefield, M.A., Loken, B. & Hornik, R.C. (2010). Use of mass media campaigns to change health behaviour. The Lancet, Vol. 376, No. 9748, Oct 2010, 1261-71, 0140-6736.

Witte, K., Allen, M. (2000). A meta-analysis of fear appeals: implications for effective public health campaigns. *Health Educ Behav*, Vol. 27, 2000, 591–615.

Woods, D.R., Davis, D., & Westover, B.J. (1991). "American Responds to AIDS": Its content, development process, and outcome. *Public Health Reports*, Vol. 106, No. 6, 1991, 616-622.

5

The Unresolved Issue of the "Terminal Disease" Concept

Sergio Eduardo Gonorazky
Hospital Privado de Comunidad de Mar del Plata, Argentina

1. Introduction

1.1 Prefatory emarks

"I have already told you with what care they look after their sick, so that nothing is left undone that can contribute either to their case or health; and for those who are taken with fixed and incurable diseases, they use all possible ways to cherish them and to make their lives as comfortable as possible. They visit them often and take great pains to make their time pass off easily; but when any is taken with a torturing and lingering pain, so that there is no hope either of recovery or ease, the priests and magistrates come and exhort them, that, since they are now unable to go on with the business of life, are become a burden to themselves and to all about them, and they have really out-lived themselves, they should no longer nourish such a rooted distemper, but choose rather to die since they cannot live but in much misery; being assured that if they thus deliver themselves from torture, or are willing that others should do it, they shall be happy after death: since, by their acting thus, they lose none of the pleasures, but only the troubles of life, they think they behave not only reasonably but in a manner consistent with religion and piety; because they follow the advice given them by their priests, who are the expounders of the will of God. Such as are wrought on by these persuasions either starve themselves of their own accord, or take opium, and by that means die without pain. But no man is forced on this way of ending his life; and if they cannot be persuaded to it, this does not induce them to fail in their attendance and care of them: but as they believe that a voluntary death, when it is chosen upon such an authority, is very honourable, so if any man takes away his own life without the approbation of the priests and the senate, they give him none of the honours of a decent funeral, but throw his body into a ditch."[1] Sir Thomas More (1516)

In 1977, Leon Eisenberg suggested a distinction should be made between the terms "disease" and "illness" (Eisenberg, 1977): *"The dysfunctional consequences of the Cartesian dichotomy have been enhanced by the power of biomedical technology. Technical virtuosity reifies the mechanical model and widens the gap between what patients seek and doctors provide. Patients suffer "illnesses"; doctors diagnose and treat "disease". Illnesses are experiences of discontinuities in states of being and perceived role performances. Diseases, in the scientific paradigm of modern medicine, are abnormalities in the function and/or structure of body organs and systems. Traditional healers also redefine illness as disease: because they share symbols and metaphors consonant with lay beliefs, their healing rituals are more responsive to the psychosocial context of illness...When physicians dismiss illness because ascertainable "disease" is absent, they fail to meet their socially assigned responsibility. It is essential to reintegrate "scientific" and "social" concepts of disease and illness as a basis for a functional system of medical research and care."*.

---

[1] Direct quotations appear in italics.

Allan Young (Young, 1982) draws a further distinction between "disease", "illness" and "sickness": *"DISEASE retains its original meaning (organic pathologies and abnormalities). ILLNESS is essentially the same, referring to how disease and sickness are brought into the individual consciousness. SICKNESS (…) is redefined as the process through which worrisome behavioral and biological signs, particularly ones originating in disease, are given socially recognizable meanings, i.e. they are made into symptoms and socially significant outcomes. Every culture has rules for translating signs into symptoms, for linking symptomatologies to etiologies and interventions,and for using the evidence provided by interventions to confirm translations and legitimize outcomes. The path a person follows from translation to socially significant outcome constitutes his sickness. Sickness is, then, a process for socializing disease and illness"*. These ideas were later reinstated by other authors and publications, such as The Hastings Center Report: The Goals of Medicine. Setting New Priorities (Callahan et al., 1996). In this document, "disease" is defined as a physical or mental dysfunction, based on a deviation from the statistical standard, which causes impairment or increases the probability of an early death; "illness" is understood as an individual's subjective perception that his or her physical or mental wellness is either altered or absent, affecting the ability to perform normal daily activities as a consequence; "sickness" is the social perception of an individual's health status, usually, an external perception that this individual has physical or mental difficulties.

The different realities of patients, their families, physicians and society at large, which will be discussed below, lead us to consider an anthropological perspective in which the medical point of view of **terminal disease** is integrated with another that takes into account the suffering patients and their families undergo (**terminal illness**) and with the polymorphous interpretation made by the family and society (**terminal sickness**).

If we consider that the meaning of a word is made up of the set of relations (both situational and paradigmatic) reflected in that word, and that those relations are built all through the history of mankind and each individual's own history, we should understand that it is not possible to provide univocal answers in the case of such an expression as "terminal disease", which carries multiple meanings with it.

The medical description of terminal disease, the suffering patients and their families undergo, and the view society holds are often mutually and internally contradictory. The situation arising out of this is both complex and dynamic, hence the need for a dialogue focused on the suffering endured by the "protosufferers" (patients and next of kin) when it comes to making decisions involving them.

The meaning of terminal disease should ultimately be a single, non-reproducible, contextualized construction, one which embodies the dialectic contribution made by the various agents involved.

The purpose of this paper is to question the pretended univocity of the definition of terminal disease as it is understood from an exclusively unidimensional approach (the medical one), definition which, from a functional point of view, turns out to be a rigid concept that imposes itself over the needs of patients, their families, and even healthcare workers.

It should be borne in mind that the definition of terminal disease is not intended to be solely descriptive, but, as it is later observed, it has a determining functional nature. Based on it, it could be determined whether a particular treatment is futile or not, or if therapeutic

obstinacy or neglect is evidenced, or whether those who are close to the patient (next of kin, caregivers and therapists) are respectful of the patient's dignity.
It could be said that decision-making from a functional perspective frequently fails to overtly specify whether a given disease is terminal or not. However, an in-depth look into the matter reveals that it does so implicitly, in so far as it considers whether the implementation of measures which will unnecessarily prolong life and/or the suffering of patients and their families is unsubstantial or not.
The concept of terminal disease will be discussed all through this paper; however, it is convenient to clarify *ad initio* that, in fact, there are no terminal diseases but terminal patients, and this is precisely the main guiding principle behind this work. Reification of the concept of terminal disease, disregarding the terminal patient, frees many from the burden of disentangling the complex, dynamic nature of each situation in particular and the commitment which that entails.

2. Terminal disease, terminal illness and terminal sickness

2.1 Terminal disease or the medical point of view

The definition of terminal disease is seemingly simple, clear and univocal. The Spanish Society of Palliative Care (Sociedad Española de Cuidados Paliativos [SECPAL, n.d.]), for example, provides the following definition:
"In the case of terminal diseases, a number of elements should be present. These elements are important not only to consider a terminal disease as such but also to determine the most suitable therapy.
The key elements are:
1. *Presence of advanced, progressive, incurable disease.*
2. *Reasonable unresponsiveness to the specific treatment.*
3. *Presence of multiple, changing, severe symptoms or problems of multifactorial origin.*
4. *Great emotional impact on the patient, the family and healthcare workers, closely related to the implicit or explicit immediacy of death.*
5. *Life expectancy of six months or less.*

This complex situation requires the uninterrupted provision of appropriate care and support.
End-stage CANCER, AIDS, motor neuron disease, specific organ system failure (kidney, heart, liver failure, etc.) meet these criteria to a greater or lesser extent. Traditionally, providing adequate care to end-stage cancer patients has been the raison d'etre of Palliative Care.
It is ESSENTIAL not to consider a potentially curable patient as terminally ill."
Some of the controversial aspects of this definition will be discussed below. It is worth pointing out, however, that this definition is not to be rejected entirely. In fact, it could be accepted as a guideline, but not as a dogma that should be asserted over concrete decisions.

2.1.1 How advanced, incurable and progressive a disease should be to be considered terminal

2.1.1.1 Advanced disease and life expectancy

An 84-year-old male patient has a 10-year history of dementia. For the last three years, he has been bedridden, unable to walk, with incontinence of bowel and bladder. His ability to communicate is nearly lost (he occasionally answers "yes" or "no" to questions), he does not react to simple commands, and he rarely recognizes loved ones. He does not present swallowing difficulties but is unable to feed himself (he requires help from a caregiver). Could this patient be considered terminally ill?

In his statement for the Association of Alzheimer Disease, SG Post expresses that *"the advanced stage of dementia includes a loss of all or nearly all ability to communicate by speech, inability to recognize loved ones in most cases, loss of ambulation without assistance, incontinence of bowel and/or bladder, and some weight loss due to swallowing difficulties. The advanced stage is generally considered terminal, with death occurring on average within two years."* (Post, 2007).

The preceding definition extends life expectancy from the maximum of six months, as stated by the Spanish Society of Palliative Care, to an average of two years. This evident inconsistency of criteria shows us that the definition of the concept from the medical perspective is not univocal.

At the age of 42, Stephen Jay Gould, the famous paleontologist, was diagnosed with an abdominal mesothelioma and was informed that the median mortality after discovery was 8 months. In his article "The Median isn't the Message", Gould explains why it is the variance more than the mean, or the median in his case, what should be taken into account to establish a disease prognosis. The reason he gives is that the most common statistical measures of central tendency (either the mean or the median) are useful only to define a Platonic state but not the hard reality of the dispersion of results (Gould, 1985). Gould died at the age of 62.

Defining how advanced a disease is by establishing a period of time which is not only arbitrary but dubious as an estimate seems to be far from functional when it comes to making the kind of decisions we are concerned with. In other words, as it was once expressed by Sir William Osler (Osler, n.d.), *"Medicine is a science of uncertainty and an art of probability"*.

2.1.1.2 Incurable, untreatable and disease-modifying drugs

In medicine, it is well-known that incurable is not synonymous with untreatable. Also, for certain diseases, there are therapies which, without being necessarily palliative, modify disease progression without curing it. In other words, disease progression in a group of subjects receiving a new drug may be statistically better relative to a particular aspect when compared to an untreated group.

The fact that a disease is incurable but its progression may be slowed down creates a grey area between "curable and incurable". Disease-modifying drugs are useful but they do not cure.

Furthermore, certain measures considered therapeutic or even curative in some cultures are not accepted in others. A clear example is the rejection of blood transfusion by Jehovah's Witnesses.

2.1.1.3 Lack of primary injury progression is not synonymous with lack of disease progression

Non-progressive secondary injuries may put a patient at such a risk that, in the event of complications, they may cause his or her death.

Patients with severe sequelae, such as irreversible permanent vegetative state following anoxic or traumatic brain injury, who exhibit no progression of their primary brain injury, may be maintained in that state through intensive care procedures. These procedures are usually implemented to prevent the occurrence of complications or to reverse them if they

occur. Yet, in settings with less sophisticated means, patients are expected to progress towards death. Anencephaly could be mentioned as another example of nonviable disease, possibly comparable to an irreversible vegetative state; it is terminal but it does not meet the progressiveness criteria required in the definition.
In spite of the lack of primary injury progression, there could be modifications which may improve or worsen the clinical condition, thus challenging the univocal definition of the term "progressive disease".
Furthermore, there are dimensions in the progression of a disease which cannot be seen from an exclusively biological perspective, such as the social and psychological impact that failure of recovery has on patients, their families and even the community (and this impact can certainly be progressive). In other words, there may not be an "unfavourable" progression in biological terms but there could be one from a psychological and/or social point of view.

2.1.2 Discussion

While a two-valued logic provides us with safe, clear definitions (advanced vs. not advanced, progressive vs. non-progressive, incurable vs. curable), our patients' individual situations, seen from a medical perspective, challenge us to adhere to a multi-valued, even fuzzy, logic, in which "things are to the extent they are, and things are not to the extent they are not", and in which "nothing exists by itself but in relation to other things".
If we understand that there are no diseases but patients, that there are no absolute, timeless realities but concrete, historical circumstances in which individuals live, get sick and die, the criteria to define a disease as advanced, progressive or incurable vary, and, as we have already mentioned, they need to be specified by medical professionals considering each individual case.

2.2 Terminal illness or the patient's perspective

Recently published news articles in Argentina (Carbajal, 2011a, 2011b, 2011c, 2011d, 2011d), described the situation of a 19-year-old girl (MG) who had been diagnosed with neurofibromatosis type I (Von Recklinghausen disease). The girl considered she had an "advanced" form of the disease. She was bedridden and had severe shortness of breath; however, she was in full possession of her mental faculties. "*It is not fair to live like this. Nearly all of my body is numb, and whatever I feel is painful. I can't even hold a cup in my hand, and I'm forced to lie down all the time. I choke, I can't breathe. This is not a life worth living; I don't want to go on like this. But they don't understand, they think one can always pull through. But I can't bear it any longer, I simply can't*", one of the articles transcribed. Despite her medical condition, MG was lucid and was very clear when expressing her position. Physicians considered that hers was not a terminal disease; nonetheless, the patient wanted to be given sedatives to induce unconsciousness and stop feeling pain.
The case became known to the public. Melina, that was her name, was apparently sedated in the end, and died a few days after the media published her case (Carbajal, 2011e, 2011f).
Ramón Sampedro was a patient who was not considered terminal from a medical point of view. He was quadriplegic due to a traumatic cervical spine injury, and was bedridden for more than 30 years as a consequence of this. In his "Letters from Hell", where he claimed to be living in, he expressed (Sampedro, 2004), (translation is mine):
"To no avail, I say to them: No!, I am dead!,

I tell them I can't speak like them
Because it is absurd to speak as human beings do
And they don't let me be, either dead or alive
These crazy, freaked-out nuts"

A different situation is that of Stephen Hawking's, who could find his purpose in life despite having a progressive disease and being severely disabled. Yet, no comparison between these two patients' moral values is intended, this last example has been introduced to show that personal experiences with a particular medical condition vary greatly.

In his 1845 short story, "The Facts in the Case of Mr. Valdemar" (Poe, 1845), Edgar Allan Poe presents a visionary metaphor of today's intensive care units with their intervened deaths which is worth commenting on. Mr. Valdemar, who is *"in articulo mortis"*, accepts to undergo an experimental hypnotic technique and he is suspended between life and death for a period of seven months. During that time, he is not allowed to die but he cannot be awakened either. The objective of the investigator carrying out the experiment is to find out up to what extent or for how long, the hypnotic process would be able to prevent death from occurring. During the 7-month experiment, Mr. Valdemar is visited by physicians and friends and receives continuous nursing care. All through this process, however, Mr. P (the mesmerist) is unable to make decisions. It is Mr. Valdermar himself who, given the investigator's inability, begs: *"For God´s sake! -quick!-quick!–put me to sleep-or, quick!– waken me!–quick!–I say to you that I am dead."*.

In light of a helpless but grandiose medicine, which does not allow either to live or to die, it is the undead who demands changing the status quo.

JV, a 38-year old male patient who suffered from amyotrophic lateral sclerosis, was fully aware of his disease and its prognosis. Percutaneous gastrostomy for enteral feeding was suggested when he was still able to undergo the procedure, but he rejected it. He also expressly refused in writing to receive invasive or non-invasive ventilatory support of any kind. He was later hospitalized due to an infectious complication. At that moment, he was unable to express himself orally (he communicated what he wanted to say by pointing at letters on a sign with his right index finger). To our surprise, when his wife asked him whether he still rejected ventilatory support, despite not being dyspneic at that time, he reproached her for such a question because it seemed to suggest she wanted him to die. Then, he indicated that he obviously wanted to be provided with ventilatory support if it was required. A few days later, it was necessary to implement the support. The patient survived 4 months in the intensive care unit and finally died.

In 2008, the case of a 13-year-old girl named Hannah Jones became known to the public. She had previously suffered from leukemia and refused to have a heart transplant to treat a chemotherapy-induced cardiomyopathy (BBC News, 2008). Her attending physicians sought court intervention to force her to undergo surgery. The media informed that physicians recommended the transplant as the only solution available, but they could not guarantee survival after the surgery. And, if she survived, her leukemia could relapse and her new heart would last ten years at the most. Hannah decided that she had suffered long enough and told her physicians that she preferred to spend the rest of her life without having to go through another traumatic treatment. Her parents were supportive of her decision, but the hospital where she was being treated in Herefordshire interfered with Hannah's decision. Physicians warned Hannah's mother, Kirsty (a nurse), that they would apply for a court order at the High Court in London to remove the child's custody from them. The following day a child protection officer visited Hannah at home. Nobody knows what Hannah said to the officer, but, a few hours later, the Hospital Legal Department withdrew the legal action. *"The girl is firm in her decision to refuse surgery"*, said the child protection officer. *"It is incredible that such a young person who has gone through so many things has the courage to defend her rights"*, her father Andrew proudly said.

Hannah did not have what in medical terms would be considered a terminal disease; however, she made the decision to refuse the suggested treatments with apparent autonomy and competence. She had already decided that her illness was terminal. She could have been wrong, but so could have been her physicians thus prolonging her suffering.

Dr Tony Calland, chairman of the British Medical Association's ethics committee, is quoted in the same BBC News article: *"a child of Hannah's age was able to make an informed decision to refuse treatment". Dr Calland said he understood why a doctor might have taken this action. He said: "I think some doctors take the view that they must intervene and they are making that decision in what they see as the best interests of the patient. But of course best interests of patients is not just the best medical interests - it's the overall holistic interests of the person in general." He added: "I think obviously a child of 13 with these circumstances should be perfectly capable of making the decision and particularly when supported by the parents."*.

In the city of Mar del Plata, Argentina, a patient was admitted to the General Acute Care Hospital (Hospital Interzonal de Agudos) with a history of diabetes and gangrene in the right foot. Above-knee leg amputation was performed on August 9, 1995 after obtaining consent from the patient (he had denied consent previously). On August 16, 1995 he was diagnosed with necrosis of the left first and fourth toes, cellulitis and edema involving the entire foot were also observed. On August 23, 1995 he was diagnosed with vascular ischemia of the left lower limb. Below-knee amputation was indicated, but the patient refused to undergo this procedure. The following was documented with respect to his refusal: *"The patient refuses to receive treatment, his decision being entered into his medical record. Considering that the patient is lucid, we deem it advisable to notify the Direction in the event of a legal issue."*. The patient was perfectly lucid and fully aware that he was putting his life at risk. The Hospital Ethics Committee stated that patient autonomy should be respected. However, court intervention was sought, and the judgment was granted in favour of the patient and his decision (Hooft, 1995).

As we have already mentioned, a typical example in which the concept of "terminality" differs between patients and physicians is that of Jehovah's Witnesses. A Jehovah's Witness patient who presents with hemorrhage caused by a treatable condition prefers to refuse blood transfusion and die rather than violate his or her religious beliefs for a treatment not considered as such.

Autonomous and competent patients who refuse a particular treatment and put their lives at risk when making such a decision provide their own concept of "terminality", different from their physicians' concept.

The poet (Victor Jara) expresses *"life is eternal in five minutes"*. A few days or hours stolen from death may be enough for some patients to reconcile with their loved ones or to say goodbye to them. Conversely, a few minutes or hours, or sometimes months or years, may be tormentous for other patients because of the physical, mental and/or moral suffering they have to endure during that time. Those who find meaning in the agony of the last moments of life are no better than those who no longer find a reason to go on living.

2.2.1 Discussion

In any case, patients themselves are the ones who have to endure suffering. Our role as family members, friends and healthcare providers is to cooperate with them in the construction of their own meaning of life and death, as long as they allow us to do so.

2.3 Terminal sickness or the perspective of the family, caregivers, next of kin, society and the state

There is a large number of well-known cases published in the medical literature or by the media in which patients and/or their families have spent long years in distress struggling to have an illness recognized as terminal in order to allow the sufferer to die with dignity and loved ones to mourn their loss.

The hegemonic line of thought, however, considers death as a failure that should be delayed as long as possible. Sufferers (patients and/or their families) are thus severed from the decision-making process, and medicine, the courts and religious institutions are allowed to exercise their power over other people's bodies even if, after a long pilgrimage, sufferers are granted what they have asked for.

We have already commented on situations in which patients refused treatments which they considered futile or required measures to be taken so that they could die with dignity. We also examined the case of a patient who, having an illness which his physicians considered had reached its end-stage, first refused and then asked for support measures.

Greater is the complexity of the cases in which patients are unable to express themselves and it is their family who ask for withdrawal of life-sustaining measures in the absence of the patients' explicit statement of their will to do so.

Patients in an irreversible permanent vegetative state are not considered terminally ill in the applicable definitions. Due to their brain injury, these patients have neither self-awareness nor awareness of the surroundings. They do not feel pain but they are able to breathe autonomously. They may have some reflex activity, including eye movements, grimacing and grunting. They are unable to take food or fluids by mouth and they require tube feeding for nutrition and hydration. The sleep-wake cycle is preserved and, if they are provided with adequate care, they do not look critically ill at first sight. A distinction should be made, however, between the irreversible permanent vegetative state and the potentially reversible persistent vegetative state. After coming out of a coma due to brain injury, a patient progresses to a vegetative state if sufficient sparing of the brain stem allows for preservation of his or her autonomic functions. Recovery from a vegetative state is unlikely after three months if brain damage is anoxic or a year if brain damage is traumatic; in those cases, the vegetative state is said to be permanent. "Vegetative" does not mean that the patient is a vegetable but that the so-called vegetative functions are preserved (breathing, heart rate, body temperature control, blood pressure, gastrointestinal motility, etc.) (The Multi-Society Task Force on PVS, 1994a, 1994b). The vegetative state must be distinguished from the minimally conscious state, in which the patient shows minimal self-awareness and awareness of the surroundings.

Our purpose is to show that these medical conditions are seen from different perspectives by families, physicians, the courts and society at large. Some of them consider that these patients are terminally ill and that they are being subjected to futile treatments, whereas others see them as living patients who are comparable to other disabled individuals and whose life should be sustained regardless of their families' wish or the wish they may have expressed when they were competent.

In 1975, 21-year-old Karen Ann Quinlan suffered a cardiopulmonary arrest after ingesting a combination of alcohol and tranquilizers. She subsequently went into a permanent vegetative state and was placed on mechanical ventilatory support. Hers was the first case in which parents requested withdrawal of the ventilator. Physicians turned down the request, so Mr. and Mrs. Quinlan resorted to the courts. New Jersey Supreme Court authorized the family's request relying on the substituted judgment standard, which is intended first to determine the individual's own needs and wishes and then to decide on how to proceed once his or her personal value system is known. In Quinlan's case, the court sought to protect the autonomy of an individual who was unable to defend it on her own by honouring her parent's opinion (Beauchamp, Childress, 1999). Additionally, as Annas clearly recalls: *"Since the court believed that the physicians were unwilling to withdraw the ventilator because of the fear of legal liability, not precepts of medical ethics, it devised a mechanism to grant the physicians prospective legal immunity for taking this action. Specifically, the New Jersey Supreme Court ruled that after a prognosis, confirmed by a hospital ethics committee, that there is "no reasonable possibility of a patient returning to a cognitive, sapient state," life-sustaining treatment can be removed and no one involved, including the physicians, can be held civilly or criminally responsible for the death."* (Annas, 2005).

Once ventilatory support was withdrawn, Karen continued breathing on her own and lived for another 9 years (10 years since she had suffered the cardiopulmonary arrest) still sustained by tube feeding. Her parents did not consider requesting discontinuation of artificial feeding (Kinney et al, 1994), which could mean that Karen's parents considered that the need for ventilatory support indicated that her condition was terminal, while the other life-sustaining measures placed her in a different situation.

Nancy Cruzan's case provides us with another context. Nancy was in a permanent vegetative state as a result of a car accident she had had in 1983 (Annas, 1990). She required tube feeding but not ventilatory support. When her parents were certain that she would not recover, they requested discontinuation of the treatment stating that this was Nancy's desire as expressed by her in the past. Physicians did not accept treatment withdrawal, but the trial court authorized it. On appeal, the Supreme Court of Missouri reversed the trial court judgment and so did the U.S. Supreme Court (it was the first time that the U.S. Supreme Court had heard a case like this). Among the reasons provided, it was stated that even though a patient had the right to refuse treatment, the same decision made by surrogates on behalf of a previously competent patient could not be accepted. It was also expressed that the State should in principle favour the preservation of life and that the patient's decision as to the withdrawal of treatment should be practically indubitable (halfway between what society considers in that situation and what the law considers beyond any reasonable doubt). This last requirement limited the decision-making capacity of Nancy's parents, who loved her beyond doubt.

A new petition was submitted to the Supreme Court of Missouri, and the court rejected it again stating that there was no clear and convincing evidence that Nancy would have refused tube feeding had she been alive. It was also added that artificial nutrition and hydration were considered ordinary treatment procedures which should be provided under any circumstances, and that the State's interest in preserving life was absolute and unconditional. The State Court also expressed that although the patient is in an irreversible vegetative state, ***"She is not dead. She is not terminally ill. Medical experts testified that she could live another***

thirty years"[2] (Cruzan vs. Hamon, 1989). The U.S. Supreme Court, in turn, pointed out that tube feeding was **an extraordinary treatment procedure which could be discontinued** and that if there was enough evidence of the patient's wishes, artificial feeding could be removed. It also expressed that even though the State of Missouri should set the standard to discern what the patient's wishes were, it did not have the absolute right to deny refusal of treatment. In light of new evidence provided by Nancy's friends and acquaintances with respect to what her wishes would have been in her situation, the Court of Missouri authorized the removal of artificial nutrition and hydration. The treatment was discontinued on December 15, 1990 and Nancy died 12 days later (Cruzan vs. Director, 1990).

Although the definition of terminal disease was not the main discussion in this case, as seen above, it is explicitly mentioned by the Supreme Court of Missouri: ***"She is not terminally ill"***.

Dissenting opinions as regards Nancy's state were expressed by the U.S. Supreme Court Justices and the President of the Supreme Court of Missouri, which are worth transcribing (Cruzan vs. Director, 1990).

Justice Brennan from the U.S. Supreme Court, with whom Justices Marshal and Blackmun joined, expressed the following (bold emphasis is mine):

"*Medical technology has effectively created a* ***twilight zone of suspended animation where death commences while life****, in some form, continues. Some patients, however, want no part of a life sustained only by medical technology. Instead, they prefer a plan of medical treatment that allows nature to take its course and permits them to die with dignity.*"

"Nancy Cruzan has dwelt in that twilight zone for six years... The Court would make an exception here. It permits the State's abstract, undifferentiated interest in the preservation of life to overwhelm the best interests of Nancy Beth Cruzan, interests which would, according to an undisputed finding, be served by allowing ***her guardians to exercise her constitutional right to discontinue medical treatment****. Ironically, the Court reaches this conclusion despite endorsing three significant propositions which should save it from any such dilemma. First, a competent individual's decision to refuse life-sustaining medical procedures is an aspect of liberty protected by the Due Process Clause of the Fourteenth Amendment.* ***Second, upon a proper evidentiary showing, a qualified guardian may make that decision on behalf of an incompetent ward****. Third, in answering the important question presented by this tragic case, it is wise "'not to attempt, by any general statement, to cover every possible phase of the subject.'". Together, these considerations suggest that Nancy Cruzan's liberty to be free from medical treatment must be understood in light of the facts and circumstances particular to her. A grown woman at the time of the accident, Nancy had previously expressed her wish to forgo continuing medical care under circumstances such as these. Her family and her friends are convinced that this is what she would want. A guardian ad litem appointed by the trial court is also convinced that this is what Nancy would want. Yet the Missouri Supreme Court, alone among state courts deciding such a question, has determined that an irreversibly vegetative patient will remain a passive prisoner of medical technology -- for Nancy, perhaps for the next 30 years."*

Justice Stevens, in turn, extensively quotes Judge Blackmar from the Supreme Court of Missouri who explained that decisions about the care of chronically ill patients were traditionally private: "*I would not accept the assumption, inherent in the principal opinion, that, with our advanced technology, the state must necessarily become involved in a decision* ***about using extraordinary measures to prolong life. Decisions of this kind are made daily by the patient***

[2] Hereinafter bold emphasis is mine.

or relatives, on the basis of medical advice and their conclusion as to what is best. Very few cases reach court, and I doubt whether this case would be before us but for the fact that Nancy lies in a state hospital. *I do not place primary emphasis on the patient's expressions, except possibly in the very unusual case, of which I find no example in the books, in which the patient expresses a view that all available life supports should be made use of. Those closest to the patient are best positioned to make judgments about the patient's best interest."*

"Judge Blackmar then argued that Missouri's policy imposed upon ***dying individuals*** *and their families a controversial and objectionable view of life's meaning: "****It is unrealistic to say that the preservation of life is an absolute, without regard to the quality of life.*** *I make this statement only in the context of a case in which the trial judge has found that there is no chance for amelioration of Nancy's condition. The principal opinion accepts this conclusion.* ***It is appropriate to consider the quality of life in making decisions about the extraordinary medical treatment.*** *Those who have made decisions about such matters without resort to the courts certainly consider the quality of life, and balance this against the unpleasant consequences to the patient. There is evidence that Nancy may react to pain stimuli. If she has any awareness of her surroundings, her life must be a living hell. She is unable to express herself or to do anything at all to alter her situation.* ***Her parents, who are her closest relatives, are best able to feel for her and to decide what is best for her. The state should not substitute its decisions for theirs. Nor am I impressed with the crypto-philosophers cited in the principal opinion, who declaim about the sanctity of any life without regard to its quality.*** *They dwell in ivory towers.""*

"Finally, Judge Blackmar concluded that the Missouri policy was illegitimate because it treats life as a theoretical abstraction, severed from, and indeed opposed to, the person of Nancy Cruzan, adding that "the Cruzan family appropriately came before the court seeking relief. The circuit judge properly found the facts and applied the law. His factual findings are supported by the record and his legal conclusions by overwhelming weight of authority. The principal opinion attempts to establish absolutes, but does so at the expense of human factors. In so doing it unnecessarily subjects Nancy and those close to her to continuous torture which no family should be forced to endure."

Justice Stevens, in turn, pointed out that *"It is perhaps predictable that courts might undervalue the liberty at stake here. Because death is so profoundly personal, public reflection upon it is unusual. As this sad case shows, however, such reflection must become more common if we are to deal responsibly with the modern circumstances of death.* ***Medical advances have altered the physiological conditions of death in ways that may be alarming: Highly invasive treatment may perpetuate human existence through a merger of body and machine that some might reasonably regard as an insult to life rather than as its continuation. But those same advances, and the reorganization of medical care accompanying the new science and technology, have also transformed the political and social conditions of death: People are less likely to die at home, and more likely to die in relatively public places, such as hospitals or nursing homes(…).*** *The trial court's order authorizing Nancy's parents to cease their daughter's treatment would have permitted the family that cares for Nancy to bring to a close her tragedy and her death. Missouri's objection to that order subordinates Nancy's body, her family, and the lasting significance of her life to the State's own interests. The decision we review thereby interferes with constitutional interests of the highest order(...).It seems to me that the Court errs insofar as it characterizes this case as involving "judgments about the 'quality' of life that a particular individual may enjoy. "* ***Nancy Cruzan is obviously "alive" in a physiological sense. But for patients like Nancy Cruzan, who have no consciousness and no chance of recovery, there is a serious question as to whether the mere persistence of their bodies is "life" as that word is commonly understood, or as it is used in both the Constitution and the Declaration***

of Independence. The State's unflagging determination to perpetuate Nancy Cruzan's physical existence is comprehensible only as an effort to define life's meaning, not as an attempt to preserve its sanctity(...)."

In their words, these judges forestall several of the theses put forward in this document: the irreducibility of life to its mere biological nature, the need to consider such aspects as quality of life, the ability to stop the progression of a severe medical disease through technology (a disease which would be otherwise terminal) but, at the same time, the inability to reverse the condition, the fact that these cases are usually settled in a different way when decision-making occurs within the family circle (Nancy's case reached the U.S. Supreme Court because she was hospitalized in a state hospital).

A very different case (the reverse of the preceding one) is that of Helga Wanglie, an 86-year-old patient who died after being in a vegetative state for more than a year (Miles, 1991). At the age of 85, she was hospitalized with symptoms of shortness of breath caused by chronic bronchiectasis. She required emergency intubation. During hospitalization, she acknowledged discomfort and occasionally recognized her family. Five months later, she was referred to a chronic care facility after several unsuccessful attempts to withdraw ventilatory support. A week later, she experienced a cardiopulmonary arrest, from which she was successfully resuscitated. She was then transferred to an intensive care unit, where she was diagnosed with hypoxic-ischemic encephalopathy. Physicians suggested removing the ventilator first a month and then two months after diagnosis. They did not believe that ventilatory support would benefit the patient in any way. The family, however, rejected this suggestion saying that doctors should not play God and that Helga would not be better off dead. They also added that she had not expressed any decisions with respect to such a situation. Ten months after her first admission and five months after the cardiopulmonary arrest, Helga was still unconscious and supported by a ventilator. A medical consultant whose opinion was requested at that time considered that the patient was at the end of her life, and that mechanical ventilation was not beneficial for the patient, that it would not cure her lung condition and that she would not survive without it. However, because ventilation could prolong life, it could not be considered futile. The conflict between the family and the hospital, which held that it was not obliged to provide non-beneficial medical treatment, was finally taken to court. It was first determined that the hospital had no financial interesting in withdrawing treatment since expenses were covered by Medicare for the first hospitalization and by a private insurance for the second one. The trial court also appointed the patient's husband as the person who could best represent her interests. In the light of uncertainty about its legal obligation, the hospital decided to continue providing the treatment. However, Mrs. Wanglie died of septicemia three days after the court ruling.

The debate that followed was largely focused on discussing that while there is general agreement that patients may refuse treatment, it is arguable whether they or their families have the right to claim for any kind of medical treatment, regardless of its efficacy, additionally bringing up the issue of fair distribution of healthcare resources into the discussion.

What was interesting about the court decision was that it asserted the family's right to make decisions on behalf of an incompetent patient (Angell, 1991). However, it did not bring into consideration the discussion about the contents of their decision and its eventual futility.

From the physicians' point of view, Helga was terminally ill. The family, however, did not seem to consider the concept of terminality as a point of discussion. What mattered to them was that the patient was alive and that her state was better than being dead.

"For the first time in the history of the United States, Congress met in a special emergency session on Sunday, March 20, to pass legislation aimed at the medical care of one patient – Terri Schiavo. President George W. Bush encouraged the legislation and flew back to Washington, D.C., from his vacation in Crawford, Texas, so that he could be on hand to sign it immediately. In a statement issued three days earlier, he said: "The case of Terri Schiavo raises complex issues(. . . . Those who live at the mercy of others deserve our special care and concern. It should be our goal as a nation to build a culture of life, where all Americans are valued, welcomed, and protected – and that culture of life must extend to individuals with disabilities." (Annas, 2005) This is how Annas describes the shock produced by the decision of the courts of Florida to authorize withdrawal of artificial nutrition and hydration from Terri Schiavo, a patient who was in a permanent vegetative state.

In 1990, when she was 27 years-old, Terri had a cardiac arrest, which was probably caused by hypokalemia induced by an eating disorder. She progressed to a permanent vegetative state due to the resulting hypoxic-ischemic encephalopathy and she required tube feeding placement. Eight years later, her husband requested legal authorization to discontinue tube feeding. A judge found that there was clear and convincing evidence that Terri was in a permanent vegetative state and that had she been able to decide on her own, she would have chosen to discontinue the treatment. The Appellate Court affirmed the judgment and the Supreme Court of Florida declined to review it. The situation was somehow similar to that after the final decision in Nancy Cruzan's case.

However, the case became more complex and sparked nationwide debate and international attraction when Terri's parents claimed that there was evidence of treatment which would help her recover from her condition. This claim was refuted by three of the five experts asked to examine the patient (two appointed by Terri's husband, two by her parents and one by the trial court judge). The Supreme Court of Florida refused to hear an appeal again on the grounds that the parents had no standing to bring it. The State Legislature, in turn, passed a bill which gave Governor Jeb Bush the authority to order the reinsertion of the feeding tube (it had been removed after the court decision), which was reinserted as ordered. The Supreme Court of Florida declared that the law was unconstitutional and the U.S. Supreme Court refused to hear an appeal brought by the Governor. The trial court judge finally ordered the tube to be withdrawn on March 18, at 1 p.m.

Amidst death threats against one of the judges, and after another unsuccessful attempt by the Florida Legislature to pass a new bill aimed at restoring Terri's tube feeding, the U.S. Congress met in an emergency session, interrupting their Easter recess, in order to pass a bill which would allow Terri's parents to bring an appeal. In spite of this, Terri's parents could not modify the court decision and Terri finally died on March 25, 2005.

In this particular case, the concept of terminal disease was not openly discussed. However, it could be said that it was implicitly present in more than one aspect of the debate. The possibility of maintaining a patient in a permanent vegetative state, "suspended" for an indefinite period of time as opposed to an advanced cancer patient, led some people to consider Terri as a terminally ill patient whose life was being artificially sustained, while others believed that she was not actually terminally ill. In the first case, tube feeding was considered futile, a measure which undermined the patient's dignity and whose withdrawal would allow for her condition to follow its natural course; in other words, it would allow the patient to die. In the second case, the treatment was deemed vital since its discontinuation would lead to the patient's death (she would be killed instead of being allowed to die). Those who argued for the withdrawal believed that the patient's wishes, or the wishes of those who represented her interests, would be violated if treatment was withheld; while those who opposed discontinuation considered treatment withdrawal as an offense against life.

In the debate held in the U.S. House of Representatives, several of its members showed crass ignorance of what an irreversible vegetative state is. Furthermore, some members who are also physicians offered their opinions about Terri's condition without conducting their own examinations (Quill, 2005).

The media, in turn, showed people, some of them were children, trying to bring Terri a glass of water, claiming that she was being starved to death and dehydrated (this shows that most people ignored the patient's real condition – she was unable to swallow and feel hunger or thirst).

A similar case was debated in Argentina, though it did not have the same impact as Terri's case in the United States. A female patient (MdelC) had been in a permanent vegetative state under her husband's care for two years. She progressed to that state after suffering heart failure when giving birth to her fourth child (all the children were under the father's care after that tragic event). In 2000, the patient's husband (AMG) petitioned the court for withdrawal of tube feeding, but her parents objected to the request.

In his critical review of the decision adopted by the courts of the Province of Buenos Aires (Argentina) with regard to this case, Dr. Carlos Gherardi clearly shows how ignorance and prejudice may lead to unfounded decisions (Gherardi, 2007). It is worth quoting what he wrote in the introduction to his review: *"We should start by transcribing the description of the patient provided by the Counsel for Minors and Incompetent Persons, which was repeatedly quoted in the relevant judgments: "I was really surprised because I did not find what I had expected. Based on the diagnosis, I thought I would find a physically impaired person, who would be completely unable to move, asleep, dishevelled, and connected to a mechanical respirator and machines controlling her heart rate, but the truth is that I found a woman with a very good physical appearance. She was breathing on her own and there were no machines controlling her. She only has a feeding tube which provides her with nutrition and hydration. I was really shocked to see her blink, she looked towards different places, she coughed and moved when doing so, and she made some facial gestures." The Counsel requested the petition to be dismissed "in limine" on the grounds of the defense of the right to life and because he considered that if the petition were sustained, it would eventually constitute neglect followed by death or aggravated homicide. In his argumentation, the Counsel makes reference to the Creator and the Parable of the Talents. He concludes that: "the hope for a Miracle should never be abandoned. Love and faith will always dwell in a heroic heart. And, waiting for God's time, which we know is different from man's time, is an act of heroism.".*

This unusual account, made by the only court officer who actually saw the patient, seems to be referring to an individual in a nearly normal condition when, in fact, the patient is a person who has tragically and irreversible lost all cognitive activity, and who does not exhibit the essential communicative skills and affective expression inherent to a person's identity. It is quite clear that this account had an impact on the judges and that it was considered reliable by them, since it was frequently quoted by the Court Attorney and some of the judges when providing the reasons for their votes. The probably erroneous perception of those who had to decide on such a complex and debatable issue may have been enhanced by the fact that none of them actually saw the patient and that they did not take into account the evidence provided by the various witnesses (family members, professionals, priests). Even though there was no procedural obligation, nothing prevented the judges from hearing the witnesses' statements, which would have contributed to their knowledge of the case. It is hard to believe that none of the judges felt the moral obligation to see the patient or meet her husband and children to evaluate the situation of the family."

Dr. Gherardi adds that *"the patient's husband expressed that he did not know what her preferences were with respect to life-sustaining measures. However, two people who were close to the patient, one of them was a psychologist, stated that the patient had previously told them that if she had been in such a condition, she would not have wished to be kept alive. These statements were not taken into account by the judges and they were not accepted as witnesses, and neither were others who offered their testimony."*.

The courts not only rejected the evidence provided by a psychologist and one of the patient's friends about her preferences, but it also based its considerations on an erroneous interpretation of the purpose of medicine ("to defend life at all costs"), the patient's medical condition, the situation the family was going through, and the suffering endured by those who took care of the patient, especially her husband. One of the judges (who never actually saw the patient) reveals an absolute lack of respect for the patient and her caregivers when he appeals to a possible miracle and calls for heroism while waiting for God's time. Should not therapeutic obstinacy be considered as an example of man's challenge to God's time?

Regardless of technological advances and the development of new goals, just as before, today's medicine will seldom cure, will often provide relief and will always have to comfort. It is not its objective to defeat death, because human beings are doomed to die. It should try to avoid early death but it should also allow patients to die in peace. And, it should not defend life at all costs since, in doing so, it would fall into such a negative value as therapeutic obstinacy. Allowing a dying person to die is not the same as killing him or her. By showing respect for a dignified death, we are also dignifying life. We dignify others when we consider them as persons, when we respect them, listen to them, watch them, talk to them. In the abovementioned case, regardless of the adopted decision, the judges showed a clear lack of respect for the patient's dignity in their failure to see or listen. With their behaviour, they ultimately showed the opposite side of therapeutic obstinacy: neglect.

3. Conclusion

We usually define "terminal disease" as a pathological condition that cannot be cured and, in spite of the treatments applied, it will end up in the death of the patient in a short period of time, i.e. 6 months. We consider that this definition is unilateral (made up by physicians). We propose that the real meaning should come up as a construction based on the dialogue between patients, their families, caregivers and healthcare workers. In addition, this process should be developed by incorporating the cultural concepts of the society in which each individual lives. The aim of this construction is to show that the meaning of "terminal disease" is not unique but multidimensional, since it can change depending on the circumstances.

4. Acknowledgement

The author would like to express his gratitude to the Ethics Comitte of the Hospital Privado de Comunidad de Mar del Plata (Private Hospital of the Community of Mar del Plata) for letting me be a member of it, to Dr Jorge Manzini for his teachings and his critical review of the manuscript, and to Anna Banchik for her providing me part of the bibliography. This work was financially supported by the Fundación Médica Mar del Plata (Mar del Plata Medical Foundation).

5. References

Angell, M. (1991). The case of Helga Wanglie. A new kind of "right to die" case. *N Engl J Med.*, Vol.325, No.7, (August 1991), pp 511-2, ISSN 0028-4793

Annas, GJ. (1990). Nancy Cruzan and the right to die. *N Engl J Med.*, Vol.323, No.10, (September 1990), pp. 670-673, ISSN 0028-4793

Annas, GJ. (2005). "Culture of life" politics at the bedside--the case of Terri Schiavo. *N Engl J Med.* Vol.352, No.16, (April 2005), pp. 1710-1715, ISSN 0028-4793

BBC News. (2008) Girl wins right to refuse heart (11 November 2008). Available from http://news.bbc.co.uk/2/hi/uk_news/england/hereford/worcs/7721231.stm (accessed 05 March 2011)

Beauchamp, TL. & Childress, JF. (1999). *Principios de Ética Médica*, Masson, S.A., ISBN 84-458-0480-4, Barcelona, Spain

Callahan, D. et al. (1996) The goals of medicine. Setting new priorities. *Hastings Cent Rep.*, Vol.26, No.6, (November-December 1996), pp.S1-27,1996. ISSN 0093-0334

Carbajal, M. (2011a). Pagina 12. La niña que pelea por una muerte digna. Edition 19 february 2011. Available from http://www.pagina12.com.ar/diario/sociedad/3-162653-2011-02-19.html (accessed 8 March de 2011)

Carbajal, M. (2011b).Pagina 12 El dictamen del Comité de bioética. Edition 28 february 2011. Available from http://www.pagina12.com.ar/diario/elpais/subnotas/163187-52260-2011-02-28.html (accessed 8 March de 2011)

Carbajal, M. (2011c).Pagina 12 Quiero transitar lo último que me queda en paz. Edition 28 february 2011 Available from http://www.pagina12.com.ar/diario/elpais/1-163187-2011-02-28.html (accessed 8 March 2011)

Carbajal, M. (2011d).Pagina 12. Una visión desde la bioética. Edition 28 february 2011. Available from http://www.pagina12.com.ar/diario/elpais/subnotas/163187-52259-2011-02-28.html (accessed 8 March de 2011)

Carbajal, M. (2011e).Pagina 12 La chica que peleó por una muerte digna. Edition 2 march 2011. Available from http://www.pagina12.com.ar/diario/sociedad/3-163303-2011-03- 02.html (accessed 8 March de 2011)

Carbajal, M. (2011f).Pagina 12 La espera de Melina. Edition 2 march 2011. Available from http://www.pagina12.com.ar/diario/sociedad/subnotas/163303-52292-2011-03-02.html (accessed 8 March 2011)

Cruzan v. Harmon (1989), 760 S.W.2d 408, 411 (Mo. 1989) in Cruzan, By Her Parents And Co-Guardians V. Director, Missouri Department Of Health Supreme Court Of The United States 497 U.S. 261 June 25, 1990, Decided. Available from http://law2.umkc.edu/faculty/projects/ftrials/conlaw/cruzan.html (accessed 19 March 2011)

Cruzan, By Her Parents And Co-Guardians V. Director (1990), Missouri Department Of Health Supreme Court Of The United States 497 U.S. 261 June 25, 1990, Decided. Available from http://law2.umkc.edu/faculty/projects/ftrials/conlaw/cruzan.html (accessed 19 March 2011)

Eisenberg, L. (1977). Disease and illness. Distinctions between professional and popular ideas of sickness. *Cult Med Psychiatry*. Vol.1, No.1, (April 1977), pp. 9-23, ISSN (electronic): 1573-076X

Gherardi, CR. (2007) *La Ley* Actualidad . Vol. LXXI, No.245, (December 2007), pp. 1-3, ISSN 0036-1636

Gould, S. (1985) The Median isn´t the Message. Available from http://www.phoenix5.org/articles/GouldMessage.html (accessed 27 march 2011)

Hooft, P. (1995). Juzgado de Primera Instancia en lo Criminal y Correccional N° 3, Mar del Plata, setiembre 18 de 1995.-"Dirección del Hospital Interzonal General de Agudos (HIGA) de Mar del Plata s/ Presentación" (firme), In: Cuestiones bioéticas en torno a la muerte, T Zamudio (Ed), *Cuadernos de Bioética*. Ed. Ad Hoc. ISSN 0328-8390. Buenos Aires, Argentina. Available from http://www.muerte.bioetica.org/juris/fallos5.htm (accessed 08 November 2009)

Kinney, HC.; Korein, J.; Panigrahy, A.; Dikkes, P. & Goode, R. (1994) Neuropathological findings in the brain of Karen Ann Quinlan. The role of the thalamus in the persistent vegetative state. *N Engl J Med.*, Vol.330, No.21, (May 1994), pp. 1469-1475, ISSN 0028-4793

Miles SH. (1991). Informed demand for "non-beneficial" medical treatment. *N Engl J Med.*, Vol.325, No.7, (August 1991), pp. 512-515, ISSN 0028-4793

More, T. (1516) "*Utopia*". Transcribed from the 1901 Cassell & Company Edition by David Price, Project Gutenberg Ebook Utopia Available from http://www.gutenberg.org/files/2130/2130-h/2130-h.htm (accessed 27 March 2011)

Osler, W. (n.d.). Available from http://en.wikiquote.org/wiki/William_Osler (accessed 27 March 2011)

Poe, EA. (1845). The Facts in the Case of M. Valdemar. From *The Works Of Edgar Allan Poe*, Vol. II A.C. Armstrong & Son, New York, 1884. Available from http://www.taalfilosofie.nl/bestanden/bar_analyse_valdemar_eng_poe_tekst.pdf (accessed 27 March 2011)

Post, SG. (2007), The Aging Society And The Expansion Of Senility: Biotechnological And Treatment Goals, In: *The Oxford Handbook of Bioethics*, B.P. Steinbock (Ed), 304-323, Oxford University Press Inc, ISBN 978-0-19-927335-5, New York, USA

Quill, TE. (2005). Terri Schiavo--a tragedy compounded. *N Engl J Med.*, Vol.352, No.16, (April 2005), pp. 1630-1633, ISSN 0028-4793

Sampedro Ramón (2004). *Cartas desde el Infierno*. Editorial Planeta, S.A, ISBN: 9788408056324, Barcelona, Spain

SECPAL (n.d.) *Guía de Cuidados Paliativos*. Available http://www.secpal.com/guiacp/index.php?acc=dos (accessed 6 March 2011)

The Multi-Society Task Force on PVS. (1994a) Medical aspects of the persistent vegetative state (1). *N Engl J Med.*, Vol.330, No.21, (May 1994), pp. 1499-1508, ISSN 0028-4793

The Multi-Society Task Force on PVS. (1994b) Medical aspects of the persistent vegetative state (2). *N Engl J Med.*, Vol.330, No.22, (June 1994), pp. 1572-1579, ISSN 0028-4793

Young, A. (1982) The Anthropologies of Illness and Sickness. *Annual Review of Anthropology,* Vol.11, (1982), pp. 257-285, ISSN: 0084-6570

6

Tolerance to Tick-Borne Diseases in Sheep: Highlights of a Twenty-Year Experience in a Mediterranean Environment

Elisa Pieragostini, Elena Ciani,
Giuseppe Rubino and Ferruccio Petazzi
University of Bari
Italy

1. Introduction

The European landscape is characterised by a range of diverse farming systems. These relate not only to varied geographical environments and animal genetic resources, but also to different social and cultural contexts for farming and food production. This diversity is unique to Europe and, among the European countries, Italy is the home for a great variety of native breeds because of its complex orography and its long boot shape with very different climatic conditions from north to south. In the 1980's, two of us moved from northern Italy to Apulia and soon came to appreciate the differences between the biotic and abiotic features of northern environment and the Apulian one. One of the most impressive differences were the enzootic tick borne diseases (TBD) and the related responses of the animals. As a consequence, much of our professional life has been devoted to the challenges posed by the diseases and to the study of the genetic peculiarities of native breeds both *per se* and in terms of their tolerance to TBD.

This report is a review of the results obtained in a 20-year experience investigating the haematological features and tolerance to tick-borne diseases in Mediterranean native sheep breeds - mainly Apulian native breeds - compared to exotic breeds under various experimental conditions. In the wake of William Thomson (Lord Kelvin), a pioneer in thermodynamics and electricity, who said in 1891 that when you can measure what you are speaking about, and express it in numbers, you know something about it, but when you cannot measure it, your knowledge is of a meager and unsatisfactory kind, the central concept or research theme that guided all our research efforts stems from the notion that direct measurement of disease phenotypes and/or physiological features such as the hematological pattern provides a direct assay for measuring disease changes and the attitude of a genetic pool in facing disease. The work is concerned with the following main issues:

- Haematological pattern of Apulian native sheep breeds
- Breeds and tolerance to TBD in Apulia
- Response to experimental anaemia
- Response to *Anaplasma ovis* infection in experimentally infected sheep.

2. Haematological pattern of Apulian native sheep breeds

In Apulia, the region covering the heel of the boot-shaped Italian peninsula, the rather harsh conditions of the soil and climate and the selective pressure of endemic haemotropic parasites have yielded genetic pools that are generally rustic and tolerant to the diseases caused by haemotropic parasites. An evaluation of the local genetic resources to explore their potential for sustainable and profitable genetic development programs is based on the knowledge of the physio-pathological features of blood according to species, breed and animal.

2.1 The Apulian sheep native breeds

Altamurana and Leccese, the latter also known as Moscia Leccese, are two ancient dairy breeds native to Apulia whose origins are not fully known. It is thought that they developed from an Asian breed, particularly from a Zackel type stock. They are rough wooled, well suited to life in harsh and semiarid conditions and they make good use of marginal pastures. Both breeds are seriously endangered. Though not as endangered as the former two breeds, Gentile di Puglia sheep may be considered, according to Alderson (2009), at risk of extinction because of their numerical scarcity and population trends. Yet, the Gentile di Puglia is classified as one of the main fine-wooled ovine breeds. The origin of the breed can be traced back to ancient Roman times when the soft fleece of an Apulian sheep, the Tarentine breed, was used to make the *togas* of important Roman citizens. According to William Youatt (1867), the Tarentine breed "had gradually spread from the coast of Syria and the Black Sea, and had now reached the western extremity of Europe. Many of them mingled with and improved the native breeds of Spain, while others continued to exist as a distinct race; and, meeting with a climate and a herbage suited to them, retained their original character and value, and were the progenitors of the Merinos of the present day."

2.2 Adult haematological pattern

Table 1 has been compiled from the existing repertoire of haematological values obtained analysing the blood of Apulian sheep; it reports least-square means (LSM) and standard error (SE) of haematological data obtained by analysing blood samples collected in population surveys of Gentile di Puglia and Leccese (Pieragostini et al., 1994; Pieragostini, 2006). Samples for Altamurana sheep were obtained from 58 purebred ewes ranging from 2-6 years of age and bred on an experimental farm near Bari (Pieragostini et al., 1999). Comparison with the literature (Jain, 1993), where range and medians are available, is also shown. On the basis of the normal probability plot, our data appear to follow a normal distribution where the median equals the mean.

When compared to normal blood values for sheep in the literature (Greenwood, 1977; Jain, 1993), the blood of Apulian sheep appears to be characterized by fewer erythrocytes that are normal in size and have higher haemoglobin content. This phenomenon typically seems to reflect a Mediterranean/North-African ovine blood picture (Pieragostini et al., 1994). The decreased PCV values correspond to lower blood viscosity and thus greater availability of water, which seems to be of particular adaptive significance in habitats characterized by an arid climate like Apulia (Ariely et al. 1986). The fact that some blood factors are related to the suitability of the breeds under particular environmental conditions was suggested long ago (Cresswell & Hutchings, 1962).

	Altamurana		Gentile di Puglia		Leccese		Jain (1993)	
Parameter	LSM±SE	N	LSM±SE	N	LSM±SE	N	range	median
RBC ($10^6/\mu l$)	8.3±0.13	58	9.4±0.06	263	8.3±0.14	145	9 - 15	12
Hb (g/dl)	9.8±0.11	58	10.4±0.25	263	9.3±0.32	996	9 - 15	11
PCV (g/dl)	30.6±0.33	58	30.6±0.16	263	29.5±0.11	996	26 - 45	34
MCV (fl)	37.9±0.52	58	32.8±0.13	263	36.4±0.59	145	28 - 40	34
MCH (pg)	12.2±0.15	58	11.2±0.05	263	11.6±0.21	145	8 - 12	10
MCHC (g/dl)	32.2±0.16	58	34.1±0.44	263	32.4±0.36	996	31 - 34	32
WBC ($10^3/\mu l$)	7.4±0.20	58	8.4±0.16	178	7.8±0.19	145	4 - 12	8

Table 1. Least-square means (LSM) and standard error (SE) of haematological data from adult animals belonging to native Apulian sheep breeds. RBC, Red Blood Cells; Hb, Haemoglobin; PCV, Packed Cell Volume; MCV, Mean Corpuscular Volume; MCH, Mean Corpuscular Haemoglobin, MCHC, Mean Corpuscular Haemoglobin Content; WBC, White Blood Cells; N, Number of animals.

Comparison of the data in table 1 shows that the haematological patterns in the three breeds are broadly the same. Gentile sheep seem to exhibit slight differences from the other two breeds, particularly as to the erythrocyte count, the mean corpuscular volume (MCV) and the mean corpuscular haemoglobin (MCH); in fact they are apparently the most European among the three. The traditional breeding sites of Gentile and Leccese differ substantially; one is in the southern part and the other in the northern part of Apulia, which is 500 Km long extending from the 39° to the 42° parallel. The Altamurana breeding site is in the Murgia uplands, in the central portion of Apulia. Its location in a rather harsh environment, together with the common origin of the two breeds, may account for the fact that Altamurana is closer to Leccese than to Gentile (Tab.1). However, a non-negligible point is that the physiological pattern characterizing the Altamurana and the Leccese breeds differs considerably from that of the Gentile di Puglia, as they belong to the group of dairy breeds while the Gentile is a fine wool and meat-producing sheep.

2.3 Lamb haematological pattern

Although the paucity of data in the literature concerning the haematological picture of lambs is scarce, general and particular information is available on the developmental pattern of their haematological values. The development of haematological picture of Altamurana lambs was investigated to assess the normal blood parameters and check the first occurrence in the blood smears of endemic endoerythrocytic parasites (Pieragostini et al., 2000). Standard haematological values were calculated for 22 Altamurana lambs controlled from birth to 18 months of age The values recorded in the neonatal period were strongly affected by birth weight. As clearly shown in table 2, the haemoglobin concentration (Hb), packed cell volume (PCV) and white cell count (WBC) exhibited significant age-dependent variations, particularly Hb % and PCV decreased while WBC increased.

Over weeks 1-5, red cell indices mainly followed the same trends as the Hb and PCV. Over the first four months, the RBC values on average remained unchanged at approximately 9 million/µl but then decreased. Starting from the fifth month, overall mean values were practically the same as in adults.

Age	Haematological parameters						
	RBC ($10^6/\mu l$)	Hb (g/dl)	PCV (g/dl)	MCV (fl)	MCH (pg)	MCHC (g/dl)	WBC ($10^3/\mu l$)
	LSM±SE	LSM±SE	LSM±SE	LSM±SE	LSM±SE	LSM±SE	LSM±SE
2 days	9.6±0.9	13.0±1.0	42.0±4.1	43.7±3.0	13.5±0.9	31.1±1.34	4.5±1.0
7 days	8.7±1.1	12.6±0.9	39.7±1.9	46.2±6.0	14.7±2.2	31.7±1.17	5.4±1.6
15 days	9.0±0.9	12.5±0.7	39.5±2.0	44.1±2.8	14.0±0.5	31.7±1.5	5.6±2.8
21 days	9.4±0.8	11.6±0.7	35.7±1.5	38.2±3.32	12.4±1.0	32.5±2.1	5.3±1.7
30 days	9.2±1.2	11.2±0.5	35.4±1.9	38.7±4.9	12.4±1.5	31.7±1.4	6.1±2.5
45 days	9.9±1.2	10.8±0.8	35.5±2.0	36.1±3.8	11.0±1.4	30.5±1.9	7.5±2.1
2 months	9.8±0.8	10.7±0.4	34.9±2.1	35.6±3.0	10.9±0.9	30.6±1.3	7.8±1.7
3 months	9.3±0.8	10.5±0.4	32.7±1.4	35.4±3.1	11.4±1.0	32.2±0.9	6.8±1.8
4 months	9.1±1.2	10.3±0.6	32.6±1.9	36.2±3.1	11.4±1.0	31.5±0.8	8.1±2.0
7 months	7.8±0.5	9.1±0.5	29.9±1.4	38.4±1.3	11.7±0.6	30.6±0.8	7.9±1.9
9 months	7.9±0.7	9.4±0.8	30.1±1.3	38.1±2.6	11.9±0.9	31.2±1.5	7.3±1.4
12 months	7.5±0.3	9.4±0.5	28.5±1.5	38.0±2.1	12.4±0.6	32.8±1.3	8.9±1.4
15 months	7.6±0.4	9.3±0.4	28.4±1.5	37.5±2.5	12.2±0.7	32.7±1.3	8.8±1.4
18 months	7.8±0.3	9.3±0.3	28.6±0.7	36.8±1.0	12.0±0.5	32.6±0.7	8.6±1.4

Table 2. Least-square means (LSM) and standard errors (SE) of haematological values recorded for 22 Altamurana lambs controlled from birth to 18 months of age. Modified from Pieragostini et al. (2000). RBC, Red Blood Cells; Hb, Haemoglobin; PCV, Packed Cell Volume; MCV, Mean Corpuscular Volume; MCH, Mean Corpuscular Haemoglobin, MCHC, Mean Corpuscular Haemoglobin Content; WBC, White Blood Cells.

Considering that reference data are mainly from breeds originally selected in northern European countries, when a comparison was made between 12 month-old Altamurana lambs and their northern counterparts, the erythrocytes of the Altamurana were fewer (7.5 *versus* 11.8 millions/µl) but bigger (38.0 ft *versus* 26.5 ft) and full of haemoglobin (12.4 pg *versus* 9.3 pg). This is the same phenomenon encountered in Mediterranean/North-African ovine blood picture as well as in the native Apulian adults.

The overall pattern is suggestive of erythrocyte physiological effectiveness, which was confirmed by the perfect physical development of the subjects examined in this study. In the blood smears obtained at seven months of age, namely in full spring when lambs start to graze pastures, endoerythrocytic enzootic parasites (*Theileria* spp. and *Anaplasma* spp.) were recorded and then became a constantly occurring phenomenon as will be documented in the following sections.

3. Breeds and tolerance to TBD in Apulia

Tick-borne diseases are of global importance to human and animal health and welfare. They are also responsible each year for dramatic economic losses which comprise direct losses from death of animals, loss of productivity and indirect losses due to the costs of control measures. In 1979, the amount of losses were estimated to be globally USD 7 billion (McCosker, 1979), but several reports on the economic costs of specific tick-borne diseases indicated that the earlier report is an underestimate (Jongejan & Uilenberg, 2004). There is a wide portfolio of measures which could be used to control tick-borne diseases among which both husbandry practices and host-related factors such as age, innate tolerance and breed are of great importance. Breeds whose historical breeding site is situated under the latitude of 41° show the ability to thrive in areas where tick borne diseases (TBD) are common. This trait, which can be defined as tolerance to TBD, is associated with the ability to resist the development of anemia in the face of infection.

A review on host resistance to tick borne diseases is documented in cattle (Correia de Almeida Regitano & Prayaga, 2010). As for other species, the case of the tolerance to tick-borne diseases shown by the sheep and horse native to Apulia is emblematic (Pieragostini & Petazzi, 1999; Rubino et al., 2006). In southern Italy, and particularly in Apulia, pyroplasmosis represents a longstanding and heavy burden for every type of livestock farm (Ceci & Carelli, 1999). Previous work performed on Gentile di Puglia sheep found that blood smears for parasite detection revealed an overall positivity rate of 93% for tick borne parasites (TBP) (Pieragostini et al, 2006). This high TBP positivity rate associated to normal blood values highlighted the tolerance of the native sheep towards TBP infection and accounted for endemic TBD.

3.1 Tick borne diseases in Apulian native sheep: A low income disease

According to Townsend & Thirtle (2001), studies of the rates of return to research have usually been based on the implicit assumption that if there were no research, then there would be neither growth nor decline in output or productivity. In the case of livestock, particularly in those areas characterized by a sub-tropical disease ecology, the assumption is especially unreasonable. It ignores the losses that would have occurred in the absence of livestock health research, resulting in an underestimation of the rates of return. The financial impact of a range of clinical and subclinical diseases and mortalities on farms is difficult to assess because there are insufficient accurate survey data on their prevalence causes or production losses on a national basis. Thus demonstration of the economic advantage of animal health is one of the relevant issues in animal production. Pieragostini et al. (1996) carried out a four year study to check the economic and zoonotic importance of TBD on sheep farms.

To this purpose sheep belonging to breeds tolerant to TBD systematically underwent one prophylactic treatment with diminazene aceturate (Berenil, Hoechst, AG, Germany) in full spring before the mating season. Table 3 shows the results obtained. The comparison between the reproductive values in the treated sheep and in an untreated control group highlighted significant differences in fertility and fecundity, with the group of treated sheep that were more fertile and fecund. Pyroplasmosis, even though unapparent, represents an important cause of perturbation of animal welfare. The authors estimated relevant (≈30%) economic losses in non treated animals, thus defining pyroplasmosis as a "low income disease".

Parameter	Altamurana		Leccese		Total	
	T (N =149)	NT (N = 259)	T (N = 49)	NT (N = 89)	T (N = 198)	NT (N = 348)
Fertility (%)	93[a]	65[b]	86[a]	62[b]	91[A]	64[B]
Prolificacy (%)	139	131	144	142	138	134
Fecundity (%)	132[a]	89[b]	119[a]	90[b]	128[A]	89[B]

Table 3. Least-square means of the reproductive parameters in Altamurana and Leccese sheep and in the whole sample (Total), as a function of the prophylactic treatment against pyroplasmosis with diminazene aceturate (T = treated, NT = not treated). Modified from Pieragostini et al. (1996). Means within rows with different letters significantly differ: capital letters: $P < 0.001$; small letters: $P < 0.05$.

3.2 Breed sheep and TBD

It is now generally acknowledged that importing exotic breeds can result in activities within the livestock sector that are uneconomic and/or have a negative impact on the environment. In many cases these activities are subsidized or otherwise provided for by development programs such as the case of Apulia which was documented in a study assessing attempts to introduce highly productive north European sheep breeds to Apulia (Pieragostini & Petazzi, 1999). The investigation analyzed data concerning the incidence and severity of pyroplasmosis in the five years spanning 1980-1984 on an experimental farm situated on the Murgia uplands in the province of Bari. The farm contained sheep belonging to gene pools of different geographical origin (Apulian, Italian island and north European breeds) or genotype classification (pure breeds or crossbreds) (Fig. 1).

The northern Finnish, Friesian and Romanov breeds were very susceptible to the disease; conversely, the native Apulian breeds showed very low rates of morbidity and mortality, followed in turn by breeds like Sardinian and Comisana, whose native areas have climatic and pedological characteristics similar to those of Apulia (Fig. 2). It is also worth noting that while the native and island breeds were regularly taken out to graze, the north European breeds were kept constantly under cover to reduce the likelihood of encountering ticks.

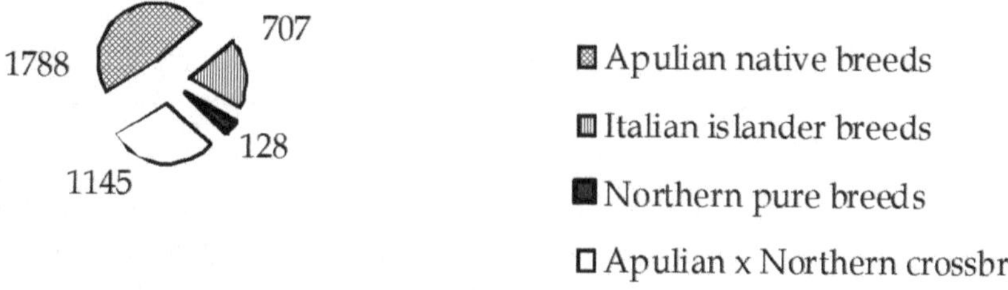

Fig. 1. Size of the investigated samples, clustered as sheep ecotypes. Modified from Pieragostini & Petazzi (1999).

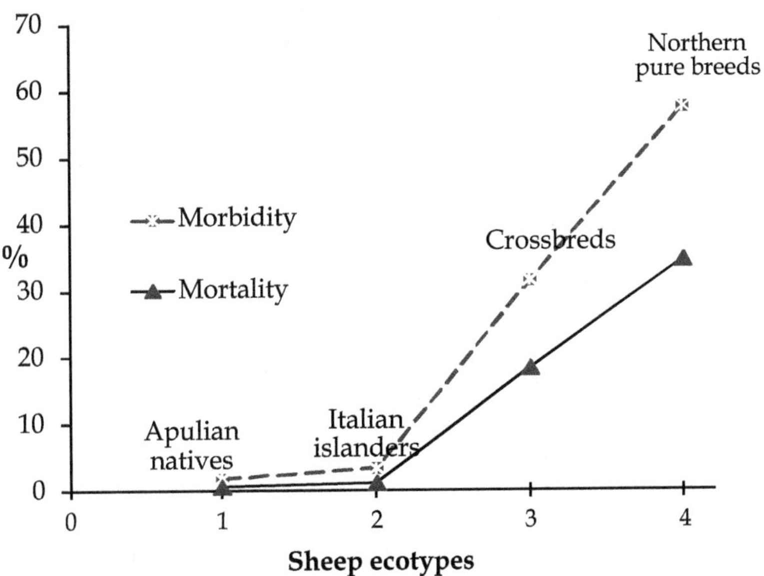

Fig. 2. Graphical representation obtained by processing morbidity and mortality data evidencing the influence of genotype on tolerance to pyroplasmosis in sheep living in Apulia. 1, Apulian native breeds (Altamurana, Gentile di Puglia and Leccese); 2, Italian islander breeds (Comisana and Sardinian); 3, Crossbreds (Finnish x Altamurana, Finnish x Leccese, Friesian x Altamurana, Friesian x Leccese; Romanov x Altamurana, Romanov x Leccese); 4, Northern pure breeds (Finnish, Friesian and Romanov). Modified from Pieragostini & Petazzi (1999).

A further element to consider is that attempts to improve the productivity of Apulian breeds by crossing them with the above exotic breeds failed because of the high mortality in generations F1 and F2, almost solely due to TBD. Though the mortality rates in crossbred animals were lower than those registered in the respective parental pure breeds, the number of individuals killed by the impact with endoerythrocytic pathogens was in any case too high (Fig. 2).

Pathogens were not accurately classified since the study analyzed data from farm records in which the veterinarians' diagnosis at death, due to TBD, always mentioned pyroplasmosis. The cases, which we were able to observe, concerned five Romanov sheep and seven Suffolk (occasionally found in the course of time and seriously ill prior to our visit). Examination of the animals always revealed classic symptoms of babesiosis and this was confirmed once the blood samples taken at the same time were analyzed. The haematological situation showed severe microcytic and hypochromic anaemia and *Babesia ovis (B. ovis)* was consistently identified in the blood smears.

By contrast, among the resilient breeds of sheep, the animals infected with pyroplasmosis showed only a state of discomfort which usually does not last more than few days and is characterized by a brief rise in temperature, slight dejection in the form of a tendency to move away from the flock, loss of appetite which might also be very transitory, translucent mucosae, slightly blueish against a pale background and in a few cases subicteric.

3.3 Piroplasmosis in naturally infected tolerant sheep

Resistance is a dynamic process of parasite regulation by the host. The pathogen must penetrate host cell barriers in sufficient numbers, attack target cells and replicate. Sub-clinical or clinical expression of the disease is dependent on the pathogen's virulence and the interaction between pathogen and host characteristics. Particularly, the phenomenon of tolerance to tick borne pathogens (TBP) is closely linked to a particular type of anaemia which is generally the symptom *par excellence* of the disease. In the tolerant animals, as shown in a study carried out on Altamurana sheep, this takes a benign macrocytic and hyperchromic form. A comparison of the haematological parameters of healthy sheep with those of sick sheep in table 4 showed that the latter presented a numerical deficiency of red blood cells that was compensated by the fact that the mean corpuscular volume (MCV) increased by about 50% as did the mean corpuscular haemoglobin (MCH). The results shown in table 4 did not stem from a dedicated investigation because the haematologic alterations were met with by chance when investigating on the functional effect of a rare alpha globin gene variant. At sampling, the affected sheep did not show any patent signs of the disease and thus only the haemocromocytometric parameters, the related observation of blood films and the results of the osmotic fragility test led to classifying the sampled animals in healthy and affected. Observation of blood films in this study and in other subsequent occasional analyses on Apulian sheep in similar conditions, highlighted that in most cases there were mixed infections in which *Anplasma* spp. and/or *Theileria* spp. and/or *Babesia* spp. occurred at the same time (Fig. 3). *B. ovis* was consistently present in the blood films of the affected animals with visible symptoms of haematuria. This fact, taken together with the evidence from tests on Romanov sheep infected and killed by babesiosis, convinced us that *B. ovis* was one of the causes of the pathogenetic activity in Apulian sheep, and certainly in non-native breeds. However, diseases often occur in clusters of time (years, seasons, production cycles, etc.) and space (herd, pasture, farm, region, etc.) and the prevalence of this pathogen was never the target of a dedicated epidemiological investigation.

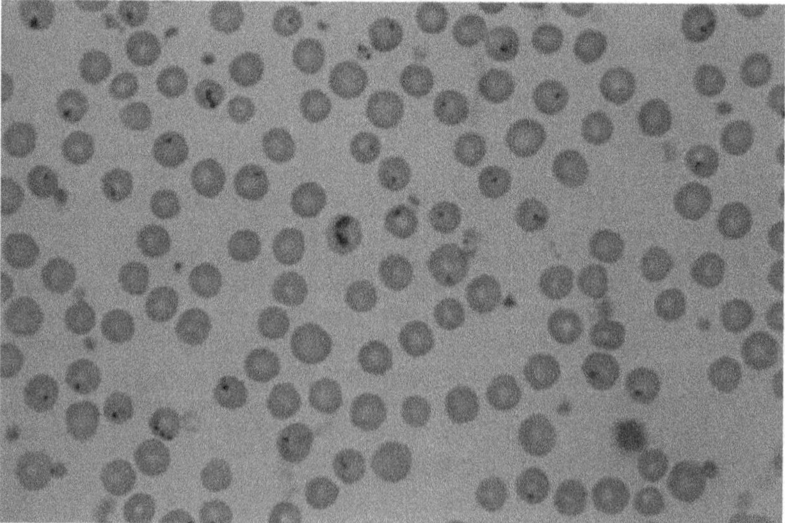

Fig. 3. Blood film showing a mixed infection of *Anaplasma* spp. and *Babesia ovis*.

Haematological parameters	Samples		Significance
	Healthy (N =22)	Affected (N =28)	
RBC ($10^6/\mu l$)	9.5±0.19	6.3±0.70	**
Hb (g/dl)	9.9±0.18	9.2±0.50	*
PCV (g/dl)	32.3±0.55	30.3±0.50	**
MCV (fl)	34.3±1.43	48.7±1.29	**
MCH (pg)	10.4±0.46	15.2±0.42	**
MCHC (g/dl)	30.5±0.44	31.2±0.40	n.s.
WBC ($10^3/\mu l$)	9.6±0.40	9.5±0.37	n.s.
MCF (g%NaCl for 50% haemolysis)	0.72±0.02	0.82±0.03	**

Table 4. Comparison of the haematological parameters recorded in healthy and affected Altamurana sheep (mean values ± standard errors). Modified from Pieragostini & Petazzi, 1999. (RBC=Red Blood Cells; Hb=Haemoglobin %; PCV= Packed Cell Volume; MCV= Mean Corpuscular Volume; MCH=Mean Corpuscular Haemoglobin, MCHC=Mean Corpuscular Haemoglobin Content; WBC=White Blood Cells; MCF=Mean Corpuscolar Fragility) $*P<0.05$;$**P<0.01$; n.s.= not significant.

3.4 Anaplasmosis in naturally infected splenectomized sheep

Anaplasmosis is one of the most important tick-borne diseases of ruminants worldwide. The disease is caused by infection of animals with the obligate intraerythrocytic bacteria *Anaplasma* spp. which is classified in the family *Anaplasmataceae*, order *Rickettsiales* (Dumler et al, 2001). This section includes some experiences with sheep splenectomy and describes disease onset and course in eight splenectomized TBD-tolerant sheep that were naturally infected with piroplasms. Though the trials had been performed in different time periods, the results obtained were very similar and the facts surrounding the experiments gave us both general and specific insights into the field of splenectomy of carrier sheep from areas where endoerythrocytic parasites are endemic.

Particularly in the first trial, the surgical operation had two purposes: a) to evaluate the rôle of the spleen as a filter-pad to check parasites and as modulator of the direct response to anemia; b) to obtain a high number of parasites in the blood to prepare a local specific antigen.

The following trials were mainly related to the need to obtain *A. ovis* which was isolated from splenectomized sheep allowed to be naturally infected pasturing in tick areas.

Splenectomy was slightly traumatic for all the subjects and 24 hours after the surgical operation the sheep showed normal functions. The sheep were identified with female names for easier checking. Clinical evaluation was done on a daily basis and rectal temperatures were recorded every morning for 12 weeks post splenectomy. Blood and serum samples were routinely collected twice a week during the observation period. Haematological variables were evaluated using a haematology analyzer. The erythrocyte fragility test was performed by exposing erythrocytes to hypotonic saline solutions decreasing by 0.02% starting from 0.86%. Parasites in the blood were checked by Giemsa staining every 3 days. During the acute phase of the disease, the most important haematological values, erythrocyte fragility and parasitaemia were monitored daily. In the case of Gilda, Lina and Zoppina, which were part of the experiment to check the response to *A. ovis* infection of

different sheep breeds, described in section 5, parasite density was estimated on thin blood film and expressed as the percentage of parasitized red blood cells.
Fifteen days after the splenectomy, the general situation worsened and the animals became anorexic, staggering with a severe anaemia and dehydration. At the same time the RBC, Hb% and PCV values dropped (Tab. 5), and a number of organisms started appearing in the blood films (Rosalba showed a carpet of *A. ovis*; Stella a great deal of *A. ovis*; Lisa and Lola a great deal of *A. ovis* and a few *Babesia* spp.; Claretta a great number of *Theileria* spp.). Rosalba and Stella died of severe anaemia respectively 24 hours and 4 days after the diagnosis despite specific drugs and whole blood trasfusions with blood drawn from a donor subject. Claretta, Lisa and Lola showed less violent initial symptoms, the anaemic crisis was less severe and following a therapy with anti-protozoal drugs associated with desametazone they gradually began to eat and became clinically and haematologically healthy in 15-20 days. Since Lina, Zoppina, and Gilda, were included in the above cited experimental design to investigate the tolerance to *A. ovis*, they were constantly monitored and parasitaemia was recorded every two days after splenectomy. The cases of Lina and Zoppina allowed comparison between a mixed infection by *T. ovis* and *A. ovis* and an almost single infection by *A. ovis*. Interestingly, the two sheep coped differently with the infections. Though both animals were positive for *A. ovis* and *T. ovis* after splenectomy, the maximum of parasitized erythrocytes (MPE) by *T. ovis* peaked to 17% in Zoppina, while in Lina *T. ovis* caused a latent infection. Conversely, MPE by *A. ovis* in Zoppina was less than a half that of Lina (Tab. 5).

	Splenectomized sheep							
	Rosalba	Stella	Lisa	Lola	Claretta	Lina	Zoppina	Gilda
Year of splenectomy	1994	1994	1994	1994	1994	2009	2009	2010
Incubation Time (days)*	19	21	25	32	42	29	35	21
Max Temperature (C°)	39.80	39.80	39.60	39.40	39.20	39.40	39.20	39.60
Min PCV (g/dl)	7	7	10	10	11	10	11	10
PCV reduction (%)	75	74	56	55	57	61	75	60
Hb reduction (%)	73	74	58	53	52	55	72	54
Max parasitemia *A.ovis*(%)	>70	>60	n.e.	n.e.	n.e.	36	15	60
Max parasitemia *T.ovis* (%)	n.e.	n.e.	n.e.	n.e.	n.e.	3	17	2

Table 5. Summary of clinical findings recorded in eight sheep splenectomised in different time periods (n.e.=observed but not estimated; *Incubation Time=number of days from first observation of infected blood cells on stained blood smears to the peak of the disease).

Then, Lina developed the disease after an incubation period of 29 days and recovered within a month, exhibiting a slight decrease in PCV (less than 25%) on post-splenectomy day 90 due to a slight increase in parasitaemia by *A. ovis* (Fig. 4). The two sheep were transfused with blood from a healthy donor sheep and treated every two days for a week with oxytetracycline (Terramicina long acting 1000 mg) and dexamethasone (Desashock Fortdodge Animal Health S.p.a., 80mg single dose). Both Lina and Zoppina quickly recovered from the disease, reaching normal blood values within four weeks, but, one month after their recovery, they had a relapse which they coped with successfully.

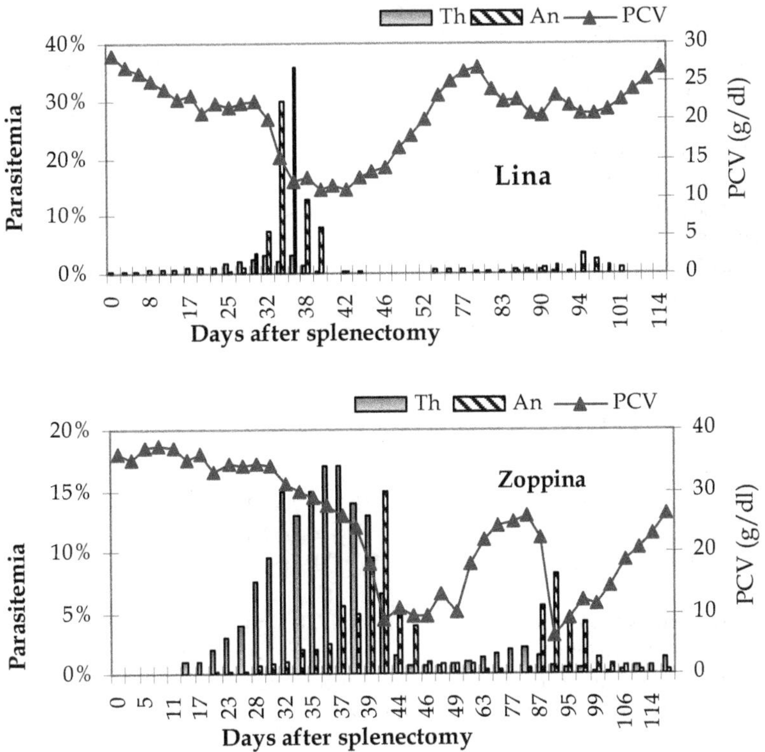

Fig. 4. Trend of PCV values and parasite densities (*An=Anaplasma ovis* and *Th=Theileria ovis*) expressed as percentage of red blood cells parasitized in Lina and Zoppina, the two splenectomized sheep monitored over a five week period after splenectomy.

During the recovery period, clinical examination revealed only pale mucous membranes. The pattern of evolution of the disease and recovery in Gilda was almost the same as in Lina except for a higher level of parasitaemia. In this instance *A. ovis* was the sole agent of the illness of our sheep. Secondly, the increase in *A. ovis* is apparently slowed down by the presence of *T. ovis* which seems to have a 'buffer effect' on the appearance of anaplasmosis but not in tempering its severity. Three points emerge from these results: i) in contrast to babesiosis and to the literature of some years ago (Radostits et al., 2000), hemoglobinuria did not occur in any of the seven severe cases of anaplasmosis; ii) treatment produced an immediate reduction in parasitaemia without leading to a complete clearance of the parasites; iii) disease relapse might be accounted for by the persistence of *A. ovis*.

Though not a novelty, in areas with enzootic erythrocytic parasitoses, even apparently healthy breeding animals may host pathogens and show tolerance and/or premunition to them without presenting with circulating parasites. This is a limit that should always be taken into account and may constitute a complication for any stress-associated situation. Anaemia secondary to anaplasmosis may evolve in a remarkably violent fashion probably due to the mechanism effected by the reticulo-endothelial system (RES) virtually with no haemolysis. In our small experience the use of desametazone had a beneficial effect as it reduced the general response to the stimulation of the pathogen and particularly macrophage activity and improved red blood cell membrane response. Several years have elapsed since the first experiment and Lola, Lisa and Claretta got back to 'normal life' and, before their death, caused by old age, they showed no signs of disease which might have been related to haematological parasitosis. As to Lina, Gilda and Zoppina, they are back in the flock following a normal breeding and reproductive cycle. With no doubt the spleen naturally acts as an immunologically active filter-pad countering even severe red blood cell deprivation; its activity is particularly prominent in the presence of antibodies given that even after splenectomy these animals were still able to resist local diseases. There are grounds to believe that the animals may have a genetically derived tolerance to such instances based on active, diffuse and efficient structural systems which do not relate to one sole organ.

4. Response to experimental anaemia

It is difficult to distinguish whether, in the case of native sheep, the slightness of the degree of anaemia should be considered the cause or the effect of tolerance. However, it is certain that these animals have an unquestionable ability to maintain a good level of homeostasis during TBD evidenced from the data shown in table 4, particularly those concerning PCV, Hb and MCHC.

To the purpose, four sheep belonging to a sensitive and non tolerant breed (Romanov), and four sheep to a sensitive but tolerant breed (Altamurana) underwent regular bleeding for seven days, stopping when the decrease of the packed cell volume ranged from 35 to 40%, the same as usually observed in clinical ovine babesiosis caused by *B. ovis* (Yeruham et al., 1998).

Over time the quantity and quality of the evolution of the haematological response were checked. The regression analyses performed to compare the two breeds with respect to the various data sets, gave the following results (Tab. 6):

- the intrabreed correlation coefficients recorded for PCV, Hb and RBC, were statistically significant only in the case of Romanov sheep, testifying to high difformity in the anaemization response between Romanov individuals, while Altamurana sheep behaved almost the same;
- the comparisons between the correlation coefficients obtained for PCV, Hb and RBC, in the two different breed groups were highly statistically significant.

Of these two points, while the latter might have been expected as the trial was based on the assumption of difference between the two breeds, the former result opens new vistas in the evaluation of the phenomenon. The low variability in the response to the anaemization exhibited by Altamurana sheep might be the result of the selection pressure acted by the constant presence of anaemizing parasites. Conversely the variability of the Romanov sheep could be taken as the individual response to the impact of an unusual stress.

As a general consideration, the two groups were composed by animals which were profoundly different and constantly on different levels from the haematological point of view. Both situations observed seemed to represent different aspects of normality, particularly the Altamurana sheep are constantly "poor" in the absolute levels of PCV, Hb and RBC and constantly "richer" regarding the derived parameters, MCV, MCH, MCHC, the latter being constantly those expressing haematological "efficiency" in the face of anaemia (Pieragostini & Petazzi, 1999). So if it is a matter of fact that from the numerical point of view, the two breeds' responses to anaemization are to a large extent not very dissimilar, the greater efficiency of the local breeds is beyond doubt. It is not to be excluded that this may be identified in their greater capacity to cope with anoxemic stress, both by the production of red globules enriched with haemoglobin and maybe also by accelerating the turnover of older and less efficient red blood cells.

Contrasts	Haematological parameters		
	RBC	Hb	PCV
Within Altamurana	n.s.	n.s.	n.s.
Within Romanov	***	***	***
Between Altamurana and Romanov	****	****	****

Table 6. Statistical significance of the differences between the correlation coefficients calculated by the regression analysis performed to compare the two breeds, Altamurana and Romanov, with respect to the hematological parameters RBC (Red Blood Cells), Hb (Haemoglobin) and PCV (Packed Cell Volume). ***$P<0.001$; ****$P<0.0001$; n.s., not significant.

The reading of these haematological aspects should be looked at without losing sight of the general aspect of the overall comparison between the two breeds. From this point of view, the considerable difference in absolute values, apparently almost negligible as regards the curve trends, becomes very striking in the comparison between the general situations of overall well-being of the two breeds compared. The Altamurana sheep continued to exhibit apparent good health when subjected to anaemization, at ease with their surroundings, ready to feed and drink. Conversely, the Romanovs exhibited a serious dulling of the senses and lack of reaction once anaemization was achieved; this necessitated support treatments with rehydrating solutions to allow them to overcome their state of anergy (Pieragostini & Petazzi, 1999). These results strongly support the hypothesis that, beyond the environmental factors such as stress, nutrition and other conditions, which in general facilitate infections (Agyemang et al., 1990; Bennison et al., 1998; Oppliger et al., 1998) and which are supposed to be particularly relevant in the case of non-native breeds, genetic predisposition plays a major role also in the pathogenesis of TBD.

5. Response to *Anaplasma ovis* infection in experimentally infected sheep

Animal well-being has become a significant concern among consumers who expect food animals to be well treated, raised in idyllic environments, and free of disease. Consumers also expect their meat products to be free of residual antibiotics and therapeutic drugs. For these reasons, new approaches or alternatives to addressing animal diseases are needed. One approach is genetic selection for animals resistant to disease, that is: an approach whose focus is on accepting certain constraints of the environment and using breeds that can cope with these constraints, as opposed to the earlier approach which focussed on changing the environment to create opportunities for exotic breeds to be productive. But identifying the phenotype for disease resistance is difficult.

As to TBD, the response is known to be under multi-factorial regulation (Horin, 1998; Aguilar-Delfin et al., 2001). As highlighted in the above section 4, the phenomenon of tolerance is a broad-based one and possibly not unrelated to the erythropoietic system in different sheep breeds or to the haemoglobin genetic systems (Pieragostini et al., 2003; Pieragostini et al., 2006).

Anyway, the success of selection for disease resistance is dependent on correctly identifying the disease agent and the phenotype for disease resistance. For example, as to TBP in small ruminants, there are several reports concerning the presence of *Babesia, Theileria,* and *Anaplasma* species infecting sheep and goats in many countries world-wide but, in many regions of the Old and the New World, the identity of the tick-borne disease agents of sheep and goats and of their vector ticks is uncertain. But perhaps, the biggest challenge of selecting for disease resistance is to accurately identify the phenotype for disease resistance and/or to have reliable genetic markers with high predictive values for a disease phenotype. Phenotypic variability induced by parasites is a matter of fact, as impressively exemplified by the high number of haemoglobinopathies in human populations living in malaria-endemic areas (Evans & Wellems, 2002).

Recalling Feynman's[1] saying that nature repeats itself at every scale, we suggested that the unusual haemoglobin polymorphism recorded in Apulian native sheep breeds and the related functional effects might have an adaptive significance, also being somehow related to the selective pressure of tick borne parasites (TBP) (Pieragostini et al., 1994; Pieragostini et al., 2003; Pieragostini et al., 2006). Based on these considerations, we aimed to define the phenotype of the tick borne diseases in different sheep breeds starting from the one caused by *A. ovis*, the most common parasite in our area as confirmed by a small survey on sheep TBP performed in 10 farms (throughout Apulia) on 240 individuals. *A. ovis* was identified in 58% of samples, followed by *T. ovis* (5.8%) and *T. annulata* (4.5%). *Theileria* spp. were present in mixed infections with *A. ovis, B. ovis* (0.9 %) or *Babesia* spp. (0.9 %). In particular the presence of *A. ovis* was confirmed by specific polymerase chain reactions (PCRs) for *Anaplasma* spp. (Stuen et al., 2003) and *A. ovis* (de la Fuente et al., 2005; de la Fuente et al., 2007). Then PCRs followed by reverse line blot hybridization of the amplified 18SrRNA gene from *Theileria* and *Babesia* species, was used to detect specific probes for *Theileria/Babesia catch all, Theileria sp1 china, Theileria sp2 chinal, T. buffely, T. annulata, T. velifera, T. taurotragi, T. mutans, T. lestoquardi, T. ovis, B. bovis, B. bigemina, B. crassa, B. motasi, B. ovis, B. major, B. divergens, T. hirci, B. sp1 (Turchey), B. sp2 (Lintan)* (Schnittger et al., 2004).

Year	Step 1	Year	Step 2
2009	Search for carriers	2010	Search for carriers
2009	Splenectomization	2010	Splenectomization
2009	Infection of 8 Suffolk and 8 Comisana characterized by normal alpha globin gene arrangements and different beta genotypes	2010	Infection of 18 Altamurana characterized by different alpha globin gene arrangements

Table 7. Experimental design.

[1] Richard Phillips Feynman (May 11, 1918 – February 15, 1988) was an American physicist who received the Nobel Prize in Physics in 1965.

Thus, a project was set up to evaluate the response to anaplasmosis in susceptible and tolerant sheep breeds including the use of haemoglobin genetic systems as genetical markers of tolerance to the disease. Summarized actions are described in table 7.

5.1 Materials and methods

5.1.1 Search for carriers and parasites

Sixty ewes were sampled from a flock extensively reared in the countryside near Bari. The flock consisted of approximately 250 heterogeneous subjects belonging mainly to TBD tolerant breeds and crossbreds. The presence of TBPs was checked in the blood samples by a PCR-based molecular approach as described above. Most of the sampled animals were found to carry *A. ovis* mixed with other TBPs. Based on the results of the flock survey and the consent given by the breeder, three ewes carrying *A. ovis* and *T. ovis* were selected and purchased. Following the experimental design (table 7) Lina and Zoppina were splenectomized in 2009 while Gilda in 2010, as described in subsection 3.4.

5.1.2 Animals

Selected animals 7/8 months of age were involved in this study. Lambs less than six months of age were purchased and housed at the Medical Clinics of the Faculty of Veterinary Medicine of the University of Bary. Upon arrival at the Faculty of Veterinary Medicine, the animals were weighed and faecal samples were obtained to establish their worm burdens. Feet were checked for foot rot. The animals were dewormed with a broad spectrum anthelmintic. All of them were then housed in a tick proof isolation unit. In particular, in 2009 the lambs were selected based on different breed and equally divided between Suffolk and Comisana.

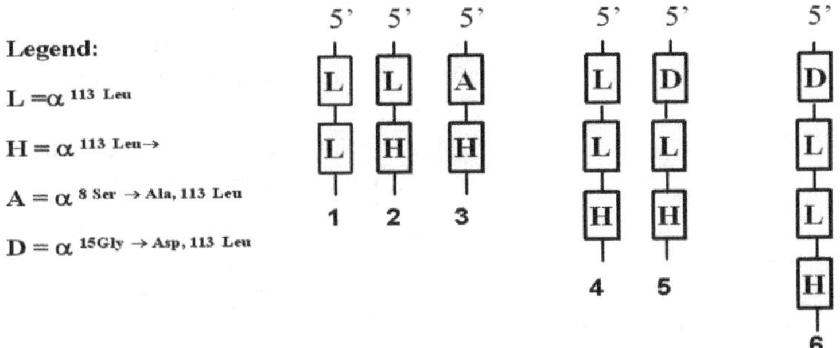

Fig. 5. Alpha-globin gene haplotypes detected so far in sheep, namely: haplotypes 1, 2 and 3 are normally duplicated (NH); haplotypes 4, 5 and 6 show extranumeral alpha gene arrangements (EH); particularly haplotypes 4 and 5 are triplicated while haplotype 6 is quadruplicated.

All the lambs were characterized by a normal duplicate alpha gene arrangement (Fig. 5) and most of them by homozigosity at the beta globin loci. Owing to high frequency of HBBA gene in the Suffolk breed, three out of the eight Suffolk lambs were HBBAB heterozygotes.
In 2010 eighteen Altamurana lambs less than six months of age, housed and treated as above described, were selected based on different alpha globin genetic arrangements. Nine lambs were homozygotes for the normal duplicate alpha gene haplotype (NH), the others carrying an extra-numeral alpha haplotype (EH) (Fig.5); most of the 18 lambs were homozygotes for the HBBB allele at the beta globin loci.

5.1.3 Experimental infection

A. ovis was isolated from one of the above splenectomized sheep. Lina was the donor for the 2009 lambs and Gilda for the 2010 lambs. Parasite density was estimated on thin blood film obtained by the buffy coat method and expressed as the percentage of parasitized red blood cells. At the peak of parasitaemia in the donor sheep (36% and 60% of red blood cells parasitized respectively), about 400 ml of blood were obtained and each lamb in the breed groups was inoculated intraperitoneally with 25 ml of infected blood.

5.1.4 Clinical observations

Clinical evaluation was done on a daily basis and rectal temperatures were recorded every morning for 8 weeks post infection. Blood and serum samples were collected twice a week during the observation period. Haematological variables were evaluated using a haematology analyzer. Parasite density was estimated on thin blood film as above described.

5.1.5 Haemoglobin phenotype

The reversible switch from haemoglobin A to C was observed in the above HBBAB Suffolk lambs. The expression of the silent gene encoding for Hb C was detected by isoelectric focusing and quantified by high performance liquid chromatography (Alloggio *et al.*, 2009).

5.1.6 Statistics

First, differences between breed groups for clinical and haematological data were assessed using analysis of variance (ANOVA) by GLM procedure (SAS, 1990). A second ANOVA was carried out only for the Altamurana group, considering the interaction between the alpha globin type (2 levels: NH and EH) and each clinical variable. The last ANOVA was carried out only for the Suffolk group considering the interaction with the beta globin type (2 levels: AB and BB) of the linear and quadratic regression of each haematological variable on the number of days from the infection, with three of the Suffolk that were AB compared to as many BB. This analysis was performed for the Suffolk, where, as cited above, both AB and BB genotypes were found, whereas only BB animals occurred in the Comisana.

5.2 Results and discussion

The following is an overall picture of the findings where they are reported and discussed relating to the different approaches.

5.2.1 Clinical findings

Host responses in the three experimentally infected sheep groups were first compared mainly according to typical high fever periods, microscopic observation and haematological values. *A. ovis* began to appear in the blood a week before the fever and the following records showed that the maximum of erythrocytes parasitized by *A. ovis* in any case did not exceed 2%.

All the animals developed the disease (Table 8) but symptoms varied in terms of severity and duration and none died. Fever syndrome (listlessness, anorexia, weakness, ruminal stasis, respiratory distress, increased heart and respiratory rates) and pallor of the mucous membranes were recorded in seven of the Suffolk group, in only one of the Comisana group and in none of the Altamurana.

Breed	Dose of infection	Symptoms	Need for therapeutic intervention	Morbidity	Expected Mortality
Suffolk	36%	very severe	7 out of 8 subjects	100%	87.5%
Comisana	36%	severe	1 out of 8 subjects	100%	12.5%
Altamurana	56%	mild	none	100%	0%

Table 8. Overview of responses to anaplasmosis in the three analyzed breeds.

The haematological patterns were then analyzed in detail comparing the intra breed variations between the different physiopathological moments - normal health status (time 0=T_0), acute phase (time 1=T_1) recovery phase (time 2=T_2) - and the between breed variations intra physiopathological moments (table 9). Finally, clinical parameters, such as incubation time (I.T) after infection, temperature peak (T.P.), percentage decrease in haematocrit (Δ HCT), percentage decrease in haemoglobin content (Δ Hb) expressed as gr Hb/dl blood, percentage decrease in red blood cells (Δ RBC) were evaluated for each breed (Table 10).

Breed	Parameter	T_0			T_1			T_2		
		Mean	SD		Mean	SD		Mean	SD	
Suffolk	PCV (g/dl)	31.9	± 2.8	a	12.7	± 2.7	A	23.9	± 2.3	a
	Hb (g/dl)	11.5	± 1.0	a	4.7	± 0.7	A	7.7	± 0.7	a
	RBC (10^6/μl)	12.5	± 1.2	A	4.5	± 0.8	a	7.2	± 1.0	
	MCV (fl)	25.0	± 1.0	A	32.3	± 1.6	A	33.3	± 3.0	A
	MCH (pg)	9.2	± 0.3	B	10.5	± 0.6	A	10.7	± 0.6	A
	MCHC (g/dl)	36.8	± 1.0	A	32.5	± 1.2		32.3	± 0.8	
	WBC (10^3/μl)	8.6	± 1.1		10.9	± 2.4		0.3	± 1.1	a
Comisana	PCV (g/dl)	35.0	± 2.4	b	11.3	± 2.7	A	26.2	± 1.7	b
	Hb (g/dl)	12.6	± 1.0	b	4.7	± 0.5	A	8.6	± 0.7	b
	RBC (10^6/μl)	11.9	± 1.3	A	5.1	± 0.8	a	6.9	± 0.7	
	MCV (fl)	29.7	± 2.3	B	29.1	± 3.2	B	38.4	± 3.2	B
	MCH (pg)	10.7	± 0.7	A	9.4	± 1.1	B	12.5	± 0.9	B
	MCHC (g/dl)	35.9	± 1.3	A	32.1	± 0.4		32.5	± 1.0	
	WBC (10^3/μl)	10.1	± 2.7		7.5	± 1.4		10.4	± 2.9	b
Altamurana	PCV(g/dl)	31.2	± 3.2	a	21.6	± 3.1	B	25.8	± 2.4	b
	Hb (g/dl)	0.4	± 1.0	C	7.1	± 1.0	B	8.2	± 0.8	b
	RBC (10^6/μl)	9.4	± 1.0	B	6.2	± 1.0	b	7.1	± 0.8	
	MCV (fl)	33.2	± 1.9	C	34.7	± 1.7	C	36.6	± 2.0	B
	MCH (pg)	10.6	± 0.5	A	11.4	± 0.5	C	11.6	± 0.5	B
	MCHC (g/dl)	31.7	± 0.7	B	32.8	± 0.9		31.9	± 1.0	b
	WBC (10^3/μl)	10.1	± 2.6		9.6	± 2.0		10.1	± 1.4	B

Table 9. Haematological parameters assessed for the three analyzed breeds, namely normal health status before infection (time 0=T_0), during the acute phase (time 1=T_1) and during the recovery phase (time 2=T_2). Means within columns with different letters significantly differ: capital letters: $P < 0.01$; small letters: $P < 0.05$.

As already reported, none of the animals had more than 2% erythrocytes parasitized by *A. ovis*. This confirms the role the spleen plays in the phagocytosis and clearance of parasitized erythrocytes; otherwise only splenectomized sheep showed significant percentages of parasitized erythrocytes (table 5).
Mean parasitaemia in the single group could theoretically be inferred from the Δ RBC and conclude that the higher the Δ RBC value, the higher the suceptibility of the erythrocytes to *Anaplasma* infection. According to the results shown in table 8 depicting the response of the three breeds to infection, broken down according to the dose of infection, symptoms, need for therapeutic intervention and expected mortality, seven out of the Suffolk group recovered after being treated every two days for a week with oxytetracycline and dexamethasone whereas seven subjects of the Comisana group recovered from clinical anaplasmosis with no drug treatment other than a single dose of dexamethasone. The highest degree of tolerance was observed in the Altamurana group where all the subjects showed only mild alteration of behaviour and basic life functions. Comparison of the haematological patterns of the three breeds at T_0 in table 10 revealed that, in normal health conditions, the differences which may be noticed are consistent with those of earlier studies described in section 2, indicating that both environmental and productive specialization seem to account for the different physiological results.
Hence the Altamurana breed is characterized by significantly lower RBC and Hb values and by significantly higher MCV, MCH and MCHC values than Suffolk, a northern meat breed, while Comisana, a Mediteranean dairy breed has intermediate values. At T_1 and T_2 the same variation pattern may be observed, that is:

- haematologically, *A. ovis* infection does not seem to seriously affect Altamurana whose response may be described as a moderate normochromic normocytic anemia followed by a normochromic macrocytic pattern representing an active regeneration phase.
- conversely, the Suffolk and Comisana animals exhibited a violent response to *A. ovis* with a severe anaemia. The hyperchromic and macrocytic anaemia in the Suffolk was followed by a slow regeneration and the hypochromic normocytic anaemia of the Comisana by an active regeneration phase, similar to the Altamurana pattern, as documented by the high MCV values.

The results shown in table 10 confirmed the differences among the three breeds both in terms of quantitative (Altamurana *vs* Suffolk) and temporal (Comisana *vs* Suffolk) variation in haematological parameters. While Suffolk animals displayed the most severe reduction in the number of erythrocytes and haemoglobin content, Altamurana was characterized by a more controlled response, with only a minor and more gradual decline in RBC and Hb values. Comisana experienced a more severe reduction in the number of erythrocytes than did Suffolk, though the decline in RBC values was not accompanied by a decrease in the total haemoglobin content as severe as that observed in Suffolk. This could be due to the significantly higher MCH values characterizing the Comisana haematological pattern as compared to the Suffolk.
Considering the overall responses shown in table 8 and detailed in table 9 and 10, there is no doubt that we are dealing with very different animal groups exhibiting different physiopathological phenotypes where a healthy haematological picture plays a relevant role.

Breed	I.T (days)	T.P. (°C)	ΔHCT (%)	ΔHb (%)	ΔRBC (%)
Suffolk	24.2[A]	40.5[A]	65.4[A]	60.2[A]	60.3[A]
Comisana	38.8[B]	39.9[B]	57.7[B]	56.9[A]	55.9[A]
Altamurana	25.3[A]	39.9[B]	19.2[C]	19.8[B]	33.7[B]

Table 10. Clinical parameters assessed for the three breeds analyzed at the peak of the disease, namely incubation time (I.T) after infection, temperature peak (T.P.), percentage decrease in haematocrit (ΔHCT), percentage decrease in haemoglobin content (ΔHb), percentage decrease in red blood cells (ΔRBC).

5.2.2 Functional effect of beta globin genes on the recovery from anemia

As to the functional effect of beta globin genes on the recovery from anemia, Figure 6 shows the results of the analysis performed in the Suffolk, where both AB and BB genotypes were found.

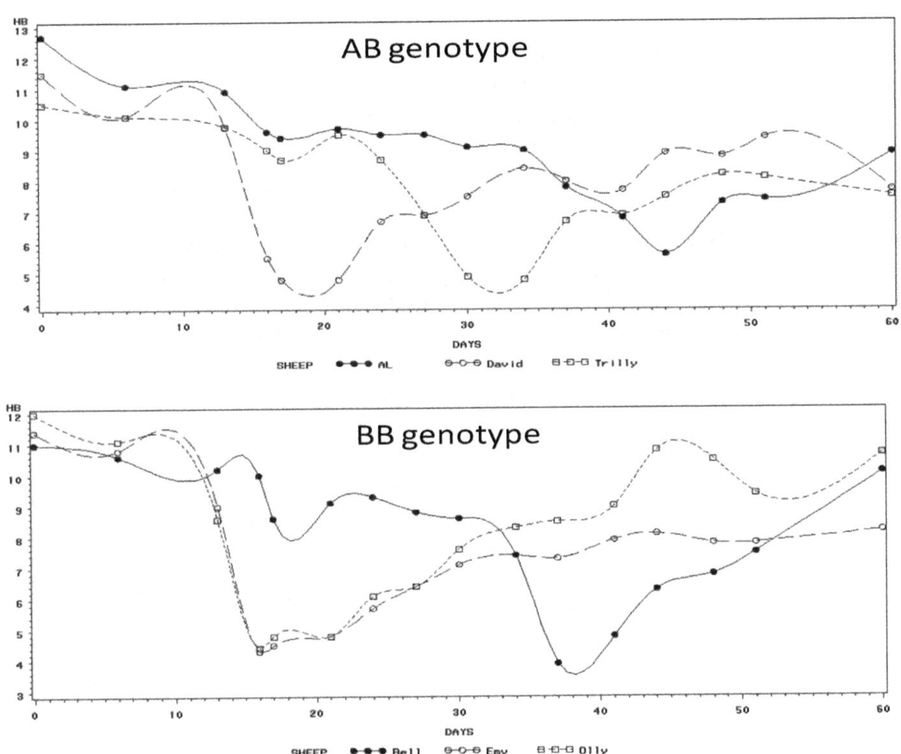

Fig. 6. Trend of Haemoglobin (Hb, g/dl) as a function of the number of days from the infection (DAYS) for the haemoglobin genotypes AB and BB (Modified from Alloggio et al. 2009).

Goats and some sheep under conditions of erythropoietic stress (anaemia) or hypoxia, synthesize a juvenile haemoglobin (Hb) type, Hb C, where β-globin is encoded by the silent gene *HBBC*. Anaemia causes a change in the type of circulating haemoglobin only in sheep carrying βA-globin haplotype, where Hb A is replaced by Hb C. Pioneered by the work of van Vliet and Huismam (1964), the Hb C in Caprini species has been thoroughly studied and particularly the mechanism of reversible switching has triggered focused research in the 70's (Nienhuis and Anderson, 1972; Nienhuis and Bunn, 1974). Little information is available on the effect of Hb A replacement by Hb C. Owing to the high oxygen affinity of Hb C (Huisman and Kitchens, 1968), the reversible switch from Hb A to Hb C may be considered a way to cope with the reduced amount of oxygen available at higher altitudes and thus suggest a positive effect on the fitness of mountain Caprini. Conversely, in the case of erythropoietic stress, it was suggested (Pieragostini et al., 1994; Pieragostini et al., 2006) that Hb C might negatively affect peripheral oxygen delivery and worsen the clinical picture of sheep breeds native of areas with endemic haemotropic pathogens. Hence, in the present case, the *conditio sine qua non* for checking the effect of beta globin genotype was the detection of Hb C switched on in AB individuals following a strong erythropoietic stress. As an example, figure 6 also shows the different trend after infection (days = 0) of the Hb content for the AB and BB ewes. Apart from individual differences observed in reaching the lowest Hb values, the recovery was always faster in BB sheep, as also indicated by the significantly higher quadratic regression coefficient of Hb for BB *vs* AB genotype (0.0045 *vs* 0.0027, $P < 0.03$). The different behaviour of one of the three heterozygous subject (Figure 6) may be justified by its less severe haematological picture due to a lower anoxaemic stress, also confirmed by the lack of the Hb A to Hb C switch in the same animal.

5.2.3 Functional effect of alpha globin system on the response to the anaplasmosis

As mentioned before, the extra numeral alpha globin haplotypes (EH) were suggested to be related to the host's response to TBDs. The unusual frequency of EH recorded in southern Italian sheep breeds and the peculiar haematologic pattern exhibited by the EH homozygous subjects may be taken as evidence of a selective advantage of the corresponding phenotypes in endemic TBD areas. Individuals carrying extra alpha-globin genes exhibit an overall blood picture mimicking a thalassaemia-like syndrome. In greater detail, when the erythrocytes of EH homozygotes were compared with those of NH individuals, the former had fewer erythrocytes that were bigger in size and had a higher Hb content and a greater erythrocyte osmotic fragility. These changes in EH homozygotes were assumed to produce an unfavorable environment for the parasites.

Thus, the trial checked this hypothesis as the different haematological patterns and the accelerated turnover of erythrocytes of EH individuals compared to the NH ones were expected to produce differences in the spread of the pathogen into the host blood.

Unfortunately a relevant element of prejudicial questions to obtain maximum results was the fact that only EH heterozygotes were present in the Altamurana group, since no homozygous lambs were found during the population survey. In normal health conditions, such as those recorded in the experience reported by Pieragostini et al. (2003), the EH heterozygotes showed an intermediate pattern, between that of EH homozygotes and that of NH homozygotes (Pieragostini, unpublished data).

The second relevant element was the level of response which undoubtedly is a limiting factor in checking the results.

Thirdly, owing to experimental constraints, the sample size was of nine subjects per each alpha haplotype group. Hence, based on these considerations, we could not expect striking results as to the functional effect of the alpha globin gene arrangements, except in the case of a strong interaction with the response to experimental infections. Despite our hopes, our concerns were well-founded because all the above elements of prejudicial questions affected the results.

α-globin gene arrangements	N	T.P. (°C)	PCV (g/dl)	Hb (g/dl)	RBC (10^6/μl)	MCV (fl)	MCH (pg)	MCHC (g/dl)	WBC (10^3/μl)
NH	9	40.1 A ± 0.18	25.9 ± 1.55	8.1 ± 0.89	7.8 ± 0.85	33.1 ± 1.03	10.4 ± 0.51	31.4 ± 0.51	10.3 ± 1.29
EH	9	39.8 B ± 0.12	26.3 ± 1.18	8.5 ± 0.39	8.0 ± 0.31	33.7 ± 0.73	10.6 ± 0.43	31.4 ± 0.47	10.5 ± 1.17

Table 11. Temperature peak and haematological parameters assessed during the acute phase of the disease, for the two Altamurana groups classified on the basis of the α-globin gene arrangement. Means within columns with different letters significantly differ; capital letters: $P < 0.01$.

Altamurana subjects exhibited a very mild symptoms and no patent differences could be recorded in terms of haematological pattern between the EH and NH individuals within the Altamurana group. The EH group had a temperature peak that was significantly lower ($P < 0.001$) than that of the NH group. This suggested that the level of response to infection in the EH group was lighter than in the NH group (Table 12). Morever, as shown in table 11, though no significance was attained by the ANOVA when the mean values of the haematological parameters of the two groups were compared, a univocal trend emerged whereby the RBC, PCV and Hb values in the EH group decreased less than in the NH group. These two phenomena seem to indicate a milder *Anaplasma* infection in EH subjects than in the NH individuals.

6. Conclusions

Several examples of breed-related tolerance to diseases have been reported worldwide but often the claims made for specific breeds have not been subject to scientific investigation. As to small ruminants, only tolerance to Heartwater (Cowdriosis) has been documented for Damara, a South African native sheep breed (Commission on Genetic Resources for Food and Agriculture, 2007). This report extends our knowledge about tolerance to tick borne diseases. The main findings can be summarized in the following points:

- Tolerance to piroplasmosis is documented for Apulian (Altamurana, Gentile di Puglia and Leccese) and Italian islander (Comisana and Sarda) sheep breeds.
- Non-tolerance to piroplasmosis is documented for Finnish, Friesian and Romanov breeds.
- Suffolk breed is shown to be not tolerant to anaplasmosis.
- Different physiological pattern and environment of origin may explain breed-specific haematological characteristics.
- Altamurana sheep breed is tolerant to anaemia *per se.*
- The response of Altamurana to simultaneous *B. ovis* and *A. ovis* infection results in a mild anaemia.
- There seems to be confirmatory evidence that haemoglobin genetic systems underlie the host response in the acute phase of disease and in recovery.

7. Aknowledgements

The earlier experiences reported in this work were supported by Bari University and/or the Italian Ministry for University and Research. The last section is part of a project sponsored by the Italian Ministry for Agriculture, Food and Forestry Policies (MIPAAF) for the improvement of animal breeding by means of molecular genetics (SELMOL). As far as the expert identification of TBP, the Authors are deeply endebted to Dr. Alessandra Torina head of the national reference laboratory for *tick-borne* diseases (C.R.A.BA.R.T.- Istituto Zooprofilattico Sperimentale della Sicilia "A. Mirri", Palermo, Italy). The authors are grateful to Dr. Rosanna Lacinio for the quality of her technical support at the haematology laboratory of the Veterinary Clinic of Bari University along years of collaboration. The authors are also grateful to Dr. Athina Papa for her accuracy in revising the English of the manuscript.

8. References

Aguilar-Delfin, I., Homer, M.J., Wettstein, P.J. & Persing, D.H. (2001). Innate resistance to Babesia infection is influenced by genetic background and gender. *Infection and Immunity*, Vol. 69, No. 12, December 2001, pp. 7955-8. ISSN 0019-9567

Agyemang, K., Dwinger, R.H., Touray, B.N., Jeannin, P., Fofana, D. & Grieve, A.S. (1990). Effects of nutrition on the degree of anaemia and liveweight changes in N'Dama cattle infected with trypanosomes. *Livestock Production Science,* Vol. 26 No. 1, September 1990, pp. 39-51, ISSN 0301-6226

Alderson, L. (2009). Breeds at risk: Definition and measurement of the factors which determine endangerment. *Livestock Science,* Vol. 123, No. 1, July 2009, pp. 23-27, ISSN 1871-1413

Alloggio, I., de Ruvo, G., Torina, A., Caroli, A., Petazzi, F. & Pieragostini E. (2009). Reversibile switch from haemoglobin A to C in sheep and recovery from anemia following experimental infection with *Anaplasma ovis. Italian Journal of Animal Science,* Vol. 8, No. S2, January 2010, pp. 27-29 ISBN/ISSN 1594-4077

Ariely, R., Heth, G., Nevo, E. & Hoch, D. (1986). Haematocrit and haemoglobin concentration in four chromosomal species and isolated population of actively speciating subterranean mole rats in Israel. *Experientia,* Vol. 42, No. 4, April 1986, pp. 440-443, ISSN 0014-4754

Bennison, J.J., Clemence, R.G., Archibald, R.F., Hendy, C.R.C. & Dempfle, L. (1998). The effect of work and two planes of nutrition on trypanotoleralt draught cattle infected with *Trypanosoma congolense. Animal Science,* Vol. 66, No. 3, June 1998, pp. 595-605, ISSN 1806-2636

Ceci, L & Carelli, G. (1999). Tick-borne diseases of livestock in Italy: general review and results of recent studies carried out in the Apulia region. Parassitologia. Sep; 41 Suppl 1:25-9.

Commission on Genetic Resources for Food and Agriculture, Food and Agriculture Organization of the United Nations (2007). *The State of the World's Animal Genetic Resources for Food and Agriculture.* Barbara Rischkowsky & Dafydd Pilling, eds. ISBN ISBN 9789251057629, Rome, Italy

Correia De Almeida Regitano, L. & Prayaga, K. (2010). Ticks and tick-borne diseases in cattle, In: *Breeding for Disease Resistance in Farm Animals,* Bishop, S.C., Axford, R.F.E., Nicholas, F.W. & Owen, J.B., pp. 295-314, CAB International, ISBN 978 1 84593 555 9, UK

Cresswell, E. & Hutchings, H. (1962). A comparison of production on blood values between the Romney Marsh and the Cheviot ewes in New Zealand. *Research in Veterinary Science,* Vol. 3, pp. 209–214, ISSN 00345288.

de la Fuente, J., Van Den Bussche, R.A., Prado, T.M. & Kocan, K.M. (2003). *Anaplasma marginale* msp1α genotypes evolved under positive selection pressure but are not markers for geographic isolates. *Journal of Clinical Microbiology,* Vol. 41, No. 4, April 2003, pp. 1609–1616, ISSN 0095-1137

de la Fuente J., Massung R. F., Wong S. J., Chu F. K., Lutz H., Meli M., von Loewenich F. D., Gzeszczuk A., Torina A., Caracappa S., Mangold A.J., Naranjo V., Stuen S., Kocan K.M. (2005). Sequence Analysis of the msp4 Gene of Anaplasma phagocytophilum Strains. J. Clin. Microbiol., 43, 1309–1317.

de la Fuente, J., Atkinson, M.W., Naranjo, V., Fernández de Mera, I.G., Mangold, A.J., Keating, K.A., Kocan, K.M. (2007). Sequence analysis of the msp4 gene of Anaplasma ovis strains. Vet. Microbiol. 119: 375-381.

Dumler, J.S., Barbet, A.F, Bekker, C.P., Dasch, G.A., Palmer, G.H., Ray, S.C., Rikihisa, Y. & Rurangirwa, F.R. (2001). Reorganization of genera in the families *Rickettsiaceae* and *Anaplasmataceae* in the order *Rickettsiales*: unification of some species of *Ehrlichia* with *Anaplasma, Cowdria* with *Ehrlichia* and *Ehrlichia* with *Neorickettsia,* descriptions of six new species combinations and designation of *Ehrlichia equi* and 'HGE agent' as subjective synonyms of *Ehrlichia phagocytophila. International Journal of Systematic and Evolutionary Microbiology,* Vol. 51, No. 6, November 2001, pp. 2145–2165, ISSN 1466-5026.

Evans, A. G. & Wellems, T. E. (2002). Coevolutionary genetics of *Plasmodium malaria* parasites and their human hosts. *Integrative and Comparative Biology,* Vol. 42, No. 2, April 2002, pp 401–407, ISSN 1557-7023.

Greenwood B. (1977). Haematology of the sheep and the goat, In: *Comparative Clinical Haematology*, Archer R.K., Jeffcott L.B., pp.305-308, Blackwell Scientific Publications, ISBN 0 632 00289 1, Oxford, UK .

Horin, P. (1998). Biological principles of heredity of and resistance to disease. *Revue scientifique et technique*, Vol. 17, No. 1, April 1998, pp. 302-314, ISSN 0253-1933.

Huisman, T.H. & Kitchens, J. (1968). Oxygen equilibria studies of the haemoglobins from normal and anemic sheep and goats. *American Journal of Physiology*, Vol. 215, No. 1, July 1968, pp. 140-146, ISSN 0002-9513

Jain, N.C. (1993). *Essential of Veterinary Haematology*. Lea & Febiger, ISBN 081211437X, Philadelphia, PA.

Jongejan, F. & Uilenberg, G. (2004). The global importance of ticks. *Parasitology*, Vol. 129, No. S1, October 2004, pp. S3–S14, ISSN 0031-1820

McCosker, P.J. (1979). Global aspects of the management and control of ticks of veterinary importance, In: *Recent Advances in Acarology*, Rodriguez, J.G., pp. 45–53, Academic Press, ISBN 0125922027, New York

Nienhuis, A. W. & Anderson, W. F. (1972). Haemoglobin switching in sheep and goats: change in functional globin messenger RNA in reticulocytes and bone marrow cells. *Proc. Natl. Acad. Sci.*, Vol. 69, No. 8, August 1972, pp. 2184-2188, ISSN 1091-6490

Nienhuis, A.W. & Bunn, H.F. (1974). Haemoglobin switching in sheep and goats: occurrence of haemoglobins A and C in the same red cell. *Science*. Vol. 185, No. 9, August 1974, pp. 946-948, ISSN 0036-8075

Oppliger, A., Clobert, J., Lecompte, J., Lorenzon, P., Boudjiemadi, K. & John-Alder, H.B. (1998). Environmental stress increases the prevalence and intensity of blood parasite infection in the common lizard *Lacerta vivipara*. *Ecology Letters*, Vol. 1, No. 2, September 1998, pp. 129-138, ISSN 1461-0248

Pieragostini, E., Dario, C. & Bufano, G. (1994). Haemoglobin phenotypes and hematological factors in Leccese sheep. *Small Ruminant Research*, Vol. 13, No. 2, March 1994, pp. 177-185, ISSN 0921-4488

Pieragostini, E., Dario, C., Petazzi, F. & Bufano, G. (1996). La piroplasmosi negli ovini pugliesi: una malattia da scarso reddito. Nota III. Profilassi e performance riproduttive. *Proceedings of the XIII International Congress of Mediterranean Federation for Ruminant Health and Production*, Murcia (Spain), 27-28 May 1996.

Pieragostini, E. & Petazzi, F. (1999). Genetics and tolerance to tick borne diseases in South Italy: experience in studying native Apulian and exotic sheep breeds. *Parassitologia*, Vol. 41, No. S1, September 1999, pp. 89-94, ISSN 0048-2951

Pieragostini, E., Petazzi, F. & Rubino, G. (1999). Haematological values in Apulian native sheep breeds. *Proceeding of the VII International Congress of Mediterranean Federation for Ruminant Health and Production*, ISBN/ISSN: 972-8126-05-0, Santarem, Portugal, 22–24 April 1999

Pieragostini, E., Petazzi, F., Rubino, G., Rullo, R. & Sasanelli, M. (2000). Switching emoglobinico, quadro ematologico e primo incontro con i parassiti endoeritrocitari enzootici in agnelli autoctoni pugliesi. *Obiettivi e Documenti Veterinari.* Vol. 7/8, pp. 31-40, ISSN 0392-1913.

Pieragostini E, Petazzi F, Di Luccia A. 2003 The relationship between the presence of extra alpha-globin genes and blood cell traits in Altamurana sheep. Genetic Selection Evolution, Vol. 35 No. 1, July 2003, pp. S121-133, ISSN 0999-193X.

Pieragostini, E., Rubino, G., Bramante, G., Rullo, R., Petazzi, F. & Caroli, A. (2006). Functional effect of haemoglobin polymorphism on the haematological pattern of Gentile di Puglia sheep. *Journal of Animal Breeding and Genetics,* Vol. 123 No. 2, April 2006, pp. 122-130, ISSN 0931-2668

Rubino, G., Cito, A.M., Lacinio, R., Bramante, G., Caroli, A., Pieragostini, E. & Petazzi, F. (2006). Hematology and some blood chemical parameters as a function of tick-borne disease (TBD) signs in horses. *Journal of Equine Veterinary Science,* Vol. 26, No. 10, October 2006, pp. 475-480, ISSN 0737-0806

Radostits, O. M., Arundel, J. H. & Gay, C.C. (2000). *Veterinary medicine: a textbook of the diseases of cattle, sheep, pigs, goats and horses* (9th ed.). W. B. Saunders & Co. ISBN 0702026042, Philadelphia, PA.

SAS, 1990: SA/Stat User's Guide, Version 6, 4th ed. SAS Institute Inc., Cary, NC.

Sayin, F., Dyncer, S., Karaer, Z., Cakmak, A., Yukary, B.A., Eren, H., Deger, S. & Nalbantoglu S. (1997). Status of the tick-borne diseases in sheep and goats in Turkey. *Parassitologia.* Vol. 39, No. 2, June 1997, pp. 153-156, ISSN 0048-2951

Schnittger, L., Yin, H., Qi, B., Gubbels, M.J., Beyer, D., Niemann, S., Jongejan, F., Ahmed, J.S. (2004). Simultaneous detection and differentiation of Theileria and Babesia parasites infecting small ruminants by reverse line blotting. Parasitol Res, 92:189-96.

Stuen, S., Nevland, S. & Moum T. (2003). Fatal cases of tick-borne fever (TBF) in sheep caused by several 16S rRNA gene variants of Anaplasma phagocytophilum. *Annals of the New York Academy of Sciences,* Vol. 990, June 2003, pp. 443-444 ISSN 1749-6632

Townsend, R.F. & Thirtle, C.G. (2001). Is livestock research unproductive? Separating health maintenance from improvement research. *Agricultural Economics,* Vol. 25, No. 2-3, October 2001, pp. 177-189, ISSN 0019-5014

van Vliet, G. & Huisman, T.H.J. (1964). Changes in the haemoglobin types of sheep as a response to anemia. *Biochem. J.* Vol. 93, No. 2, November 1964, pp. 401–409, ISSN 0264-6021

Whitelock, J.H. (1963). The influence of heredity and environment on maximum haematocrit values in sheep. *Cornell Veterinarian,* Vol. 53, October 1963, pp. 534–550, ISSN 0010-8901

Yeruham, I., Hadani, A. & Galker, F. (1998). Some epizootiological and clinical aspects of ovine babesiosis caused by *Babesia ovis.* A review. *Veterinary Parasitology,* Vol. 74, No. 2-4, January 1998, pp. 153-63, ISSN 0304-4017

Yin H & Luo J. (2007). Ticks of small ruminants in China. *Parasitol Res.,* Vol. 101, No. 2, September 2007, pp S187-189, ISSN 0932-011.

Youatt, W. (1867). *Sheep: their breeds, management, and diseases*. Orange Judd & Co., New York.

7

Prolactin and Schizophrenia, an Evolving Relationship

Chris J. Bushe[1] and John Pendlebury[2]
[1]*Eli Lilly and Company Ltd, Basingstoke,*
[2]*Ramsgate House, Manchester*
UK

1. Introduction

Prolactin is a polypeptide hormone originally discovered from the crop glands of pigeons in 1933 (Riddle et al, 1933; Bushe and Pendlebury, 2010), however there was some scepticism that prolactin even existed in humans until the 1970s as human prolactin was considered identical to growth hormone (GH). During the 1970s, the development of radioimmunoassay techniques allowed the isolation of prolactin and its subsequent measurement (Kohen and Wildgust, 2008). Since that time, awareness of the consequences of hyperprolactinaemia in psychiatry has been less than rapid despite clear evidence that many psychotropic agents, in particular antipsychotics, elevate prolactin levels to some degree in many patients. As a result, prolactin monitoring is not commonplace and many clinicians remain unsure of its utility. In part, this may relate to lack of knowledge regarding pathological endpoints caused by hyperprolactinaemia.

In the last decade, however, awareness has begun to emerge of the potential consequences of untreated hyperprolactinaemia including short-term adverse events of sexual dysfunction, amenorrhoea and infertility and longer term consequences that may include bone fractures and breast cancer. This has been due in part to a number of reviews focussing on the potential consequences of hyperprolactinaemia and the relatively high prevalence of this adverse event (Haddad and Wieck, 2004; Bostwick et al, 2009; Bushe and Pendlebury, 2010),). In 2008 the first set of prolactin monitoring guidelines was published and more recent data have begun to evaluate the use of specific polypharmacy to reduce prolactin levels (Peveler et al, 2008). There remain, however, many unanswered questions; most relate to the need to establish the true incidence of longer term sequelae of hyperprolactinaemia and to the simple question- what level of prolactin actually carries consequences and when? When one considers that prolactin has at least 300 biological actions it may be that this diversity of function will lead to research that further defines the precise role of and subsequent pathology induced by hyperprolactinaemia (Fitzgerald and Dinan, 2008).

2. Prolactin – What do we know about the hormone?

2.1 Structure and release

Prolactin, a polypeptide hormone that binds to prolactin receptors, is considered part of the Class 1 cytokine receptor family present in various organs including pancreas, liver, uterus and prostate and consequently may have some immunological activity. It is predominantly synthesised and secreted from the lactotroph cells of the anterior pituitary (Fitzgerald and Dinan, 2008). Lactotrophs form around 20-50% of the cellular population of the pituitary with those in the more inner zones being more responsive to dopamine. Structurally, prolactin is a single chain of 199 amino-acids containing six cysteine residues and three disulfide bonds with 40% homology between the genes encoding prolactin and GH (Fitzgerald and Dinan, 2008).

Prolactin is released from the anterior pituitary in a pulsatile manner and has a half life of around 50 minutes (Citrome, 2008). It peaks around 10 times per day in young adults (Holt, 2008) with a marked circadian rhythm highest during sleep and reaching a nadir during waking hours. Time of measurement is thus important to standardise and is best undertaken before drug dosing in a fasting state in the morning, although this is not always pragmatic in schizophrenia due to the nature of the illness. Measurement of levels during the day needs to be relatively precise as stress factors, exercise and eating can alter levels. In addition, there appears to be an annual circadian variation though with little clinical relevance. Garde et al (2000) reported that prolactin was highest in healthy female subjects in March-May (153 mIU/L) and lowest in September-November (98 mIU/L) (Garde et al, 2000).

Increasingly other confounding factors are being recognised that potentially also affect prolactin levels and any clinical interpretation of abnormality. For example, fluctuating prolactin levels have been found to be greater over the 24-hour period after dosing with perospirone than with either risperidone or olanzapine, despite the magnitude of hyperprolactinaemia being greater with risperidone (Yasui-Furukori et al, 2010). Recent data are supportive of current smokers taking antipsychotics having both a lower mean prolactin level (odds ratio [OR] 2.3, 95% confidence interval [CI] 1.2-4.7, p=0.002) and a lower prevalence of hyperprolactinaemia (Mackin et al, 2010) and other data are supportive at a minimum that is true in females (Ohta et al, 2011). This may be a critical confounder in schizophrenia where almost all patients smoke and indeed smoke more cigarettes than smokers in the general population. Other confounders are much better recognised with a study of 154 schizophrenia patients taking 6mg risperidone reporting that prolactin levels correlate with gender (higher in females), age (lower in older patients) and smoking status (p<0.01) based on a multiple regression analysis (Ohta et al, 2011).

Control of prolactin secretion from the anterior pituitary is predominantly under the control of dopamine released via hypothalamic dopaminergic neurons, the tuberoinfundibular and tuberohypophyseal dopaminergic neurones (Holt, 2008). Dopamine is transported from the hypothalamus to the anterior pituitary via the long hypophyseal portal vessels and inhibits the high basal secretory tone of the lactotroph. This high basal secretory activity is unique amongst endocrine cells. The released prolactin regulates the dopamine synthesis from the hypothalamus via a feedback loop.

The mechanism whereby prolactin is elevated by D2 blockade remains undetermined. However, the most likely explanations relate to speed of D2 dissociation and the ability of the antipsychotic to cross the blood brain barrier (Bushe et al, 2010), with drugs dissociating slowly being associated with greater prolactin elevation. In contrast, quetiapine, an example of an antipsychotic with fast dissociation, has low rates of prolactin elevation being associated with central D2 occupancy that falls from initial blockade of 60-70% at 2 hours post-dosing to around 30% at 24 hours.

3. Measurement of prolactin and definition of hyperprolactinaemia

Units of measurement have the potential to cause some confusion as US and EU data are often presented in ng/ml whereas most UK data are in mIU/L. Conversion rates from ng/ml to mIU/L are not standardised and vary between 21.2 and 36 dependent on the assay employed (Bushe et al, 2008). Furthermore, clinical reports do not always report either the normal range utilised or sometimes the units of measurement (McEvoy et al, 2007).

Definitions of hyperprolactinaemia vary depending upon the upper limit of normal (ULN) for the local assay. Normal ranges for females tend often to be around 30% higher than males, with some laboratories also reporting separate ranges for premenopausal and postmenopausal females. In the psychiatric literature, some of the highest ULNs for females are around 700 mIU/L and, for males, 500 mIU/L (Bushe and Shaw 2007), with lowest ULN at 300 mIU/L for females (Meaney et al, 2004). The Maudsley guidelines 10th edition (Taylor et al, 2009) gives fairly specific advice on blood sampling (1 hour after waking or eating) and cites normal ranges in both ng/ml and mIU/L. In their view, the ULN for females is <530 mIU/L and for males is <424 mIU/L; re-testing is advised if the prolactin level is between 530-2120 mIU/L.

There is currently also no specific definition for an elevated prolactin level that may be regarded as clinically non-significant and when we published our original data set there was no specific guidance to either diagnose or grade level of severity of hyperprolactinaemia (Bushe/Shaw 2007). Thus, we created three specific grades of hyperprolactinaemia: slightly elevated (<1000 mIU/L), significant elevation (1001-2000 mIU/L) and severe elevation (>2000mIU/L). This was based on empirical judgement and not with relation to specifically defined outcomes. In general terms, prolactin levels <2000 mIU/L may be due to a medication effect but other causes can include microprolactinoma, pituitary stalk compression, renal failure or hypothyroidism (Holt, 2008). The literature currently reports that macroprolactinomas are the most common cause of prolactin levels >2120 mIU/L in the general population (Bushe et al, 2010) although other authors propose higher levels (3180 mIU/L) at which hyperprolactinaemia can be assumed to be caused by a macroprolactinoma (Holt, 2008).

When evaluating hyperprolactinaemia it is also critical to understand the incidence or prevalence of hyperprolactinaemia from the patient perspective as opposed to a mean level from a cohort. Recent data are now tending to more commonly include both variables (Mackin et al, 2011) whereas in our 2008 review of this topic we reported that though 60% of studies reporting prolactin data included some degree of categorical analysis, this was seen mainly in the naturalistic studies (88%) rather than the randomised controlled trials (42%) (Bushe et al, 2008).

4. Consequences of hyperprolactinaemia

Many of the longer term definitive outcomes associated with elevated prolactin remain unknown. Recent findings of prolactin receptors in atherosclerotic plaques in coronary arteries of healthy subjects indicate a possible role of prolactin even in coronary artery disease (Reuwer et al, 2009). There are, however, three areas of pathology that would seem to be closely linked to elevated prolactin, sexual function, bone loss and cancer and these can be considered as short- and longer term potential adverse events.

4.1 Short term consequences of hyperprolactinaemia

4.1.1 Sexual function

Sex hormone dysregulation may be the underlying cause of both acute and longer term adverse events associated with hyperprolactinaemia as prolactin has a significant effect on sex hormone regulation and prolactin levels in patients treated with antipsychotics are inversely related to steroid sex hormone concentrations (Smith, 2002). However, the absolute link between prolactin and sexual dysfunction is complex. The relative short-term consequences of hyperprolactinaemia are well described and, in addition, to sexual dysfunction include menstrual disturbances, acne, infertility, galactorheoa and gynaecomastia although prevalence rates were until recently not well reported. In 2011, the European First Episode Schizophrenia Trial (EUFEST) study of first episode schizophrenia patients reported that sexual dysfunction was very common at baseline (Malik et al, 2011) and although often attributed to antipsychotics this is not the complete picture as smoking, physical illness, depressive and negative symptoms may also be relevant (Malik et al, 2011). Over the 1-year study, changes in prevalence of sexual dysfunction were small and varied little between antipsychotics despite hyperprolactinaemia being very common and moderately severe (Kahn et al, 2008). The authors concluded that their data emphasized that schizophrenia the illness was a key influence on sexual dysfunction although hyperprolactinemia undoubtedly plays an additional role (Malik et al, 2011). There is also an important investigational aspect to consider. In most antipsychotic studies previous medication prior to study entry is either inadequately or incompletely described, which makes interpretation of variables such as prolactin and sexual dysfunction complex. It is possible that changes measured during the trial may relate to the removal of a previous antipsychotic. As such the only data that can give a true baseline are data in treatment-naïve subjects from studies such as EUFEST. Not all data, however, are consistent with this view that prolactin may play a smaller role in sexual dysfunction than expected (Knegtering et al, 2008). For example, in a 6-week, open label study including 264 patients treated with antipsychotics, prolactin-raising antipsychotics were linked with significantly more sexual-related adverse events than patients treated with prolactin-sparing antipsychotics. The authors concluded that around 40% of emerging sexual adverse events in schizophrenia are attributable to prolactin (Knegtering et al, 2008). The importance of seeking overt symptomatology however is that it offers the opportunity to measure prolactin as many guidelines have previously not suggested prolactin measurements until the presence of relevant symptoms. The literature is fairly conclusive that sexual dysfunction is not always regarded as an important aspect to discuss with patients in routine clinical practice.

4.2 Longer term consequences of hyperprolactinaemia

4.2.1 Bone

Data on hyperprolactinaemia and bone loss have appeared during the last decade predominantly due to the work of Veronica O'Keane. Her group systematically followed the link between hyperprolactinaemia and sex hormones (males and females) and then between hyperprolactinaemia and bone loss. Some studies suggest that even relatively short periods of hyperprolactinaemia can have significant adverse effects on bone density (Meaney and O'Keane, 2007; O'Keane, 2008). Young women may be particularly susceptible to hyperprolactinaemia, and osteoporosis and osteopenia may develop in the first 8 years of antipsychotic treatment (Meaney and O'Keane, 2007; O'Keane, 2008). Of more concern is the finding that deterioration can be measured over a single year and essentially cannot be prevented (Meaney and O'Keane, 2007; O'Keane, 2008). A second set of key epidemiological studies evaluating fractures in large UK cohorts was published suggesting that hip and other bone fractures are a sequelae of mental illness and its treatment. Howard reported that hyperprolactinaemia and prolactin-elevating antipsychotics have been associated with a doubling of the risk of hip fracture in schizophrenia patients in a large UK study (OR 2.6, CI 2.43-2.78) (Howard et al, 2007). A second study also using the UK General Practice Research Database (GPRD) reported that in women the highest relative risk of fracture in a mentally ill population were in the youngest cohorts, whereas in males the greatest risks were seen in older age (Abel et al, 2008). The results showed that the relative risk (RR) of any fracture was increased more than double in females with psychotic disorders (RR 2.5: CI 1.5-4.3) but that even greater risk was measured in the cohort aged 45-74 years with psychotic disorders, with a relative risk in women of RR 5.1 (CI 2.7-9.6) and in males RR 6.4 (CI 2.6-16.1) when looking specifically at hip fractures (Abel et al, 2008). This risk may be seen to an even greater extent in males than females (Howard et al, 2007) and is present after adjusting for the other risk factors for osteoporosis highly prevalent in a cohort of patients with severe mental illness (poor diet, low exercise rates, increased alcohol consumption and decreased sunlight exposure). Other data however are needed for other fracture sites (radius and vertebrae) together with some indication as to whether it is the cumulative length of hyperprolactinaemia that is crucial (a sort of area under the curve measurement) or the effect of a critical peak level of prolactin. Recent data in non-schizophrenic males with prolactinoma reported that using DEXA scanning of the lumbar spine vertebral fractures were diagnosed in 37.5% of patients compared with 7.8% of controls ($p<0.001$) (Mazziotti et al, 2011) and that these developed independently of hypogonadism.

4.2.2 Possible association with cancer

A recent systematic review concluded that breast cancer is significantly increased in females with schizophrenia but the data have simply not been published to establish the degree of the putative role of prolactin in this increased risk (Bushe et al, 2009). A number of epidemiological studies have reported data over the last 25 years but it is only in the last few years that clarity has emerged. The importance of systematic review in addressing a clinical question is clear. In this case, when studies with adequate powering and follow up undertaken in an age group where cancer developed (>50 yrs for breast cancer predominantly) are considered, the results were clear. The specific relevance of breast cancer is that it is the most common cancer in women in the UK, it accounts for 23% of all female cancer cases worldwide, there is a lifetime risk of 1 in 9 in the general population and this risk is increasing (Bushe et al, 2010). A recent meta-analysis that included fewer studies than our systematic review (Catts et al, 2008) reported a 12% increased risk (Standardised Incidence Ratio [SIR] 1.12, 95% CI 1.02-1.23) with a more recent UK study reporting an increased risk of 52% in schizophrenia adjusting for recognised confounders such as poverty (Hippisley-Cox et al, 2007). One can only speculate over the role of prolactin and mammary carcinogenesis, however in animal toxicity and molecular studies, it has been recognised over many years (Harvey 2008) that there is a very strong association. The US Nurses' Health Study evaluated prolactin samples from 32,826 patients with normal prolactin levels during the period 1989 to 1990 and these subjects have been extensively followed over 20 years, providing conclusive evidence linking prolactin and breast cancer in the general population. Many of their study reports suggest prolactin levels to be linked to the risk of breast cancer development both in pre- and postmenopausal women (Tworoger and Hankinson, 2006; Tworoger et al, 2007). An example of these data found prolactin levels in the upper quartile of normal to be associated with an increased risk compared to the lower quartile of normal (OR 1.34, 95% CI 1.02-1.76) (Tworoger et al, 2007). Any definitive link, however, has yet to be established in schizophrenia and bipolar disorder.

A large retrospective cohort study of 52,819 females receiving antipsychotics and 55,289 control women reported a 16% increased risk of breast cancer (Wang et al, 2002) with a dose response relationship suggesting a greater risk of breast cancer with increased doses of antipsychotic. Regardless of relationship with prolactin, identical breast cancer screening should be encouraged in all schizophrenia subjects as in the general population. Screening rates for schizophrenia patients are very low compared with the general population for an illness that is very common (lifetime prevalence 1 in 9 and rising) and often curable (Bushe et al, 2010).

Hyperprolactinaemia has also been linked to pituitary adenomas and adenocarcinomas and putatively to prostate cancer (Harvey et al, 2008). The US Food and Drug Administration Adverse Event Reporting System pharmacovigilance database study strongly linked risperidone (adjusted reporting ratio 18.7) with the highest frequency of pituitary adenomas compared with haloperidol (5.6), ziprasidone (3.0) and olanzapine (2.3) (Szarfman et al, 2006). A recent case series is suggestive that amisulpride may also be associated with the development of prolactinomas mediated via hyperprolactinaemia (Akkaya et al, 2009).

The multiple actions of prolactin and relative lack of research into hyperprolactinaemia suggest that additional potential long-term effects may be discovered potentially in glands such as the thyroid. Recent data suggest there may be an association with autoimmune thyroiditis and in 75 schizophrenia patients, the prevalence of hyperprolactinaemia was higher in patients with thyroid autoantibodies ($p=0.045$) (Poyraz et al, 2008).

5. Relationship between serum prolactin concentration and adverse events

This is a complex question that remains totally unanswered for the potential longer term sequelae but can be partially addressed for short-term adverse events. There would seem to be two potential associations. Firstly, a chronic prolactin elevation that reaches a cumulative threshold over a longer term and secondly, a peak prolactin level that requires a trigger threshold to initiate pathology. Levels <1000 mIU/L are associated with decreased libido and infertility, 1000-1600 mIU/L with oligomenorrhoea, and >2000 mIU/L with amenorrhea and hypogonadism (Peveler et al, 2008). Hypogonadism is the main driver for bone mineral density loss and fractures although the possibility exists that prolactin may have a direct osteoclastic effect. Data on longer term prolactin levels tend not to report the associated changes in sex hormones making interpretation complex. The topic has, however, been reviewed (Bushe et al, 2008) and in cross-sectional prevalence studies that report bone mineral density loss in association with typicals or risperidone over 8-21 years, the mean cohort values ranged 908-3024 mIU/L (Bushe et al, 2010). These levels are common and are reached quickly in patients treated with risperidone and amisulpride (Bushe and Shaw 2007; Bushe et al, 2008). A small case series of patients receiving paliperidone reported hyperprolactinaemia within 3 weeks with levels ranging from 1500-3996 mIU/L (Skopek et al, 2010). Prolactin levels related to breast cancer in schizophrenia and bipolar disorder are unknown, however data are supportive of levels as low as 500 mIU/L being associated with an increased risk of breast cancer in the general population over the medium term (Tworoger and Hankinson 2006, Tworoger et al, 2007). However, it is critical to understand that whereas there is a strong link between prolactin and breast cancer in the general population, there are no data to address this topic in schizophrenia and bipolar disorder. In addition, breast cancer has very many aetiological factors that include social demographics, education, obesity and family history and the role of prolactin is simply not known.

6. How common is hyperprolactinaemia in an antipsychotic-treated cohort?

6.1 Overview

There are few cohorts where prolactin levels have been obtained in a complete cohort and rates of hyperprolactinaemia will be dependent on many factors including medication choice, gender, age and length of follow up. Data derived from epidemiological databases is also confounded by selection bias. Without knowing how many subjects were tested there is little way to put perspective around these data (Montgomery et al, 2004). A true perspective requires a complete cohort to be tested. Many other confounders will remain, however, including gender, smoking status, adherence to treatment, age and time on treatment.

Olanzapine, for example, may give a transient elevation of prolactin that reduces over the first months in some patients but during chronic administration prolactin elevation may remain (Bushe et al, 2008). Naturalistic data may thus be informative as prolactin monitoring is not routine and prevalence rates in complete populations screened will reflect previous under-diagnosis. Two recent naturalistic analyses in which asymptomatic schizophrenia populations have been screened for prolactin report similar prevalence of hyperprolactinaemia: 38% and 39% in UK (n=194) and Norway (n=106), respectively (Bushe and Shaw 2007; Johnsen et al, 2008). The UK study measured prolactin in the total population of a catchment area in Halifax receiving antipsychotics for schizophrenia or bipolar disorder. The population was clinically asymptomatic prior to the study. Hyperprolactinaemia was more common in females than males (52 vs. 26%), consistent with most other data (Bushe et al, 2008), and significantly elevated levels (>1000 mIU/L) were measured in 21% of subjects. For 13% of females and 19% of males, prolactin levels were above the normal limit but below 1001 mIU/L. Categorical rates of hyperprolactinaemia in trials range from 33 to 69% and confirm that no antipsychotic is prolactin neutral (Bushe et al, 2008). Most studies report both a higher prevalence and severity of hyperprolactinaemia in females as was the case in the Halifax study which found 13% of females had levels >2000 mIU/L compared with 2% of males (Bushe and Shaw, 2007).

6.2 Rates of hyperprolactinaemia with individual antipsychotics

The ideal studies to evaluate prolactin would be a long-term, first episode study where the confounding factor of previous antipsychotic usage would not need addressing and which included multiple treatment arms and a longer term randomised study in chronic schizophrenia. There are few such studies with the exception of EUFEST (Kahn et al, 2008) and CATIE (Lieberman et al, 2005). EUFEST was a 1-year, first episode study and CATIE, an 18-month study with multiple treatment arms. Both these studies concluded that hyperprolactinaemia was common though EUFEST failed to find a direct link between prolactin and sexual dysfunction.

The totality of the data is convincing that there is no such entity as a "prolactin-sparing" antipsychotic, however, data are sometimes complex to interpret. There are numerous confounding factors but broadly psychotropic polypharmacy, the choice and the dose of medication are relevant factors as are often the lack of reported data on previous antipsychotic treatment. Adherence is also important as many typicals are now administered by long-acting depot formulations whereas rates of non-adherence to all forms of antipsychotic are high. When these factors are compounded with other confounders (gender, age and smoking), definitive statements regarding prolactin become less precise though some conclusions can be made with reasonable certainty.

Much of the reported data tend to come from relatively short-term clinical trials, often done for drug registration purposes, or cross-sectional prevalence data. Neither data set has properly established the long-term trajectory of hyperprolactinaemia and there are no data to support the concept of regression back to baseline.

There are, however, a number of disparate data on comparable rates of hyperprolactinaemia amongst antipsychotics and the largest data sets reporting prolactin include a 6-week paliperidone study in 628 schizophrenia patients (Kane et al, 2007) and a 1-year risperidone and haloperidol in first episode psychosis study in 555 patients (Schooler et al, 2005). Cohort sizes range from <50 to 2725 (Bushe et al, 2010). There is also surprisingly little dissonance amongst the data sets despite many of the confounders already discussed. .

In summary, for individual antipsychotics the prevalence of hyperprolactinaemia is highest in risperidone, paliperidone and amisulpride-treated patients and approaches 100% in female patients (72-100%) being significantly higher than in patients treated with conventional antipsychotics (33% in a UK cohort on depot antipsychotics) (Bushe et al, 2008; Bushe and Shaw 2007). The recently licensed paliperidone, which is 9-hydroxyl-risperidone, the active metabolite of risperidone, has similar prolactin elevation to risperidone (Berwaerts et al, 2010).

Clinicians have been aware for many years that risperidone is associated with hyperprolactinaemia, however there has been less clarity regarding whether hyperprolactinaemia with risperidone is more prevalent than with conventional antipsychotics. A key study was a long-term, randomised clinical trial (RCT) in first-episode psychosis with subjects randomised to risperidone or haloperidol and a median treatment-length of 206 days (Schooler et al, 2005). This study reported significantly higher rates of hyperprolactinaemia (74% vs. 50%) and mean prolactin levels in the risperidone cohort than the haloperidol cohort. CATIE also reported significantly greater prolactin elevation with risperidone than perphenazine (Lieberman et al, 2005) though only mean changes in individual drug cohorts were reported, not categorical numbers of patients with hyperprolactinaemia.

Although conventional antipsychotics were for a long time regarded as almost uniformly being associated with hyperprolactinaemia, the data are not supportive of this conclusion and recent data on conventional antipsychotics suggest significantly lower prevalence rates of 33-35% in a depot-treated population (Bushe and Shaw, 2007). In part, this may relate to dosing issues. For example, Asian populations using higher doses of haloperidol (15-16mg) than typically used in Europe, have prevalence rates of hyperprolactinaemia (60-66%) approaching those of risperidone and amisulpride (Bushe et al, 2010). Supportive of this dosing issue is the excellent study from Kleinberg in approximately 2000 patients which concluded that although risperidone was associated with higher rates of hyperprolactinaemia compared with 10 mg haloperidol, no comparative differences emerged with 20mg haloperidol (Kleinberg et al, 1999). Doses of haloperidol currently used are more reflective of studies such as EUFEST, in which the maximum permitted dose was 4 mg.

Our own naturalistic series concluded that hyperprolactinaemia with oral risperidone was indeed almost 100% in females and between 63-100% in males (Bushe et al, 2008). Similar levels of hyperprolactinaemia are measured with amisulpride though data in large cohorts is lacking other than from EUFEST (Bushe et al, 2008). Depot formulations of risperidone may have a lower prevalence of hyperprolactinaemia relating to dose (53-67%) (Bushe et al, 2008; Bushe and Shaw, 2007). Paliperidone is the major metabolite of risperidone (9-hydroxyl-risperidone) and prolactin values are either similar or greater than those of risperidone (Berwaerts et al, 2010).

Aripiprazole is associated with the lowest rates of hyperprolactinaemia with prevalence rates of 3-5% in RCTs that increase to incidence rates of 17% in naturalistic studies (Bushe et al, 2010) .Recent data have evaluated aripiprazole as a prolactin-lowering agent when combined with haloperidol or risperidone with some success. Although studies report rapid reductions in prolactin levels after commencing aripiprazole (Shim et al, 2007), this may partially relate to removal of a previously used prolactin-elevating drug. Aripiprazole, however, in a placebo controlled trial when added to high-dose haloperidol (20-25 mg/day) in a cohort of schizophrenia patients resulted in normalisation of prolactin in 85% of subjects by 8 weeks contrasting with 3.6% of the placebo group ($p<0.001$) (Shim et al, 2007). Further research is indicated into the dosage of aripiprazole that may give maximal benefit.

For the remaining antipsychotics, hyperprolactinaemia is sometimes reported though significantly less often than for risperidone and amisulpride. Our review of the data found that for quetiapine reported rates range from 0-29% and for olanzapine from 6-40% (Bushe et al, 2008) although most studies report rates at the lower end of the spectrum. In a recent 6-month study of schizophrenia, patients randomised to quetiapine or olanzapine, 33% had hyperprolactinaemia at baseline which normalised in almost all patients as early as 14 days (Bushe et al, 2009). There were no significant differences between the drugs in changes in prolactin.

The depot formulation of olanzapine has recently been trialled in a complex, non-inferiority study compared with oral olanzapine. The quality of the data and trial design has meant that aspects such as dose response with variables such as prolactin have been investigated (Hill et al, 2011). Significant dose-related changes in prolactin were measured over the 24-week study, however it should be noted that a small mean increase in prolactin was measured only in the cohort receiving 600 mg/month (oral equivalent estimated as 20 mg/day). In this 600 mg/month cohort, 7/21 of female subjects (33%) moved from a normal into a high range level (Table 1). This emphasises the importance of analysing prolactin data not only as mean changes in a cohort but also the categorical changes to provide data that are meaningful in terms of patient outcomes (Bushe et al, 2008). This concept is also well demonstrated in the 555 schizophrenia patient study, Schizophrenia Trial of Aripiprazole (STAR), in which subjects were randomised to either aripiprazole or standard of care treatment (Hanssens et al, 2008; Kerwin et al,2007). There was a mean decrease of 34.2 mg/dl in the aripiprazole-treated cohort, however using a categorical analysis, hyperprolactinaemia was reported in 16.8% of subjects.

	300 mg/month (N=140)	405 mg/month (N=318)	600 mg/month (N=141)
Mean change (micrograms/l) (SD)	-5.61 (12.49)	-2.76 (19.02)	3.58 (33.78)

Table 1. Prolactin changes over 24 weeks with depot olanzapine at various dosages in a randomised controlled trial (Hill et al, 2011)

7. What are the current views of EU guidelines on all aspects of prolactin?

Only one set of guidelines, published in 2008, is devoted to prolactin and it provides both advice and the data and rationale behind the consensus group's conclusions (Peveler et al, 2008). Prior to this many guidelines did not give specific recommendations (Citrome et al, 2008). In general terms, other guidelines and relevant Summaries of Product Characteristics do not provide a specific monitoring schedule and tend to advocate prolactin monitoring only when symptoms are detected.

In 2006, guidelines on bipolar disorder from the National Institute of Clinical Excellence recommended limited pre-treatment monitoring of prolactin levels for risperidone with further monitoring should symptoms develop. The only other guideline to recommend pre-treatment monitoring are the Maudsley guidelines (Taylor et al, 2009). These guidelines recommend baseline prolactin monitoring, followed up at 6 and 12 months. Furthermore, the guidelines advise switching medications if hyperprolactinaemia is symptomatic or, alternatively, adding aripiprazole. The guidelines also concur broadly that hyperprolactinaemia is associated with both short- and longer term adverse events that include bone mineral density loss and a possible increase in the risk of breast cancer. The 2005 recommendations from the World Federation Society of Biological Psychiatry (WFSBP) curiously conclude that whereas prolactin elevation was frequent with amisulpride and typicals (>10%), it was measured only "sometimes" (<10%) with risperidone (Falkai et al, 2006). Current data now seems to have clarified these frequencies rather differently (Bushe et al, 2010; Bushe et al, 2008). The 2008 UK prolactin guidelines recommend prolactin monitoring in all patients pre-treatment regardless of medication and after 3 months of treatment with a stable dose, in addition to further monitoring when there are relevant clinical symptoms (Peveler et al, 2008). With a normal prolactin level there is no further need for monitoring in the absence of clinical symptoms. Significant dose change should also lead to consideration of further monitoring. These UK guidelines give a clear strategy for investigating the aetiology of hyperprolactinaemia in patients receiving antipsychotics and warn against concluding too easily that antipsychotics are responsible. A differential diagnosis must be considered but must always include a pregnancy test in females and thyroid function tests. Prolactin levels can be elevated to levels in excess of >2000 mIU/L in patients taking antipsychotics, however in any patient with prolactin elevation greater than 3000 mIU/L, a prolactinoma should be considered and referral to an endocrinologist is warranted. In the Halifax cohort we measured prolactin levels >2000 mIU/L in 13% of all antipsychotic-treated females and 2% of males. Antipsychotic cessation even for short periods has not been clinically recommended due to risk of worsening of the mental state although in theory this could be considered a diagnostic tool for patients taking oral preparations (Peveler et al, 2008).

8. The management of treatment-emergent hyperprolactinaemia

The management of treatment-emergent hyperprolactinaemia is complex and many of the issues have been considered by the 2008 prolactin guidelines who referenced previous recommendations (Serri et al, 2003). However, newer data have since emerged allowing novel potential management strategies to be considered (Peveler et al, 2008). Levels <1000 mIU/L can simply be monitored but in the presence of symptoms that suggest sex hormone deficiency, it is suggested that such levels should not be allowed to continue long-term due to the potential risk of bone mineral density loss (Peveler et al, 2008). Persistent levels >1000 mIU/L need consideration for medication change or dose reduction, if appropriate. The consensus group concluded that the use of dopamine agonists should be considered only in exceptional circumstances due to the risk of worsening the psychosis (Peveler et al, 2008). This view however is challenged by the Maudsley guidelines (Taylor et al, 2009) which advocate use of dopamine agonists if patients need to remain on the specific prolactin-elevating antipsychotic. They make an interesting observation that although the three agents cited (amantadine, cabergoline and bromocriptine) have the potential to worsen psychosis, that this has not been shown in clinical trials. Although there are many reviews relating to prolactin in the context of severe mental illness, there are currently few, if any, systematic reviews and meta-analyses. A recent systematic review that incorporated a meta-analysis compared the effects of bromocriptine and cabergoline in treating hyperprolactinaemia due to idiopathic causes and prolactinomas (Dos Santos Nunes et al, 2011). They concluded that cabergoline was significantly superior to bromocriptine in normalising both prolactin levels and resuming normal ovulatory cycles. Thus, cabergoline may potentially be the dopamine agonist of choice should this be mandated.

What is currently emerging in an early research phase is the use of specific polypharmacy designed to reduce prolactin levels whilst maintaining treatment on the original antipsychotic. There is little doubt that aripiprazole may have the lowest potential for prolactin elevation, although as we have already stated, in the STAR study 17% of patients did have hyperprolactinaemia (Kerwin et al, 2007 ;Hanssens et al, 2008) although in RCTs, the prevalence rates of 3% seem consistent (Bushe et al, 2008). The combination of adding aripiprazole to risperidone results in significant reductions in plasma concentrations of prolactin of between 35-63%, with maximal benefit measured with aripiprazole doses around 6 mg (Yasui-Furukori, 2010) and possibly doses as low as 3 mg. In 2009, the Maudsley guidelines stated their view that in the presence of symptomatic hyperprolactinaemia options included changing antipsychotics or adding aripiprazole to the existing treatment. As a strategy it is clear that there may be benefit to some patients, however aripiprazole as a partial dopamine agonist has been shown to be associated with worsening of psychosis in some patients. The complete risk-benefit equation for use of aripiprazole in this manner will require further clinical trials. Other salient issues to consider include the reality that schizophrenia the illness, and its associated symptomatology, is the cause of some of the more overt sexual dysfunction (Malik et al, 2011). Reducing prolactin may not always lead to clinical improvement. The correlation between prolactin and sexual dysfunction however is thus complex. In a case series

although all subjects had reduction in prolactin levels, only around half reported improved sexual function (Chen 2011). The reality of the situation is that individual patients will require individual solutions. A physician considering changing an antipsychotic in a stable patient must carefully balance the risks and benefits of continued treatment.
There will be patients who are clearly at high risk of prolactin-related adverse events for whom usage of potentially prolactin-elevating antipsychotics needs to be carefully considered,eg, patients with a history of breast cancer or osteoporosis. The other angle to management is to ensure high screening rates for patients at high risk of treatment-emegent osteoporosis and provision of relevant treatment to potentially reduce fracture incidence (Graham et al, 2011).

9. Hyperprolactinaemia in children and adolescents

There would seem to be an increasing usage of antipsychotic drugs in the treatment of many childhood psychiatric illnesses including attention deficit hyperactivity disorder, bipolar disorder and childhood schizophrenia. In general, it would seem that prolactin levels are elevated in children by the same antipsychotics that induce hyperprolactinaemia in adults (Rosenbloom, 2010). For example, in a recent review, 100% of a cohort of 34 children aged 5-14 years treated with risperidone had prolactin elevation(Rosenbloom, 2010). Prolactin levels were also assessed in a naturalistic study of children and adolescents receiving antipsychotics and in some cases concurrent stimulants (Penzner et al, 2009). This analysis revealed a number of interesting findings, however, the addition of a stimulant did not affect prolactin levels compared to no usage. It had been hypothesised that stimulant treatment may reduce any hyperprolactinaemia induced. Adolescents treated with olanzapine when compared to adults treated in clinical trials are also likely to have greater increases in prolactin levels.
The data on prolactin elevation and longer term outcomes in childhood is clearly complex to obtain. Data however do exist and broadly seem to mirror the findings in adults where hyperprolactinaemia is associated with decreased bone mineral density (O'Keane, 2008). A cross-sectional study of 83 boys aged 7-17 years treated for 3 years with the combination of selective serontonin reuptake inhibitors (SSRIs) and risperidone reported that after adjustments, a negative association was found between bone mineral density at the distal radius and serum prolactin level (Rosenbloom, 2010). The data furthermore was suggestive that this bone mineral density reduction may relate to a direct effect of prolactin on bone turnover as there was no relationship between testosterone levels and prolactin. The risk associated with longer term hyperprolactinaemia can be postulated to be a deleterious effect on peak bone mass attainment (Rosenbloom, 2010).
When considering their prolactin guidelines in 2008, the consensus group concluded that there were two groups in whom prolactin elevation should be avoided where possible. Firstly, in those when peak bone mass has not yet been attained, such as in children and young adults up to the age of 25 years (Peveler et al, 2008) with females being more vulnerable to the adverse effect of prolactin elevation than males. Risperidone is certainly being used in a variety of childhood psychiatric illnesses at young ages. A recent report in a small cohort of patients with conduct disorder (mean age 42 months) treated with risperidone at a mean dosage of 0.78mg/day and a maximum of 1.5mg/day (Ercan et al, 2011) found substantial increase in prolactin from a baseline mean of 5.3 ng/ml to 70 ng/ml at 8 weeks. Six of the eight children who completed the study had hyperprolactinaemia

without clinical symptoms, as stated by the authors. Studies suggest that children are more sensitive to the prolactin elevating adverse effects of antipsychotics and care is needed to keep these to a minimum (Correll, 2011). The second high risk group would include those with a relevant strong family history of breast cancer or osteoporosis.

10. Further research. What are the unanswered questions?

1. **What are the longer term trajectories of prolactin levels for patients with elevated prolactin?** Research has firmly established that hyperprolactinaemia emerges within days as a consequence of treatment and, as we have shown in a large RCT, equally rapidly reverts to normal with removal of the prolactin-elevating antipsychotic (Bushe et al, 2009). What is less well established is the trajectory of prolactin levels over a longer term period. Do they remain at the same level? Short-term RCTs are unlikely to address this issue and current data that follow patients for 1 year have only reported baseline and endpoint data, not the trajectory of the prolactin response (Schooler et al, 2005). In the absence of a proven mechanism for how and why antipsychotics elevate prolactin differentially (Bushe et al, 2010), one can only speculate.
2. **What are the longer term outcomes for patients with elevated prolactin?** Over the last 10 years patients receiving biologics to treat rheumatoid arthritis have been entered into voluntary, long-term databases that have addressed, albeit in a naturalistic manner, incidence of potentially associated adverse events (cancers, reactivation of tuberculosis (TB), serious infections). There is a need to formally determine the longer term harm of untreated hyperprolactinaemia in psychiatry. The last decade has better defined potential longer term sequelae of hyperprolactinaemia and these clearly cannot be measured within formal RCTs. In 2011, the clear options involve using either large epidemiological databases, prospectively and retrospectively or creating prospective collections of clinical data such as through usage of registers. The challenge exists in creating appropriate databases that allow long-term follow up of both prolactin levels and clinical outcomes. Certainly the data on bone fractures (Howard et al, 2007; Abel et al, 2008) has shown us the potential. The World Health Organization (WHO) initiated a number of databases to measure cancer rates in schizophrenia in the 1970s (Bushe and Hodgson, 2010) and have the knowledge and ability to conduct similar projects worldwide relating to outcomes of hyperprolactinaemia.
3. **What is and how can we measure the true risk-benefit of switching antipsychotic treatments**? There is absolute agreement that usage of drugs such as dopamine agonists have significant potential to worsen schizophrenia illness (Peveler et al, 2008). This creates a dichotomy where the clinician can reduce the dose or change the antipsychotic, or do nothing. There is no single pragmatic endpoint that captures this risk. A relatively short-term RCT (1 year or less) looking at formal changes in rating scales, remission levels or relapse rates may be helpful. At a minimum, it may tell us the psychiatric outcome of switching patients from prolactin-elevating antipsychotics compared to maintaining the status quo. It is difficult to see any individual institution or pharmaceutical company undertaking such a complex and expensive study, and the only viable option would be for larger bodies, such as the European Medicines Agency, National Institute of Mental Health or potentially WHO to undertake this work.

4. **Can genetics help us predict individual responses to potentially prolactin-elevating antipsychotics?** Data allow us to predict which antipsychotics are more likely to elevate prolactin but not with any precision. Potentially any patient given any antipsychotic may have prolactin elevation ranging from small to large. In the future, one can imagine that genetics will better help us understand which patients are more at risk of adverse events associated with individual antipsychotics and also their likelihood of a clinical response. Genetic variation is likely to contribute substantially. Certainly this work is ongoing in the area of weight change with antipsychotic treatment and we can expect that pharmacogenetics may play a critical role (Reynolds, 2007).
5. **Can antipsychotic polypharmacy be a potential treatment option?** Aripiprazole is already cited as a potential treatment option as an additive treatment in the influential Maudsley guidelines (Taylor et al, 2009). With the increasing availability of generic antipsychotic options over the next decade one can envisage a greater degree of polypharmacy similarly designed to reduce or prevent specific adverse events. Prolactin is one area where at least five established antipsychotics are cited as not usually associated with hyperprolactinaemia (Taylor et al, 2009). Such experimental combinations have not been well researched to date and will require a solid trial base before definitive conclusions can be drawn.
6. **How important is the prolactin receptor in terms of cancer?** The prolactin signalling cascade may be important in the pathology of breast and prostate cancers. The antagonism of the prolactin receptor and its pathways may also be important. As we learn the molecular and genetic perspectives of the role of prolactin and its signalling pathways, we may learn more about any potential role of antipsychotic treatments and their relevance in these pathways (Jacobson et al, 2011).

11. Conclusion

Long-term antipsychotic treatment currently represents a usual outcome for patients with schizophrenia and bipolar disorder. Hyperprolactinaemia can be measured in between 33-69% of patients in antipsychotic studies and many antipsychotics significantly elevate prolactin with no suggestion of any longer term decline in prolactin levels. Hyperprolactinaemia can no longer be regarded in any sense as a benign abnormality and it may have significant potential short- and potential longer term consequences. Whereas the short-term adverse events are more easily detectable, the potential longer term consequences may remain hidden and undetectable until a bone fracture or cancer emerges. Over the last 10 years, patients receiving biologics to treat rheumatoid arthritis have been entered into voluntary, long-term databases that have addressed, albeit in a naturalistic manner, incidence of potentially associated adverse events (cancers, reactivation of TB, serious infections). There is a need to formally determine the longer term harm of untreated hyperprolactinaemia in psychiatry. In addition, future research needs to focus on the risk-benefit for the usage of prolactin-elevating antipsychotics.

12. References

[1] Abel KM, Heatlie HF, Howard LM, Webb RT. Sex- and age-specific incidence of fractures in mental illness: a historical, population-based cohort study. J Clin Psychiatry. 2008;69:1398-403

[2] Akkaya C, Kaya B, Kotan Z, et al. Hyperprolactinemia and possibly related development of prolactinoma during amisulpride treatment; three cases. J Psychopharmacol 2009;23:723-6

[3] Berwaerts J, Cleton A, Rossenu S, et al. A comparison of serum prolactin concentrations after administration of paliperidone extended-release and risperidone tablets in patients with schizophrenia. J Psychopharmacol. 2010 Jul;24(7):1011-8

[4] Bostwick JR, Guthrie SK, Ellingrod VL. Antipsychotic-induced hyperprolactinemia. Pharmacotherapy 2009;29:64-73

[5] Bushe C, Shaw M. Prevalence of hyperprolactinaemia in a naturalistic cohort of schizophrenia and bipolar outpatients during treatment with typical and atypical antipsychotics. J Psychopharmacol 2007; 21:768-73.

[6] Bushe C, Shaw M, Peveler RC. A review of the association between antipsychotic use and hyperprolactinaemia. J Psychopharmacol 2008;22(2 Suppl):46-55

[7] Bushe C, Sniadecki J, Bradley AJ, Poole Hoffman V. Comparison of metabolic and prolactin variables from a six-month randomised trial of olanzapine and quetiapine in schizophrenia. J Psychopharmacol. 2010 Jul; 24(7):1001-9.

[8] Bushe CJ, Bradley AJ, Wildgust HJ, Hodgson RE. Schizophrenia and breast cancer incidence. A systematic review of clinical studies. Schizophr Res 2009;114:6-16

[9] Bushe CJ, Hodgson R. Schizophrenia and cancer: in 2010 do we understand the connection? Can J Psychiatry. 2010 Dec;55(12):761-7

[10] Bushe CJ, Bradley A, Pendlebury J. A review of hyperprolactinaemia and severe mental illness: are there implications for clinical biochemistry? Ann Clin Biochem. 2010 Jul;47(Pt 4):292-300

[11] Catts VS, Catts SV, O'Toole BI, Frost AD. Cancer incidence in patients with schizophrenia and their first-degree relatives - a meta-analysis. Acta Psychiatr Scand 2008;117:323-36

[12] Chen CY, Lin TY, Wang CC, Shuai HA. Improvement of serum prolactin and sexual function after switching to aripiprazole from risperidone in schizophrenia: a case series. Psychiatry Clin Neurosci. 2011; 65(1):95-7.

[13] Citrome L. Current guidelines and their recommendations for prolactin monitoring in psychosis.J Psychopharmacol. 2008 Mar; 22(2 Suppl):90-7.

[14] Correll CU. Addressing adverse effects of antipsychotic treatment in young patients with schizophrenia. J Clin Psychiatry. 2011 Jan; 72(1):e01.

[15] Dos Santos Nunes V, El Dib R, Boguszewski CL, Nogueira CR. Cabergoline versus bromocriptine in the treatment of hyperprolactinemia: a systematic review of randomized controlled trials and meta-analysis. Pituitary. 2011 Jan 8. [Epub ahead of print]

[16] Ercan ES, Basay BK, Basay O, et al. Risperidone in the treatment of conduct disorder in preschool children without intellectual disability. Child Adolesc Psychiatry Ment Health. 2011 Apr 13;5(1):10. [Epub ahead of print]

[17] Falkai P, Wobrock T, Lieberman J, et al; WFSBP Task Force on Treatment Guidelines for Schizophrenia. World Federation of Societies of Biological Psychiatry (WFSBP) guidelines for biological treatment of schizophrenia, part 1: acute treatment of schizophrenia. World J Biol Psychiatry 2005;6:132-191

[18] Fitzgerald P, Dinan TG. Prolactin and dopamine: what is the connection? J Psychopharmacol 2008;22(2 Suppl):12-19

[19] Garde AH, Hansen AM, Skovgaard LT, Christensen JM. Seasonal and biological variation of blood concentrations of total cholesterol, dehydroepiandrosterone sulfate, hemoglobin A 1c), IgA, prolactin, and free testosterone in healthy women. Clin Chem. 2000;46:551-9 Erratum in: Clin Chem 2001; 47:1877

[20] Graham SM, Howgate D, Anderson W, et al. Risk of osteoporosis and fracture incidence in patients on antipsychotic medication.Expert Opin Drug Saf. 2011 Jul;10(4):575-602

[21] Haddad PM, Wieck A. Antipsychotic-induced hyperprolactinaemia: mechanisms, clinical features and management. Drugs 2004;64:2291-314

[22] Hanssens L, L'Italien G, Loze JY, et al. The effect of antipsychotic medication on sexual function and serum prolactin levels in community-treated schizophrenic patients: results from the Schizophrenia Trial of Aripiprazole (STAR) study (NCT00237913). BMC Psychiatry. 2008 Dec 22;8:95

[23] Harvey PW, Everett DJ, Springall CJ. Adverse effects of prolactin in rodents and humans: breast and prostate cancer. J Psychopharmacol 2008; 22(2 Suppl):20-7.

[24] Hill AL, Sun B, Karagianis JL, et al. Dose-associated changes in safety and efficacy parameters observed in a 24-week maintenance trial of olanzapine long-acting injection in patients with schizophrenia. BMC Psychiatry. 2011 Feb 15;11:28.

[25] Hippisley-Cox J, Vinogradova Y, Coupland C, Parker C. Risk of malignancy in patients with schizophrenia or bipolar disorder: nested case-control study. Arch Gen Psychiatry 2007; 64:1368-76.

[26] Holt RIG. Medical causes and consequences of hyperprolactinaemia. A context for psychiatrists. J Psychopharmacol 2008;22(2 Suppl):28-37

[27] Howard L, Kirkwood G, Leese M. Risk of hip fracture in patients with a history of schizophrenia. *Br J Psychiatry* 2007;190:129-34

[28] Jacobson EM, Hugo ER, Borcherding DC, Ben-Jonathan N. Prolactin in breast and prostate cancer: molecular and genetic perspectives. Discov Med. 2011 Apr;11(59):315-24.

[29] Johnsen E, Kroken RA, Abaza M, et al. Antipsychotic-induced hyperprolactinemia: a cross-sectional survey. J Clin Psychopharmacol 2008;28:686-90

[30] Kahn RS, Fleischhacker WW, Boter H, et al. Lancet. 2008 Mar 29;371(9618):1085-97.Effectiveness of antipsychotic drugs in first-episode schizophrenia and schizophreniform disorder: an open randomised clinical trial. Lancet. 2008 29;371(9618):1085-97.

[31] Kane J, Canas F, Kramer M et al. Treatment of schizophrenia with paliperidone extended-release tablets: a 6-week placebo-controlled trial. Schizophr Res 2007;90:147-61.

[32] Kerwin R, Millet B, Herman E et al. A multicentre, randomized, naturalistic, open-label study between aripiprazole and standard of care in the management of community-treated schizophrenic patients. Schizophrenia Trial of Aripiprazole: (STAR) study. Eur Psychiatry. 2007;22:433-43

[33] Kleinberg DL, Davis JM, De Coster R et al. Prolactin levels and adverse effects in patients treated with risperidone. J Clin Psychopharmacol 1999;19:57-61

[34] Knegtering H, van den Bosch R, Castelein S, et al. Are sexual side effects of prolactin-raising antipsychotics reducible to serum prolactin? Psychoneuroendocrinology 2008;33:711-17

[35] Kohen D, Wildgust HJ. The evolution of hyperprolactinaemia as an entity in psychiatric patients. J Psychopharmacol 2008;22(2 Suppl):6-11

[36] Lieberman JA, Stroup TS, McEvoy JP et al. Effectiveness of antipsychotic drugs in patients with chronic schizophrenia. N Engl J Med 2005; 353:1209-23

[37] Mackin P, Waton A, Nulkar A, Watkinson HM. Prolactin and smoking status in antipsychotic-treated patients. J Psychopharmacol. 2011;25(5):698-703.

[38] Mazziotti G, Porcelli T, Mormando M et al.. Vertebral fractures in males with prolactinoma. Endocrine. 2011 Jun;39(3):288-93.

[39] Malik P, Kemmler G, Hummer M et al, Sexual dysfunction in first-episode schizophrenia patients: results from European first episode schizophrenia trial. J Clin Psychopharmacol. 2011 Jun;31(3):274-80.

[40] McEvoy, JP, Lieberman, JA, Perkins DO et al. Efficacy and tolerability of olanzapine, quetiapine and risperidone in the treatment of early psychosis: A randomized, double-blind 52-week comparison. Am J Psychiatry 2007; 164:1050-60

[41] Peveler RC, Branford D, Citrome L, et al . Antipsychotics and hyperprolactinaemia: clinical recommendations. J Psychopharmacol 2008;22(2 Suppl):98-103

[42] Meaney AM, Smith S, Howes OD, et al.. Effects of long-term prolactin-raising antipsychotic medication on bone mineral density in patients with schizophrenia. B J Psychiatry 2004;184:503-8

[43] Meaney AM, and O'Keane V. Bone mineral density changes over a year in young females with schizophrenia; relationship to medication and endocrine variables. Schizophr Res 2007;93:136-43

[44] Montgomery J, Winterbottom E, Jessani M et al. Prevalence of hyperprolactinemia in schizophrenia: association with typical and atypical antipsychotic treatment.J Clin Psychiatry. 2004 Nov;65(11):1491-8

[45] National Institute for Health and Clinical Excellence (NICE). Bipolar disorder. The management of bipolar disorder in adults, children and adolescents, in primary and secondary care. NICE clinical guideline 38, 2006 [cited 2011 May 14]; Available from: www.nice.org.uk/CG038

[46] Ohta C, Yasui-Furukori N, Furukori H, et al. The effect of smoking status on the plasma concentration of prolactin already elevated by risperidone treatment in schizophrenia patients. Prog Neuropsychopharmacol Biol Psychiatry. 2011;35(2):573-6.

[47] O'Keane V, Meaney AM. Antipsychotic drugs. A new risk factor for osteoporosis in young women with schizophrenia? J Clin Psychopharmacol 2005;25:26-31

[48] O'Keane V. Antipsychotic-induced hyperprolactinaemia, hypogonadism and osteoporosis in the treatment of schizophrenia. J Psychopharmacol 2008;22 (2 suppl):70-75

[49] Penzner JB, Dudas M, Saito E ,et al. Lack of effect of stimulant combination with second-generation antipsychotics on weight gain, metabolic changes, prolactin levels, and sedation in youth with clinically relevant aggression or oppositionality.J Child Adolesc Psychopharmacol. 2009 Oct;19(5):563-73

[50] Poyraz BC, Aksoy C, Balcioğlu I. Increased incidence of autoimmune thyroiditis in patients with antipsychotic-induced hyperprolactinemia. Eur Neuropsychopharmacol 2008;18:667-72

[51] Reuwer AQ, Twickler MT, Hutten BA, et al. Prolactin levels and the risk of future coronary artery disease in apparently healthy men and women. Circ Cardiovasc Genet. 2009; 2(4):389-95.

[52] Reynolds G. The impact of pharmacogenetics on the development and use of antipsychotic drugs. Drug Discov Today. 2007 Nov;12(21-22):953-9

[53] Riddle O, Bates RW, Dykshorn SW. (1933). The preparation, identification and assay of prolactin - a hormone of the anterior pituitary. Am J Physiol 1933;105:191-216

[54] Rosenbloom AL. Hyperprolactinemia with antipsychotic drugs in children and adolescents. Int J Pediatr Endocrinol. 2010;2010. pii: 159402. Epub 2010 Aug 24.

[55] Schooler N, Rabinowitz J, Davidson M, et al. Risperidone and haloperidol in first episode psychosis: A long term randomised trial. Am J Psychiatry 2005;162:947-53

[56] Serri O, Chik CL, Ur E, Ezzat S. Diagnosis and management of hyperprolactinemia. Canadian Medical Association Journal 2003;169:575-581

[57] Shim JC, Shin JGK, Kelly DL et al. Adjunctive treatment with a dopamine partial agonist, aripiprazole, for antipsychotic-induced hyperprolactinemia: a placebo-controlled trial. Am J Psychiatry. 2007;164:1404-10

[58] Skopek M, Manoj P. Hyperprolactinaemia during treatment with paliperidone. Australas Psychiatry. 2010 Jun;18(3):261-3.

[59] Smith S, Wheeler MJ, Murray R, O'Keane V. The effects of antipsychotic-induced hyperprolactinaemia on the hypothalamic-pituitary-gonadal axis. J Clin Psychopharmacol 2008;22:109-14

[60] Szarfman A, Tonning JM, Levine JG, Doraiswamy PM. Atypical antipsychotics and pituitary tumours: a pharmacovigilance study. Pharmacotherapy 2006;26:748-58

[61] Taylor D, Paton C, Kapur S. The Maudsley prescribing guidelines. 10th ed. London: Informa Healthcare; 2009

[62] Tworoger SS, Eliassen AH, Rosner Bet al. Plasma prolactin concentrations and risk of postmenopausal breast cancer. Cancer Res 2004;64, 6814-19

[63] Tworoger S, Eliassen AH, Sluss P, Hankinson SE. A prospective study of plasma prolactin concentrations and risk of premenopausal and postmenopausal breast cancer. J Clin Oncol 2007;25:1-7

[64] Tworoger SS, Hankinson SE. Prolactin and breast cancer risk. Cancer Lett 2006; 243:160-9.

[65] Wang PS, Walker AM, Tsuang MT et al. Dopamine antagonists and the development of breast cancer. Arch Gen Psychiatry 2002;59:1147-54

[66] Yasui-Furukori N, Furukori H, Sugawara N, et al. Prolactin fluctuation over the course of a day during treatments with three atypical antipsychotics in schizophrenic patients. Hum Psychopharmacol. 2010 Apr;25(3):236-42

[67] Yasui-Furukori N, Furukori H, Sugawara N, et al.. Dose-dependent effects of adjunctive treatment with aripiprazole on hyperprolactinemia induced by risperidone in female patients with schizophrenia..J Clin Psychopharmacol. 2010 Oct;30(5):596-9.

8

The Foragining Ecology of the Green Turtle in the Baja California Peninsula: Health Issues

Rafael Riosmena-Rodriguez[1], Ana Luisa Talavera-Saenz[1], Gustavo Hinojosa-Arango[2], Mónica Lara-Uc[3] and Susan Gardner[4]

[1]*Programa de Investigación en Botánica Marina, Departamento de Biología Marina, Universidad Autónoma de Baja California Sur, La Paz Baja California Sur,*
[2]*The School for Field Studies, Puerto de Acapulco s/n, Puerto San Carlos, Baja California Sur*
[3]*Depto. de Virología, Facultad de Medicina Veterinaria y Zootecnia, UADY, Mérida, Yucatán,*
[4]*Centro de Investigaciones Biológicas del Noroeste, La Paz Baja California Sur, México*

1. Introduction

Conservation of threatened species, such as the green turtle (*Chelonia mydas*), is closely related to habitat quality. In particular there are issues related to heavy metals, the presence of epibionts, parasites and fibropapiloms who might play a crucial role in the species survivorship. Heavy metals occur naturally in the environment (Sparling et al., 2000) as part of the biogeochemical cycles (Valiela, 2009), and it is often difficult to differentiate between natural and anthropogenic sources (Kieffer, 1991; Moreno, 2003). In marine systems, natural processes (e.g., upwelling, river runoff) can redistribute and concentrate heavy metals in the environment, occasionally reaching toxic levels (Sparling et al., 2000; Machado et al., 2002). The effects of these processes may vary over seasonal and spatial scales (Sawidis et al., 2001) and their understanding can aid in determining the sources as biomonitors (Szefer et al., 1998; Páez-Osuna et al.,2000), and ultimately their effects on wild life (Sparling et al., 2000; Talavera-Saenz et al., 2007). Also, they can be used for bioabsorption in contaminated waters (Kumar and Kaladharan, 2006). Caliceti et al. (2002) found a decrease in Zinc and Cadmium concentrations from the center of a lagoon, close to an industrial district, towards the Venice lagoon (Italy) openings to the sea, suggesting anthropogenic sources, while Villares et al. (2002) found that seasonal and spatial variation in metals was related to algal growth cycles and river runoff. Riosmena-Rodriguez et al. (2010) determined that heavy metals are related to the physiological features of each major analyzed taxon (green algae, red algae and seagrasses).

The processes controlling the concentration and distribution of metals in coastal environments and their consequences in the species health are poorly understood. It is generally assumed that diet is the main source of metals to sea turtles (Caurant et al., 1999; Anan et al., 2001), but little is known of the process of metal accumulation in these species because data on metal residues in most components of sea turtles' diet has been lacking. As adults, green turtles forage largely on marine algae and seagrasses with variation in the diet due to the relative availability of food types over geographic and temporal scales (Garnett et al., 1985; Brand-Gardner et al., 1999; Seminoff et al., 2002). In the process of metal bioaccumulation in marine food chains is poorly understood because very little data is available on metal concentration at different trophic levels (de la Lanza et al. 1989; Talavera-Saenz et al. 2007) or their temporal (Abdallah et al., 2006; Rodriguez-Castañeda et al., 2006) or spatial variation (Kalesh and Nair, 2006) and their effects on the photosynthetic process (Catriona et al. 2002). High concentrations of heavy metals have been found in sea turtles from many regions of the world (Storelli and Marcotrigiano, 2003). Although metal concentrations vary greatly by region and tissue type, green turtles (*Chelonia mydas*) have been found to have exceptionally high kidney cadmium concentrations. Elevated Cadmium levels have been measured in green turtles from around the world including Japan (Sakai et al., 2000; Anan et al., 2001), China (Lam et al., 2004), Europe (Caurant et al., 1999), Australia (Gordon et al., 1998) and the Arabian Sea (Bicho et al., 2006). Gordon et al. (1998) found that Cadmium concentrations in green turtles from Australia were up to three times higher than the levels reported in commercial seafood products. The presence of epibionts, parasites (internal and external) might occasionally cause the death of some marine turtles and being predecessors of fibropapiloms (Aguirre y Lutz, 2004; Work, 2000, Work *et al.*, 2005). The presence of fibropapiloms in Hawaiian waters was related with the presence of hirudineans (Díaz, *et al.*, 1992). This kind of infections are might be related with their foraging habitat and its conservation condition, their health condition to escape predators and, for the females, the fecundity reduction (Gámez et al., 2006; Alfaro, et al., 2006; Badillo, 2007).

The Baja California Peninsula serves an important role as foraging grounds for five of the world's seven sea turtle species (Gardner and Nichols, 2001). Although much of the peninsula is considered pristine, exploitation of mineral deposits has occurred since the 19th Century and concentrations of Cadmium, Zinc, Copper and Plumb in sediment and marine fauna have been observed above those in more industrialized regions (Gutiérrez-Galindo et al., 1999; Shumilin et al., 2000). In the mid 1970's, Martin and Broenkow (1975) reported that concentrations of Cadmium along the coast of the Baja California Peninsula were remarkably elevated as compared to other regions of the eastern Pacific. Sources of heavy metals in Baja California have been generally attributed to natural factors related to upwelling and the biogeochemistry of the region, however, the potential contribution from anthropogenic sources (e.g. mining and urbanization) cannot be entirely dismissed (Martin and Broenkow, 1975; Sañudo-Wihelmy and Flegal, 1996; Méndez-Rodríguez et al., 1998; Gutiérrez- Galindo et al., 1999; Shumilin et al., 2001). Rodríguez-Meza et al. (2008) developed an extensive evaluation of the heavy metals in sediments and seaweeds along ten sites in the bay. They suggested that the high levels of some heavy metals are related to terrigenous input from the arroyos and biogenic origin by the upwelling. In order to better understand the sources of heavy metals to marine species, more information is needed on metal concentrations in primary producers that make up the base of the food chain. However, few (Riosmena-Rodriguez et al., 2010) papers have approached the study of natural levels of heavy metals in seaweed communities and their temporal and spatial variation. Previous studies in Magdalena Bay, Mexico (Méndez et al., 2002; Gardner et al., 2006) have found high concentrations of metals in marine vertebrates, despite the lack of obvious anthropogenic sources. For example, Cadmium, Zinc, and Iron concentrations in the herbivorous green turtle, *Chelonia mydas,* were the highest ever reported in sea turtles globally (Gardner et al., 2006). In Magdalena Bay, like other regions of the Baja California

Peninsula (Seminoff et al., 2002), juvenile and adult green turtles preferentially consume soft red algae, especially species of Gracilaria (López-Mendilaharsu et al., 2005). Studies in Baja California have demonstrated that these same species of red algae tend to have higher enrichment factors of metals than other groups of seaweeds (Sánchez-Rodríguez et al., 2001), which could account for the high accumulation of metals in foraging green turtles in this region.

2. Materials and methods

2.1 Study area

Magdalena Bay is located on the Pacific coast of the Baja California Peninsula, Mexico between 24° 15′ N and 25° 20′ N, and 111° 30′ W and 112° 15′ W. It is a shallow lagoon protected from the Pacific by barrier islands, with high productivity resulting from seasonal marine upwelling along the coast. Diverse marine habitats within the bay include sandy bottoms and rocky margins, extensive beds of the seagrass *Zostera marina* and a diverse assemblage of macroalgae. A sea turtle refuge area known as Estero Banderitas is located within the mangrove channels in the northwest region of the Bay where green turtles reside year-round (Fig. 1). Because of the perceived importance of this area for green turtle foraging, its protection has been identified as a priority for conservation efforts (Arriaga et al., 1998; Nichols et al., 2000). Rodríguez-Meza et al. (2008) has found that the presence of heavy metals in the bay is heavily influenced by sediment type, organic material, and carbonates and concluded that there was no evidence of human impacts.

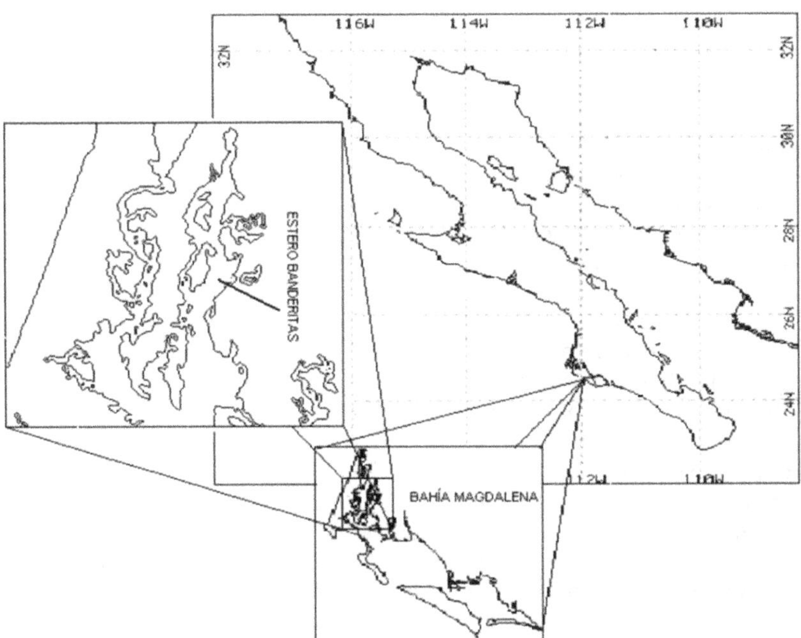

Fig. 1. Study area in Estero Banderitas (24° 50′ - 25° 00′ N and 112°08′ W) located in Bahía Magdalena, Baja California Sur, Mexico.

2.2 Marine plant collection

Three separate sampling trips were made in Estero Banderitas (November 2004, February, 2005 and April, 2005) in order to collect marine plants available during different seasons. Algae and seagrass samples were collected along the length of the mangrove channel using 16 transects of 30 m length. Every 6 m along the transects, plants were manually collected within a 25 cm2 to 1 m2 area, depending on the density of the flora at that location, for a total of 80 samples per trip. The samples were stored in labeled plastic bags and contents were separated by species using taxonomic keys (Riosmena Rodríguez, 1999). Samples were sun-dried in the field and then pressed to further remove moisture.

2.3 Sea turtle tissue collection

Liver and kidney tissues were collected from 8 dead green turtles that incidentally drowned in commercial fishing nets set in Magdalena Bay between February 2002 and April 2003. The straight carapace length of the turtles ranged from 47–77 cm, which is representative of the size range of green turtles in the region (Gardner and Nichols, 2001). The samples were collected within 24 h after the time of death from carcasses with minimal decomposition. Tissue samples were stored in plastic bags and placed on ice for transport to the laboratory where they were frozen at − 80°C until analyzed. From five turtles, intact stomachs were also collected.

2.4 Stomach content analyses

All stomach contents were collected and identified to the lowest possible taxonomic level based on published keys (Abbott and Hollenberg, 1976; Riosmena-Rodríguez, 1999). Entire sample volume and the relative sample volume of each plant species were calculated by the procedure of water displacement in a graduated cylinder. Voucher material was housed in Herbario Ficológico of the Universidad Autónoma de Baja California Sur (UABCS), La Paz, México.

2.5 Laboratory analyses

Tissue and plant samples (0.5 g) were dried in an oven at 70 °C until a dry weight was obtained. Dried samples were digested in acid-washed Teflon tubes with concentrated nitric acid in a microwave oven (CEM modelMars 5X, Matthews, NC). Samples were analyzed by atomic absorption (GBC Scientific equipment, model AVANTA, Dandenong, Australia) using an air-acetylene flame. The certified standard reference material, TORT-2 (National Research Council of Canada, Ottawa) was used to verify accuracy, and that the analytical values were within the range of certified values. All recoveries of metals analyzed were over 95%. Detection limits were: Zinc=0.0008, Cadmium = 0.0009, Mn= 0.002, Cu= 0.0025, Ni = 0.004, Fe=0.005, Pb=0.006 µg/g.

2.6 Quantitative analyses

We analyzed the data based on taxonomic group (red algae, green algae, and seagrass), season, spatial area, and dominant species. Reported statistics are medians (nN2) and ranges in µg/g on a dry weight basis. The Mann-Whitney test was used for conducting two-tailed sample comparisons of tissues for each metal separately and for comparing metals in marine plants collected in Magdalena Bay with those found in the stomach contents. The Kruskal-Wallis test was used to compare the median metal concentration across all plant species. The null hypothesis was rejected if $p \leq 0.05$. The influence of concentration differences among samples was removed by converting data to the percent contribution of each metal to the total metal signature of the individual sample. Fe was removed from these analyses because of its high Concentration and dominance of the metal signature profile. Principal Components Analysis (PCA) of the percent contribution of the metals in plants and turtle tissues. Additionally, factorial analysis was used to determine trends in the presence of heavy metals in the seaweed samples and the relative spatial and/or temporal variation. All analysis was conducted using the Statgraphics Plus software program (Version 5, Rockville, MD).

2.7 Prescence of fibropapiloms and epibionts

Monthly sampling has been develop in the Estero Banderitas and more recently in Estero San Buto as part of the monitoring efforts in was the prescence of fibropapiloms and epibionts by a physical inspection of each animal by region as head, neck, carapace, front or back fins, anus or tail. Comparative analysis was done of the proportion of animals with fibropapiloms and epibionts using the database and literature described in Lara-Uc (2011) in relation to the Bahía Madalena population information (Hinojosa-Arango unpublished data).

3. Results

3.1 Temporal and spatial variation of metal concentration in plant species

Based on our analysis, we found temporal and spatial variations in the concentration in several of heavy metals in seaweeds and seagrasses. In comparisons between the profiles of heavy metals in major plant groups, we found that Nickel differed significantly between the major groups (P=0.01), wherein seagrasses had lower concentrations (Tables 1 and 2). Analyzing all of the species (all sites combined), we found significant seasonal differences in the heavy metal concentrations with the exception of Zinc (P=0.53). Samples collected in April had a higher concentration of Cadmium (P<0.001) and Iron (P=0.002) and a lower concentration of Plumb (P<0.001) and Nickel (P=0.002) than the other months. Manganese was highest in November (P=0.049) and Copper was higher in November compared to February (P=0.01). In comparisons of the metal concentrations between plant species, the only significant differences were detected for Cadmium (p=0.009) in *Ruppia maritima* than all other species. In the case of the analysis of green algae alone, using all species combined, we found temporal significant differences of Cadmium in April (P=0.01).

In the case of other metals, we found significantly temporal differences in Plumb (Pb) concentration in *G. vermiculophylla* (P=0.02) in November but this species also had the highest concentration of Ni (P=0.03) in relation to the other species. Also, there were significant differences in the concentrations of Cadmium (P=0.001), Iron (P=0.01), and Nickel (P=0.002), while Plumb (P<0.001) and Copper (P=0.03) were significantly different than the same metals in November. In the same month, highest Nickel concentrations were recorded in *Codium amplivesiculatum*, while in April, *C. amplivesiculatum*, *Codium cuneatum*, and *Caulerpa sertularioides* from the middle region had the highest concentrations of Copper (7.3µg g−1 dw), Ni (11µg g−1 dw), and Mn (61.4µg g−1 dw), respectively. In February, like November, we had the highest Iron concentration and several species were responsible for this difference (in *H. johnstonii*; 567.5µg g−1 dw) and Zinc concentration (in *G. textorii*; 46.8µg g−1 dw). However, the lower zone had the highest concentrations of Cadmium (in *G. textorii*; 4.4µg g−1 dw) and Ni (*L. pacifica* and *Chondria nidifica*; 13.3 and 13.3µg g−1 dw). Copper (in *L. pacifica*; 2.9µg g−1 dw) and Plumb concentrations were highest in *G. andersonii* from the middle zone (3.8µg g−1 dw).

Season	Species	Cadmium	Plumb	Nickel	Manganese	Iron	Copper
November	*Codium amplivesiculatum*	0.2	1.8	8	52.9	362.2	0.9
		(nd - 0.5)	(1.3 - 2.3)	(6 - 9.9)	(42.2 - 63.5)	(349.8 - 374.7)	(0.7 - 1.2)
	Gracilaria textorii	1.5	1.4	4.8	48.5	325	1.6
		(nd - 3.9)	(nd - 1.9)	(3 - 5.1)	(45.3 - 51.1)	(100.9 - 1231.2)	(0.7 - 4.8)
	Gracilaria vermiculophylla	0.6	2.7	5.3	22.4	302.7	1.3
		(0.5 - 1.4)	(1 - 3.3)	(4.9 - 5.5)	(13 - 23.9)	(185.9 - 372.2)	(1 - 1.6)
	*Gracilariopsis andersonii**	0.5	2	5.7	28.5	195.2	2.5
		-	-	-	-	-	-
	Hypnea johnstonii	0.4	1.8	6.7	26.7	263.9	1.8
		(0.3 - 1.5)	(1.1 - 8.5)	(6 - 6.9)	(23.7 - 282.5)	(227.8 - 1424.1)	(0.9 - 4.4)
February	*Codium amplivesiculatum*	nd	0.8	6.6	12.6	190.2	0.8
			(0 - 2.3)	(6.2 - 7.3)	(12.1 - 20.4)	(189.5 - 522.7)	(nd - 1.3)
	*Codium cuneatum**	nd	1.6	5.9	17.2	241.7	0.4
		-	-	-	-	-	-
	Chondria nidifica	1	1.6	9.3	15.6	291.5	1.3
		(nd - 1.7)	(1.5 - 1.6)	(5.1 - 13.3)	(14.40- 21)	(88.8 - 557.8)	(0.2 - 1.4)
	Gracilaria textorii	3.4	1	6	49.1	139.9	0.5
		(2.7 - 4.4)	(0.7 - 2)	(4.5 - 6.2)	(43.5 - 54.8)	(81.8 - 476.3)	(0.4 - 1.2)
	Gracilaria vermiculophylla	1.1	0.8	4.3	19.3	206.2	0.6
		(1.1 - 1.6)	(0.7 - 0.9)	(3.6 - 5.1)	(14.4 - 19.5)	(139.4 - 269.9)	(0.3 - 1.6)
	*Gracilariopsis andersonii**	1.6	3.8	4.5	23.5	160.4	2.1
		-	-	-	-	-	-
	*Hypnea johnstonii**	nd	nd	11.3	20.6	567.5	nd
		-	-	-	-	-	-
	*Laurencia pacifica**	3	1.7	13.3	25.2	195.8	2.9
		-	-	-	-	-	-
	*Sarcodiotheca gaudichaudii**	0.9	1	5.4	17.2	121.8	0.1
		-	-	-	-	-	-
	*Zostera marina**	nd	2.5	3.1	78.6	51.1	0.4
		-	-	-	-	-	-
April	*Codium amplivesiculatum*	1.6	0.5	7.8	18.7	399.2	4.1
		(1.2 - 1.9)	(0.4 - 0.7)	(7.6 - 7.9)	(15.3 - 22.1)	(298.1 - 500.4)	(1 - 7.3)
	Codium cuneatum	2.1	0.3	7.1	16.7	284.3	1.2
		(1.9 - 2.2)	(0.1 - 0.5)	(3.2 - 11)	(10.5 - 23)	(141.5 - 427.1)	(0.5 - 1.8)
	Caulerpa sertularioides	2.1	0.2	2.6	34.3	374	1.8
		(1.8 - 2.3)	(nd - 0.4)	(1.8 - 3.4)	(7.3 - 61.4)	(223.9 - 524.1)	(1.1 - 2.6)
	*Gracilaria crispata**	4.6	nd	3.9	40.3	576.8	1.6
		-	-	-	-	-	-
	Gracilaria textorii	4.5	0.4	5.3	41.5	579.5	1.7
		(4.3 - 4.8)	(0.1 - 0.6)	(3 - 7.6)	(37.6 - 45.4)	(578.4 - 580.6)	(1.5 - 1.8)
	Gracilaria vermiculophylla	2.9	0.2	2.9	18.1	236.2	0.9
		(2.7 - 2.9)	(nd - 0.6)	(1.1 - 2.9)	(14.7 - 23.6)	(214.4 - 771.5)	(0.9 - 1.6)
	*Gracilariopsis andersonii**	3.8	0.1	2.3	25.5	322.3	1.5
		-	-	-	-	-	-
	*Hypnea johnstonii**	2.7	0.6	1.8	41.9	774.5	2.1
		-	-	-	-	-	-
	*Laurencia pacifica**	4.6	nd	1.9	22.9	497.6	1.8
		-	-	-	-	-	-
	Ruppia maritima	4.5	2.1	2.3	30.6	1230.2	0.5
		(2.1 - 7)	(0.5 - 3.8)	(1.7 - 2.9)	(28.6 - 32. 6)	(1017.4 - 1443)	(nd - 0.9)
	*Zostera marina**	2.2	nd	2.8	33.9	630.3	1.6
		-	-	-	-	-	-

* The values are referred to 1 specimen. nd signifies not detected.

Table 1. Temporal variation of heavy metal concentrations µg.g-1 dry weight in seaweeds and seagrasses collected at the Estero Banderitas. Values are expressed as medians and ranges given in parenthesis.

Site	Species	Cadmium	Plumb	Nickel	Manganese	Iron	Copper
Head	*Codium amplivesiculatum**	nd	2.3	6.6	20.4	522.7	0.8
		-	-	-	-	-	-
	*Chondria nidifica**	nd	1.5	5.1	14.4	88.8	0.2
		-	-	-	-	-	-
	Gracilaria textorii	1.3	1	4.5	50.1	853.7	3
		(nd - 2.7)	(nd - 2)	(3 - 6)	(45.3 - 54.8)	(476.3 - 1231.2)	(1.2 - 4.8)
	Gracilaria vermiculophylla	1.1	0.7	5	22.4	236.2	0.8
		(0.6 - 2.9)	(0.2 - 3.3)	(1.1 - 5.1)	(19.5 - 23.6)	(206.2 - 372.2)	(0.3 - 1.6)
	*Gracilariopsis andersonii**	0.5	2	5.7	28.5	195.2	2.5
		-	-	-	-	-	-
	Hypnea johnstonii	0.7	4.3	9.1	151.6	995.8	2.2
		(nd - 1.5)	(0 - 8.5)	(6.9 - 11.4)	(20.6 - 282.5)	(567.5 - 1424.1)	(nd - 4.4)
	*Ruppia maritima**	6.9	3.8	2.9	32.6	1017.4	nd
		-	-	-	-	-	-
Medium	*Coduim amplivesiculatum*	0.5	0.7	7.9	22.1	349.8	1.2
		(nd - 1.2)	(nd - 1.3)	(7.3 - 10)	(12.1 - 63.5)	(190.2 - 500.4)	(nd - 7.3)
	Codium cuneatum	0.9	1	8.4	20.1	334.4	1.1
		(nd - 2.3)	(0.5 - 1.6)	(5.9 - 11)	(17.2 - 22.9)	(241.7 - 427.1)	(0.4 - 1.8)
	*Caulerpa sertularioides**	2.3	0.4	3.4	61.4	524.1	2.5
		-	-	-	-	-	-
	*Chondria nidifica**	1	1.6	9.3	20.9	557.8	1.4
		-	-	-	-	-	-
	Gracilaria textorii	3.9	1	4.8	45.4	325	0.7
		(3.4 - 4.8)	(0.6 - 1.4)	(4.5 - 7.6)	(43.5 - 51.2)	(139.9 - 580.6)	(0.4 - 1.8)
	Gracilaria vermiculophylla	1.4	0.9	3.5	18.1	302.7	1.4
		(1.1 - 1.6)	(0.6 - 1)	(2.9 - 5.5)	(13 - 19.3)	(269.9 - 771.5)	(1 - 1.6)
	*Gracilariopsis andersonii**	1.6	3.8	4.5	23.5	160.4	2.1
		-	-	-	-	-	-
	*Hypnea johnstonii**	0.3	1.1	6.7	26.7	263.9	1
		-	-	-	-	-	-
	*Ruppia maritima**	2.1	0.5	1.7	28.6	1443	0.9
		-	-	-	-	-	-
	*Sarcodiotheca gaudichaudii**	0.9	1	5.4	17.2	121.8	0.1
		-	-	-	-	-	-
Mouth	*Codium amplivesiculatim*	nd	0.8	6.2	15.3	298.1	1
		(nd - 1.9)	(0.4 - 2.3)	(6 - 7.6)	(12.6 - 42.2)	(189.5 - 374.7)	(0.7 - 1.3)
	*Codium cuneatum**	2.2	0.1	3.2	10.5	141.5	0.5
		-	-	-	-	-	-
	*Caulerpa sertularoides**	1.8	nd	1.8	7.3	223.9	1.1
		-	-	-	-	-	-
	*Chondria nidifica**	1.7	1.6	13.3	15.6	291.5	1.3
		-	-	-	-	-	-
	*Gracilaria crispata**	4.6	nd	3.9	40.3	576.8	1.6
		-	-	-	-	-	-
	Gracilaria textorii	4.3	0.7	5.1	48.5	100.9	1.5
		(1.5 - 4.4)	(0.1 - 1.9)	(3 - 6.2)	(37.6 - 49.1)	(81.8 - 578.4)	(0.5 - 1.6)
	Gracilaria vermiculophylla	1.6	0.8	4.3	14.7	186	0.9
		(0.5 - 2.9)	(0 - 2.7)	(2.9 - 5.3)	(14.4 - 23.9)	(139.4 - 214.4)	(0.6 - 1.3)
	*Gracilariopsis andersonii**	3.8	0.1	2.3	25.5	322.3	1.5
		-	-	-	-	-	-
	Hypnea johnstonii	1.6	1.2	3.9	32.8	501.1	1.9
		(0.4 - 2.7)	(0.6 - 1.8)	(1.8 - 6)	(23.7 - 41.9)	(227.8 - 774.5)	(1.8 - 2.1)
	Laurencia pacifica	3.8	0.8	7.6	24	346.7	2.3
		(3 - 4.6)	(nd - 1.7)	(1.9 - 13.3)	(22.9 - 25.2)	(195.8 - 497.6)	(1.8 - 2.6)
	*Zostera marina**	2.2	nd	2.8	33.9	630.3	1.6
		-	-	-	-	-	-

* The values are refered to 1 specimen. nd signifies not detected.

Table 2. Heavy metal concentrations (µg.g-1 dry weight) in seaweeds and seagrasses collected in the three sites. Values are expressed as medians and ranges given in parenthesis.

Spatial differences in metal concentrations were dependent on the major taxa. In the case of seagrasses, we found a high concentration of Iron (Table 2) who was significant different from Manganese (in *Z. marina*; 78.6 µg g−1 dw) concentrations were highest in the upper zone (P=0.01) because their uneven distribution in the area. Consistent with the above analysis were the multifactorial analysis (Fig. 2) wherein the extreme values are represented by Iron and Manganese with no association among seasons or areas. In the green algae (Table 2), we were able to find many metals in the entire area, but the significant difference was found in Cadmium in April (P=0.01), when all species combined, because the low value in relation to other metals are highly concentrated. There is no consistent pattern in relation to the area of the highest concentration of any metal; they tend to present a group lower in relation to higher concentration in different areas or times (Tables 1 and 2).

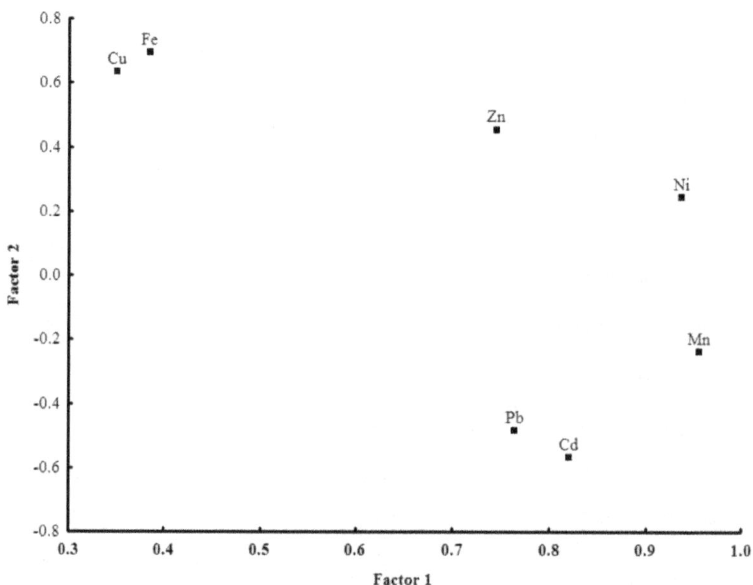

Fig. 2. Multivariate analysis of heavy metals contents in seagrasses.

This is well supported by the multivariate analysis (Fig.3) wherein most of the observed metals show a combination among them and the areas of sampling. We found an extremely high variability in the median content in the red algae (Table 2) but there were no significant differences between sites, with the exception of Zinc which was significantly higher in the upper zone (P=0.02). The highest concentration of any metal was Iron in *Hypnea johnstonii* from the upper zone (1,424.1µg g−1 dw). The highest concentration of Manganese (282.5µg g−1 dw) and Plumb (8.5) µg g−1 dw) were also detected in *H. johnstonii* from the upper zone. Similarly, Zinc (58.8µg g−1 dw) and Copper (4.8µg g−1 dw) concentrations were highest in *G. textorii* in the same zone. The highest Cadmium concentrations were measured in *G. textorii* (4.8µg g−1 dw).

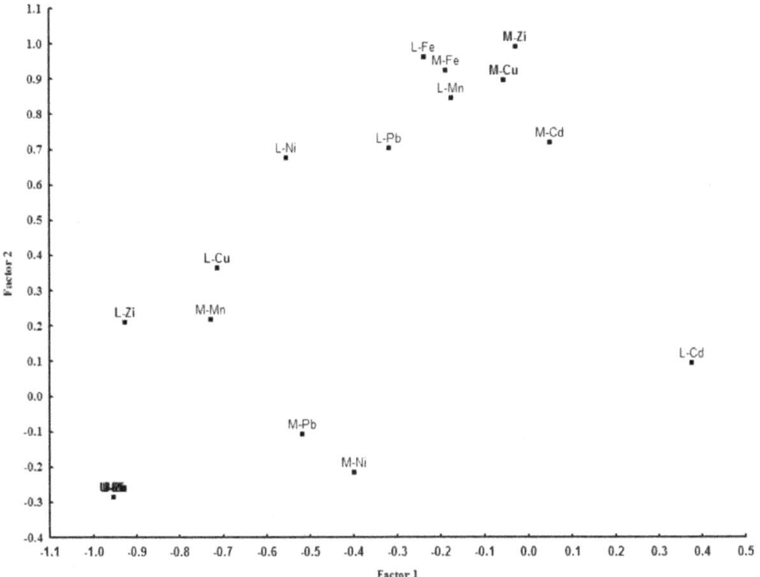

Fig. 3. Multivariate analysis of the spatial concentration of heavy metal in green algae.

Multivariate analyses show the same path in red algae (Figs. 4 and 5) with the clump of areas within metals and a group of metals with high concentration (Fig. 4) in relation to metals with low concentration (Fig. 5).

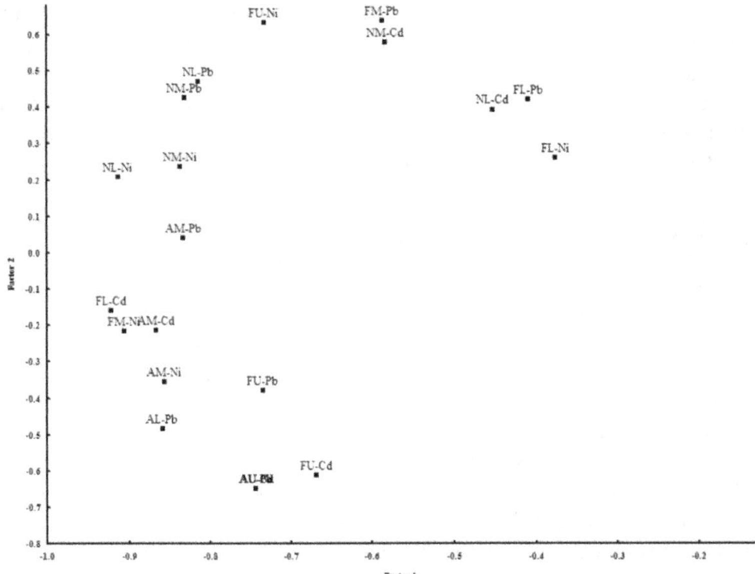

Fig. 4. Multivariate analysis of the spatial concentration of heavy metal in red algae.

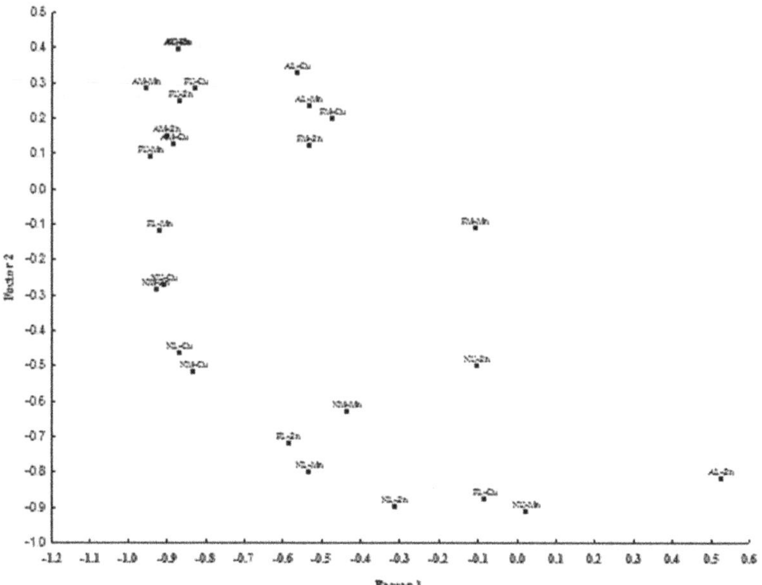

Fig. 5. Multivariate analysis of the spatial concentration of heavy metal in red algae.

3.2 Metals in sea turtle tissues, stomach contents, and plants from the bay

Concentrations of Cadmium and Zinc in flora from the sea turtle stomach contents were greater than the same species of marine plants collected in the bay ($p<0.001$ and $p=0.003$, respectively) (Figure 6). For both metals, the concentrations in sea turtle liver were not significantly different from the stomach contents. Sea turtle kidney Cadmium concentration was significantly higher than liver ($p=0.002$), while Zinc was the same in both tissues. Plumb, Manganese and Fe in flora from the stomach contents were significantly lower than in flora collected from the bay ($p<0.001$ for each) (Figure 6). The stomach contents had higher Plumb and Manganese concentrations than liver ($p=0.04$ and $p<0.001$, respectively) but were not significantly different in Fe. There were no differences in the concentrations of these metals in liver and kidney. Nickel and Copper concentrations did not differ in plants from the two sources. Nickel concentration in liver was similar to kidney concentrations, but significantly lower than the stomach contents ($p=0.005$). Copper was higher in liver than stomach contents ($p<0.001$) and higher than kidney ($p<0.001$). These same trends persisted when the data were transformed to the percent contribution of the metals in each plant species in the stomach contents as compared to the bay samples (Fig. 6). For each of the five plant species, the percent contribution of Manganese and Plumb was greater in the bay-collected plants, while Cadmium and Zinc consistently contributed more to the total metal profile in plants from the stomach contents. Fig. 7 shows the percent contribution of each metal in paired samples of liver, kidney and stomach contents (all flora combined) from the same turtles. Cadmium and Zinc contributed most to the overall metal profile in the kidney, while Copper contributed more in liver. The percent contribution of Manganese and Nickel were greatest in the plants from the stomach contents.

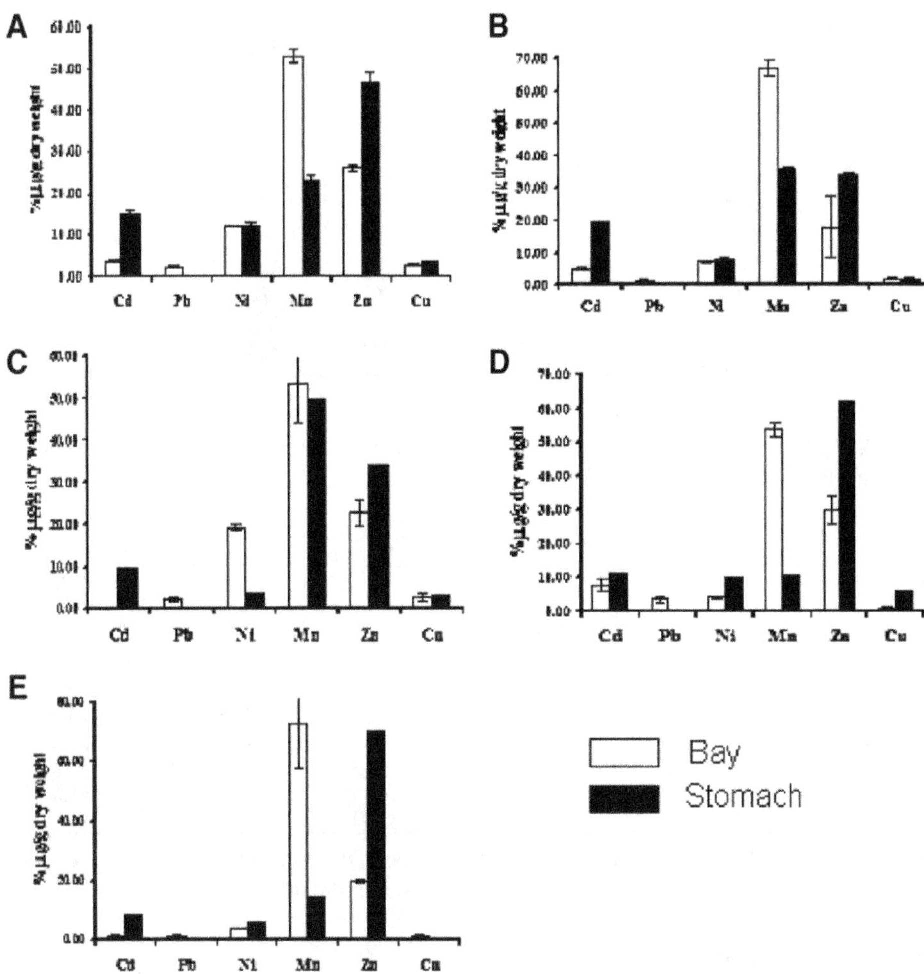

Fig. 6. Percent contribution of metals in species of marine flora collected in the Magdalena Bay and in green turtle (*Chelonia mydas*) stomach contents. A) *G. vermiculophylla,* B) *G. textorii,* C) *C. amplivesiculatum,* D) *R. maritima* and E) *Z. marina.*

Eight species of marine flora were identified within the green turtle stomach contents (Table 3). These same species were also collected from the mangrove channel of Estero Banderitas with the exception of *Neoagarddhiella baileyi, Pterocladiella capillacea* and *Ulva lactuca. Hypnea johnstonii,* which has been previously reported as a major food item in green turtle diet (López-Mendilaharsu et al., 2005), was available in the bay but not found in the stomachs of the turtles. *Gracilaria vermiculophylla* was present in 60%of the turtle stomachs analyzed and made up the greatest total percent volume (36%). Gracilaria textorii was present in the second greatest percent volume (16.5%).

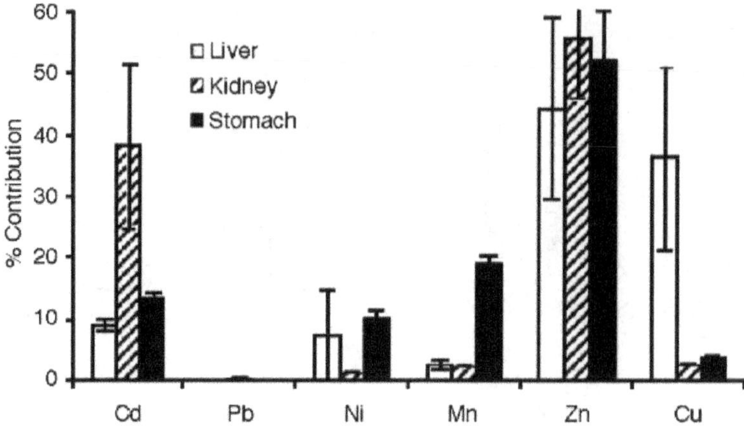

Fig. 7. Percent contribution of metals in tissues and the stomach contents of green turtles (*Chelonia mydas*) from Magdalena Bay, Mexico.

	Stomach Contents					
Species	1	2	3	4	5	TOTAL
Codium amplivesiculatum	69.1%					13.8%
Gracilaria textorii	30.9%	51.6%				16.5%
Gracilaria vermiculophylla		48.4%	33.6%		100%	36.4%
Neoagarddhiella baileyi				36.2%		7.2%
Pterocladiella capillacea				20.5%		4.1%
Rupia maritima				43.3%		8.7%
Ulva lactuca			31.8%			6.4%
Zostera marina			34.5%			6.9%

Table 3. Percent volume of macroalgae and sea grasses in the stomach contents of five green turtles (*Chelonia mydas*) collected in Estero Banderitas, Magdalena Bay, Mexico.

3.3 Principal components analysis

Principal components analysis (PCA) of the percent contribution of individual metals to the overall metal signature of each plant or tissue sample generated three principal components (PC) that explained 80.7% of the total variance in the data (50.1%, 17.6%, and 13.1%, respectively) (Fig. 8). Plots of the sample scores on the first and second principal components produced four groupings. Bay and stomach plant samples were separated by their scores on PC(1), while kidney and liver samples were separated by their scores on PC(2) (Fig. 8A). All but one of the bay plant samples obtained negative scores on PC(1), whereas plants from the stomach contents generally scored greater than 0. The loadings plot, which illustrates the influence of each metal on sample scores, indicated that the bay and stomach samples separated on PC(1) based on the dominance of the stomach samples' metal signatures by Zinc and Cadmium. The separation of liver and kidney samples appeared to be influenced by the greater contribution of Cadmium to the metal profile in kidney, and the dominance of Cu in liver samples which scored higher on PC(2) (Fig. 8B).

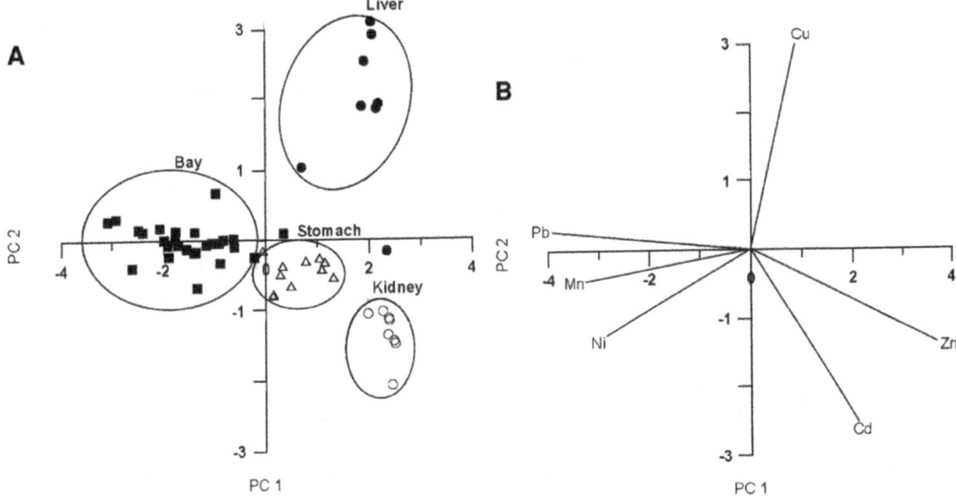

Fig. 8. A) Plot of sample scores of a Principle Component Analysis of the percent contribution of individual metals to the overall signature of marine flora from Magdalena Bay, kidney, liver and stomach contents samples from green turtles (*Chelonia mydas*). B) Loadings plot

3.4 Prescence of fibropapiloms and epibionts

In our study we found less of 1% of the animals with some fibropapiloms but at least 20% with epibionts. This is consistent with the data from Caribbean populations in where 2% had tumors present. The main observed difference was the degree of development between the populations in Bahía Magdalena (Fig. 9a) with very few in the carapace, frontal fins and head. In Caribbean populations bibber tumors (Fig. 9b) were observed and more concentrated in the head or in the frontal fins.

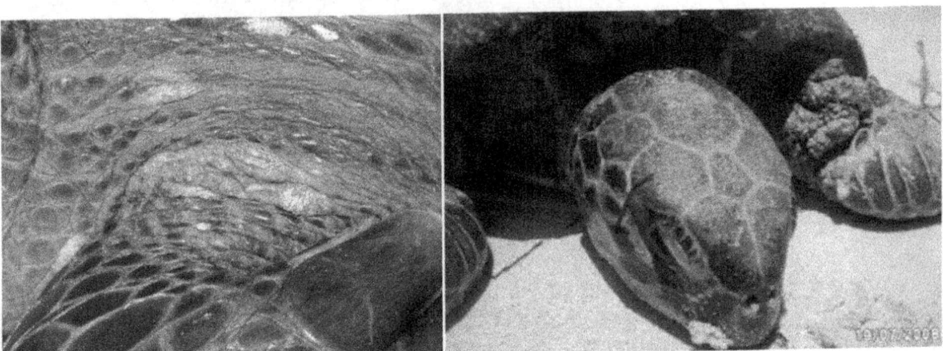

Fig. 9. A) Population in Bahía Magdalena (Fig. 9a) with very few in the carapace, frontal fins and head. B) Caribbean population's bibber tumors were observed and more concentrated in the head or in the frontal fins.

4. Discussion

Much of the literature on sea turtles has worked with absolute concentrations of metals, which is appropriate for comparisons of very similar sample types such as different sea turtle tissues or the same tissue in different sea turtle species. In the present paper we used absolute concentrations to compare metals in tissues (kidney vs. liver) and to compare metal concentrations in different plant species. However in order to better understand the source of metals to turtles in this region, the profile of all metals combined was used as an environmentally acquired marker. For this objective, we removed the influence of concentration differences among samples by converting the data to percent contribution of each metal to the total metal signature of the individual sample. This approach enabled the comparison of metal profiles across greatly different samples and was more appropriate than comparisons of absolute concentrations alone. For example, a single plant species located in two different areas will accumulate metals using the same physiological mechanisms. Therefore, a difference in metal profiles of the plant species from two different locations is an indication of differences in the availability of the metals from the environment. However, differences in the absolute concentrations of metals in plants would not necessarily indicate environmental difference because other factors might also be at play (e.g. age of the plant).

4.1 Comparison of metals in marine plant species

Metal concentrations in marine flora are controlled by both the bioavailability of metals in the surrounding water and the uptake capacity of the particular plant species. Marine algae have the capacity to accumulate trace metals several thousand times higher than the concentration in seawater (Bryan and Langston, 1992; Sánchez-Rodríguez et al., 2001). Red algae, such as Gracilaria sp tend to reflect the environmental availability of metals but have higher bioaccumulation of Cadmium, Copper and Zinc than other macroalgal groups (Sánchez-Rodríguez et al., 2001; Roncarati, 2003). These same species are a major component of the green turtle diet along the Baja California Peninsula (Seminoff et al., 2002; López-Mendilaharsu et al., 2005), and we proposed previously (Gardner et al., 2006) that their foraging habits could account for the high metal concentrations found in this population. However, comparisons across plant species in the present study suggest that species differences in metal concentrations are minimal. The only significant difference detected between plant species was that Cadmium was higher in *Ruppia maritima* than all other species, and higher in *Gracilaria textorii* than *Codium amplivesiculatum*. *R. maritima* was encountered in only one of the sea turtle stomachs analyzed, contributing a relatively small percentage of the overall diet (8.7%) in this study, and was absent from the diet of 24 green turtles analyzed in previous work (López-Mendilaharsu et al., 2005). *Gracilaria textorii* made up a larger proportion of the turtles' stomach contents (16.5%), but was similar in Cadmium concentration to most other plant species ingested by the green turtles. The results of the PCA also support this conclusion since the bay-collected plant samples grouped separately from the samples in the stomach contents despite that both groups consisted of the same five plant species.

We found significant spatial and temporal variations in heavy metal concentrations in marine plants as previous spatial studies has shown in the region (Páez-Osuna et al., 2000; Sánchez-Rodríguez et al., 2001; Rodriguez-Castañeda et al., 2006, Rodríguez-Meza et al., 2008). The high concentration of Zinc and Fe in the upper region might be related to the isolation of the site (Rodríguez-Meza et al., 2008). Heavy metal concentration was, in some cases, in the levels of toxicity. Temporal variations in metal concentrations, such as high concentrations in Cadmium and other metals observed in April, may be related to local upwelling events. Surface water Cadmium concentrations have been strongly correlated with upwelling (Lares et al. 2002) which occurs during spring and early summer off the coast of Magdalena Bay (Zaytsev et al., 2003). These levels of Cadmium in seaweeds has not been observed in the Gulf of California studied populations but strong species and spatial variations where observed (Páez-Osuna et al., 2000; Sánchez-Rodríguez et al. 2001; Rodriguez-Castañeda et al., 2006). The differences in heavy metal concentrations that we found in the seaweeds did not generally correspond with patterns of those elements previously observed in the sediment from the same region or seaweed species (Rodríguez-Meza et al., 2008), contrary to the studied sites in the Gulf of California near a mine (Rodriguez-Castañeda et al., 2006) or near industrial ports (Páez-Osuna et al., 2000; Sánchez-Rodríguez et al., 2001; Rodriguez-Castañeda et al., 2006). This finding, together with the observed species differences, suggests that the metabolic condition and life cycle stage of the individual species might influence metal uptake and accumulation (Lobban and Wynne 1981). Similarly, Riget et al., (1995) found differences between seaweed species *Ascophyllum nodosum, Fucus vesiculosus,* and *Fucus distichus*. We found lower levels of Ni and Zinc in *H. johnstonii* than in the environment as reported by Rodríguez-Meza et al., (2008). Based on our data, there are similarities between the composition and concentration of heavy metals between the plant species reviewed and the sediment; except in the case of Cu, Fe, and Mn (Rodríguez-Meza et al., 2008). All those elements are considered critical in the photosynthetic metabolism (Lobban and Wynne, 1981). We might assume that those elements are more easily assimilated by the plants because of their use in photosynthesis.

The role of seaweeds and seagrasses in coastal lagoons (like Banderitas or any other along the Baja California Peninsula) are relevant because they are feeding grounds for black turtles (*C. mydas*), loggerhead turtles (*Caretta caretta*), olive Ridley turtles (*Lepidochelys olivacea*), and hawksbill turtles (*Eretmochelys imbricata*) and migratory birds like Brant geese (*Branta bernicla*; Seminoff, 2000; Herzog and Sedinger, 2004). All of the species are included in the Mexican endangered species list (NOM ECOL 059) and on the red list in the UICN endangered species (www. uicnredlist.org). They are high productivity areas for fishing all kind of products (CONABIO, 2000; Carta Nacional, 2005). The fact that we found more significant variation in the spatial than temporal heavy metal concentrations in most of the species show that they might be constantly incorporated in the diet of many herbivorous animals (Gardner et al., 2006) with severe consequences in their health. Management strategies for these species should consider monitoring the levels of metals.

4.2 Sea turtle tissue comparisons

Pb, Cu and Mn concentrations in tissue from this study were within the range of those reported for sea turtles in other parts of the world (Lam et al., 2004; Storelli and Marcotrigiano, 2003). However, the average concentrations of Cadmium, Zinc and Ni in kidney of green turtles from Magdalena Bay were high compared to previously reports for sea turtle tissues (Sakai et al., 1995, 2000; Storelli and Marcotrigiano, 2003). Studies of loggerhead turtles (Maffucci et al., 2005) suggest that sea turtles can regulate Copper and Zinc concentrations through homeostatic processes but that Cadmium uptake is not controlled by active process and thus tissue concentrations of this metal reflect exposure. In agreement with these findings, we observed that Cadmium concentrations in green turtle liver were similar to their food and that the Cu concentration in sea turtle liver was greater than in the stomach content. Similar relationships have been observed in green turtles from Japan (Anan et al., 2001). However, contrary to the findings of Maffucci et al., (2005), Zinc concentrations in the livers and kidneys of green turtles in our study were not significantly different from their stomach contents. The distribution of metals among organs is influenced by both duration and concentration of exposure. Liver is a major site of short-term Cadmium storage, whereas during long-term exposure, Cadmium is redistributed from the liver to the kidney where it is absorbed and concentrated (Thomas et al., 1994; Linder and Grillitsch, 2000; Rie et al., 2001). Therefore a significantly greater concentration of Cadmium in green turtle kidney than liver is often observed (Storelli and Marcotrigiano, 2003; Maffucci et al., 2005; Gardner et al., 2006) and likely results from years of accumulation in this long-lived species. While kidney Cadmium concentration may serve as a good indicator for assessments of sea turtle health, liver more closely reflects the concentration of this metal in the food and so analyses of liver may provide a better indication of recent environmental exposure. Accordingly, Cadmium concentrations in the livers analyzed in the present study were not different from the food in the sea turtles' stomachs. Concentrations of Fe and Zinc in liver were also similar to the stomach contents. Whereas, Plumb, Nickel and Manganese concentrations in liver were similar to kidney, but were lower than in the stomach contents, which may indicate metabolic processing of these metals. Alternatively, Copper concentration was higher in liver than in the turtles' food and appeared to be preferentially accumulated in liver over kidney.

4.3 Metals in sea turtle stomach contents and marine plants from the bay

Two principle components, PC(1) and PC(2), explained 68%of the total variance in the data.When plotted relative to PC(1) and PC(2), the plant samples collected in the bay formed a grouping at the left side of the plot while the green turtle tissue samples and the plants from the stomach contents plotted higher on PC(1) (Fig. 4A). Examination of the loadings plot for each of the metals confirmed that samples scoring high on PC1 had signatures dominated by Cadmium and Zinc (stomach contents and kidney) or Cu (liver) (Fig. 4B). This agrees with the observation that the plants in the stomach contents contained greater percent contributions of Cadmium and Zinc than the samples collected in the bay, while Pb and Mn contributed more to the metal profiles in the bay samples as shown in Fig. 2; a tendency that was consistent in all five plant species. The metal profiles in the sea turtle tissues more closely resembled the plants in the stomach contents than the same species of plants collected within Estero Banderitas. The fact that the concentrations of Cadmium, Fe and Zinc in green turtle liver were the same as the stomach contents but different from the plants collected in the bay suggests that sea turtles collected inside of Magdalena Bay use foraging resources outside of the Estero Banderitas region. Further support of this conclusion is provided by the fact that three algal species (*N. baileyi*, *P. capillacea* and *U. lactuca*) in the stomach contents were not found in Estero Banderitas. Franzellitti et al. (2004) proposed that tissue metal profiles can be used as "environmentally acquired markers" to determine sea turtle feeding areas. Similarly, principle component analyses have been applied previously to determine sources of metals in aquatic environments (Ruiz-Fernández et al., 2001). Comparison of the metal signature profiles in plants from the bay and the sea turtle stomach contents indicate that the plant species contained inside the sea turtle stomachs originated from a location outside of Estero Banderitas, in an area where Cadmium and Zinc concentrations dominate the metal profiles in the environment. Surface water metal concentrations have been strongly correlated with upwelling events and natural components of regional biogeochemistry (Daesslé et al., 2000; Lares et al., 2002). Similar to the distribution of nutrients in the water column, metals such as Cadmium and Zinc are depleted in the surface and enriched in deeper water. Upwelling processes are an important mechanism that brings elevated concentrations of both nutrients and metals to the surface and thus available for marine floral accumulation. Therefore it is highly probable that the sea turtles collected within Magdalena Bay are utilizing foraging areas in an upwelling-rich coastal region outside of the Bay. Coastal lagoons of the Baja California Peninsula such as Magdalena Bay have been identified as priority areas for sea turtle conservation programs (Nichols et al., 2000). Long-term sea turtle monitoring studies have demonstrated high site fidelity to Estero Banderitas over time, and low emigration of sea turtles from Magdalena Bay to other coastal lagoons along the Baja California Peninsula (Grupo Tortuguero, unpublished data). Efforts to protect areas within Magdalena Bay have focused on the creation of a refuge in the mangrove channels of Estero Banderitas, in part, because of the perceived importance of this habitat for sea turtle foraging (Nichols and Arcas, 2001). However, data generated by our work suggest that sea turtles residing in Estero Banderitas are feeding in areas outside of the bay, most likely in coastal regions with high upwelling. These findings support those of López-Mendilaharsu et al. (2005) and indicate that green turtles utilize spatially distinct feeding habitats within coastal areas. Therefore, we recommend that sea turtle protected areas be designed with an appreciation of regional rather than local scales in order to protect broader foraging areas.

4.4 Fibropapiloms and epibionts

The prescence of fibropapiloms are variable from 1.4% up to 90% of the population (Herbs *et al.*, 1999, Quackenbush et al., 2001, Chaloupka et al., 2009). The observed low proportion of the green turtles in Bahía Magdalena (less than 1%) agree with a well preserved environment and less stress situation for the animals. In the case of the epibionts we found a continuously prescence of cirripedia and balanus but not a diverse fauna like in the Atlantic that even polychaetes has been reported (Lara Uc, 2011).

5. Conclusions

Conservation of threatened species, such as the green turtle (*Chelonia mydas*), is closely related to habitat quality. In particular there are issues related to heavy metals, the presence of epibionts, parasites and fibropapiloms who might play a crucial role in the species survivorship. The process of metal bioaccumulation in marine food chains is poorly understood because very little data is available on metal concentration at different trophic levels and their temporal or spatial variation and its influence in turtle health. The Baja California Peninsula, Mexico serves an important role for feeding and developing sea turtles. High concentrations of metals detected in food items (seaweeds and seagrasses) and in green turtles (*Chelonia mydas*) from Magdalena Bay prompted an investigation into the sources of metals in the region in relation to the health issues of the animals. We compared metal concentrations in sea turtle tissues in relation to plant species found in their stomach contents, and with the same species of plants collected inside a sea turtle refuge area known as Estero Banderitas and determine the health state of turtles based on our long term monitoring efforts. Our results showed that Iron, Copper, and Manganese were the most significant metals found in seagrasses, red, and green algae. We found significant more variation in temporal heavy metal concentrations in relation to the maximum abundance in the samples and spatial variation in relation to the studied taxa suggesting that herbivores' have a differential intake of the metals. Also, our results suggest that heavy metals might be incorporated regularly in the diet of many herbivorous animals with severe consequences to their health. Differences in the metal concentrations between marine plant species in relation to animal tissue were minimal. Principal components analysis of the percent contribution of individual metals to the overall metal signature of each plant or tissue sample generated three principal components that explained 80.7% of the total variance in the data. The plant samples collected within Estero Banderitas formed a separate grouping from the green turtle tissue samples and the plants from the stomach contents. The plants in the stomach contents contained greater percent contributions of Cadmium and Zinc than the plants collected inside the bay, while Plumb and Manganese contributed more to the metal profiles in the bay samples. The metal profiles in the sea turtle tissues more closely resembled the stomach contents than the same species of plants collected within Estero Banderitas, and suggest that sea turtles collected inside Magdalena Bay use foraging resources outside of the Estero Banderitas region. Green turtle from Estero Banderitas seems to be healthy at this stage in comparison with nesting areas in the Pacific and Atlantic of Mexico our data on fibropapilomas and epibionts strongly support this idea. Our data supports the suggestion that metal profiles can be used as "environmentally acquired markers" to improve our understanding of the extent of sea turtle foraging areas. Management strategies for these species should consider monitoring the levels of metals.

6. Acknowledgements

Funding for this project was provided by a grant to SC Gardner from the Consejo Nacional de Ciencia y Tecnología (Conacyt, SEP-2004-CO1-45749) and the Centro de Investigaciones Biológicas del Noroeste, S.C. (CIBNOR). The authors express their appreciation to Dr. Wallace J. Nichols, Rodrigo Rangel and the Grupo Tortuguero for their assistance in this project. We also appreciate the expertise of Dr. Samuel Chávez Rosales and Griselda Peña Armenta for their help with the quantitative analyses. This research was conducted in accordance with Mexican laws and regulations, under permits provided by the Secretaria de Medio Ambiente y Recursos Naturales (SGPA/DGVS/002-2895).

7. References

Abbott IA, Hollenberg GJ. (1976)Marine algae of California. U.S.A.: Standford University Press; 1976. 827 pp.

Abdallah AMA, Abdallah MA, Beltagy A, Siam E (2006) Contents of heavy metals in marine algae from egyptian red sea coast. Tox Env Chem 88: 9-22.

Aguirre, A.A.; Lutz, P.L. (2004), Marine turtles as Sentinels of Ecosystem Health: Is Fibropapilomatosis an indicator EcoHealth 1:275-283.

Alfaro, A. Koie, M. Buchmann, Kurt. (2006). Synopsis of infections in sea turtles caused by virus, bacteria and parasites: an ecological review. University the Copenhagen. Report.30

Anan, Y, Kunito T, Watanabe I, Sakai H, Tanabe S. (2001)Trace element accumulation in hawksbill turtles (Eretomochelys imbricata) and green turtles (*Chelonia mydas*) from Yaeyama Islands, Japan. Environ Toxicol Chem 20:2802–14.

Arriaga, CL, Vázquez-Domínguez E, González-Cano J, Jiménez-Rosenberg R, Muñoz-López E, Aguilar-Sierra V. (1998). Regiones marinas prioritarias de México. México: Comisión Nacional para el Conocimiento y uso de la Biodiversidad;. 198 pp.

Badillo, A.F.J. (2007). Epizoítos y Parásitos de la tortuga Boba (*Caretta caretta*) en el mediterráneo occidental. Tesis de Doctorado, Universidad de Valencia. 264

Bicho, R, Joaquim N., MendoncaV., AlKiyumi A., Mahmoud .IY., AlKindi A. (2006). Levels of heavy metals and antioxidant enzymes in green turtle (Chelonia mydas) in the Arabian Sea, Sultanate of Oman. Twenty sixth annual symposium on sea turtle biology and conservation. Athens, Greece: International Sea Turtle Society.

Brand-Gardner, S.J., Lanyon J.M., Limpus C.J. (1999). Diet selection by immature green turtles, Chelonia mydas, in subtropical Moreton Bay, South-east Queensland. Aust J Zool;47:181–91.

Bryan , G.W., Langston W.J. (1992). Bioavailability, accumulation and effects of heavy metals in sediments with special reference to United Kingdom estuaries: a review. Environ Pollut 76:89-131.

Caliceti, M., Argese E., Sfriso A., Pavoni B. (2002). Heavy metal contamination in the seaweeds of the Venice lagoon. Chems 47:443-454.

Carta Nacional Pesquera (2005) Carta Nacional Pesquera, SEMARNAT México D.F. 120 pp.

Caurant F, Bustamante P, Bordes M, Miramand P. Bioaccumulation of cadmium, copper and zinc in some tissues of three species of marine turtles stranded along the French Altantic coasts. Mar Pollut Bull 1999;38:1085–91.

Catriona MO, Macinnis-Ng CMO, Peter JR (2002) Towards a more ecologically relevant assessment of the impact of heavy metals en the photosynthesis of the seagrass, *Zostera capricorni*. Mar Poll Bull 45: 100-106.

CONABIO 2000. Plan Nacional sobre Biodiversidad. CONABIO México D.F. 250 pp,

Daesslé, L.W., Carriquiry J.D., Navarro R., Villaescusa-Celaya J.A. (2000). Geochemistry of surficial sediments from Sebastian Vizcaino Bay, Baja California. J Coast Res 16:1133–45.

Díaz, M.M.; Gutiérrez, B.J.; Jasso, L.D.; López, S.C.; Sarti, M.L.; Vallejo, A.C. (1992). Epibiontes y estado físico de las tortugas *Lepidochelys olivacea* y *Dermochelys coriacea* en el playón de Mexiquillo, Michoacán, durante la temporada de anidación 1988-1989; Publ. Soc. Herpetol. Mex. 19-25.

Franzellitti, S., Locatelli C.,Gerosa G., Vallini C., Fabbri E. (2004). Heavymetals in tissues of loggerhead turtles (Caretta caretta) from the northwestern Adriatic Sea. Comp Biochem Physiol C 138:187–94.

Gámez, S.V., Osorio, D.S., Peñaflores, C.S.; García, A.H.; Ramírez, J.L. (2006). Identification of parasites and epibionts in the Olive Ridley Turtle (*Lepidochelys olivacea*) that arrived to the beaches of Michoacán and Oaxaca, Mexico. *Vet. Méx.* 37:431-440.

Gardner, S.C., Nichols W.J. (2001). Assessment of sea turtle mortality rates in the Bahía Magdalena region, Baja California Sur, México. Chelonian Conserv Biol 4:197–9.

G ardner, S.C., Fitzgerald S.L., Acosta-Vargas B., Méndez-Rodríguez L. (2006) Heavy metal Accumulation in four species of sea turtles from the Baja California Peninsula, Mexico. Biomet. 19(1): 91-99.

Garnett, ST, Pirce IR, Scott FJ. The diet of the green turtle, Chelonia mydas (L.), in Torres Strait. Aust Wildl Res 1985;12:103–12.

Gordon, A.N., Pople A.R., Ng. J. (1998). Trace metal concentrations in livers and kidneys of sea turtles from south-eastern Queensland, Australia. Mar Freshw Res 49:409–14.

Gutiérrez-Galindo , E.A., Villaescusa-Celaya J.A., Arrelola-Chimal A. (1999). Bioaccumulation of metals in mussels from tour sites of the coastal region of Baja California. Cienc Mar 25:557–77.

Herbst, L.H., Jacobson E.R., Klein P. A., Balazs G., Moretti R., Brown T. and Sndberg J.(1999).Comparative Pathology and Pathogenesis of Spontaneous Experimentally Induced Fibropapillomas of Green Turtle (*Chelonia mydas*). Vet Pathol 36:551-564

Herzog, M.P., Sedinger J.S. (2004) Dynamics of foraging behavior associated with variation in habitat and forage availability in captive black brant (*Branta bernicla nigricans*) Goslings in Alaska. Auk 121:210-23.

Kalesh, NS, Nair SM (2006) Spatial and temporal variability of copper, zinc, and cobalt in marine macroalgae from the southwest coast of India. Bull Environ Contam Toxicol 76:293-300.

Kieffer, F. (1991). Metals and their compounds in the environment. Weinheim: VCH: 481 pp.

Kumar, V.V., Kaladharan P. (2006) Biosorption of metals from contaminated water using seaweed. Curr Sci 90:1263-7.

Lam, J.C.W., Tanabe S., Chan S.K.F., Yuen E.K.W., Lam M.H.W., Lam P.K.S. (2004). Trace element residues in tissues of green turtles (Chelonia mydas) from South China waters. Mar Pollut Bull 48:164–92

Lanza, G, Ortega MM, Laparra JL, Carrillo RM, Godinez JL (1989) Chemical analysis of heavy metals (hg, pb, cd, as, cr and sr) in marine algae of Baja California. An Inst Biol Univ Nac Auton Mex (Bot) 59:89-102.

Lara-Uc, M. (2011). Establecimiento de valores hematológicos y bioquímicos de las tortugas carey (*Eretmochelys imbricata*) y blanca (*Chelonia mydas*), con y sin parásitos o fibropapiloma, que anidan en Yucatán. Upublised Ph.D. thesis Universidad Autónoma de Yucatán, Merida, 105 pp.

Lares, ML, Flores-Munoz G, Lara-Lara R (2002) Temporal variability of bioavailable cd, hg, zn, mn and al in an upwelling regime. Environ Pollut 120:595-608.

Linder, G., Grillitsch B. (2000) Ecotoxicology of Metals. In: Sparling DW, Linder G, Bishop CA, editors. Ecotoxicology of amphibians and reptiles. Society of Environmental Toxicology and Chemistry SETAC press; p. 325–459

Lobban, C.S., Wynne M.J. (1981) The Biology of Seaweeds. Botanical Monographs Vol. 17. Blackwell Scientific Publications, USA,786 p.

López-Mendilaharsu, M, Gardner SC, Riosmena-Rodríguez R, Seminoff J (2005) Identifying critical foraging habitats of the GreenTurtle (*Chelonia mydas*) along the Pacific Coast of the Baja California Peninsula, México. Aqu Conserv: Mar and Fresh Ecosys 15: 259-269.

Machado, W, Silva-Filho EV, Oliveira RR, Lacerda LD (2002) Trace retention in mangrove ecosystems in Guanabara Bay, SE Brazil. Mar Poll Bull 44: 1277-1280.

Maffucci, F, Caurant F, Bustamante P, Bentivegna F. Trace element (Cd, Cu, Hg, Se, Zn) accumulation and tissue distribution in loggerhead turtles (Caretta caretta) from the Western Mediterranean Sea (southern Italy). Chemosphere 2005;58:535–42.

Martin, J.H., Broenkow W.W. (1975). Cadmium in plankton: elevated concentrations off Baja California. Science 190:884–5.

Méndez-Rodríguez, L., Acosta-Vargas B., Alvarez-Castañeda S.T., Lechuga-Devéze C.H. (1998). Trace metal distribution along the southern coast of Bahia de La Paz (Gulf of California), Mexico. Bull Environ Contam Toxicol 61:616–22.

Méndez, L., Álvarez-Castañeda S.T., Acosta B., Sierra-Beltrán A. P. (2002) Trace metals in tissues of gray whale (*Eschrichtius robustus*) carcasses from the Northern Pacific Mexican Coast. Mar Poll Bull 44, 217-221.

Moreno, M (2003) Toxicología ambiental, evaluación de riesgo para la salud humana. Mc Graw- Hill. España. 370 pp.

Nichols ,WJ, Arcas F. Third Annual Meeting of the Sea Turtle Conservation Network of the Californias (Grupo Tortuguero de las Californias). Mar Turt Newsl 2001;93:30–1.

Nichols, W.J., Bird K.E., Garcia S.(2000). Community-based research and its application to sea turtle conservation in Bahia Magdalena, BCS, Mexico. Mar Turt Newsl 89:4–7.

Páez-Osuna, F., Ochoa-Izaguirre M.J., Bojórquez-Leyva H., Michel-Reynoso I.L. (2000). Macroalgae as Biomonitors of Heavy Metal Availability in Coastal Lagoons from the Subtropical Pacific of Mexico. Bull of Env Cont Tox 64:846-851.

Quackenbush, S. L., Casey R. N., Murcek R. J., Paul T. A., Work T. M., Limpus C. J., Chaves A., duToit L., Vasconcelos P. J., Aguirre A. A., Spraker T. R., Horrocks J. A., Vermeer L. A., Balazs G. H., Casey J. W. (2001). Quantitative análisis of Herpesvirus Sequences from normal tissue and Fibropapillomas of marine Turtles with Real-Time PCR. J. Virology. 287:105-111.

Rie, M.T., Lendas K.A., Callard I.P. (2001). Cadmium: tissue distribution and binding protein induction in the painted turtle, Chrysemys picta. Comp Biochem Physiol C 130:41–51.

Riget ,F., Johansen P., Asmund G. (1995) Natural seasonal variation of cadmium, copper, lead and zinc in brown seaweed (*Fucus vesiculosus*). Mar Poll Bull 30; 409-414.

Riosmena-Rodríguez, R. (1999) Vegetación subacuatica. In: Gaytán, J.,Informe Final de Actividades del Proyecto Bahía del Rincón . UABCS-S&R. 350 pp,

Riosmena-Rodríguez, R., Talavera-Saenz A.L., Gardner S.C., Acosta-Vargas B. (2010). Heavy metals dynamics from Seaweeds and Seagrasses in Bahía Magdalena, B.C.S., México. *J. App. Phyc.* 22; 283 -291.

Rodríguez-Meza, G. D. (2005) Caracterización geoquímica de componentes mayores y elementos traza de sedimentos de los ambientes marinos costeros adyacentes a la península de Baja California. Ph D. thesis, IPN-CICIMAR.

Rodriguez-Castaneda, A.P., Sanchez-Rodriguez I., Shumilin E.N., Sapozhnikov D. (2006) Element concentrations in some species of seaweeds from La Paz bay and La Paz lagoon, south-western Baja California, México. J App Phyc 18: 399-408.

Roncarati, F. (2003). Utilizzo di macrofite marine come indicatori di stress ambientali. Thesis in Environmental Sciences. University of Bologna, Campus Ravenna, Italy.

Ruiz-Fernández, A.C., Páez-Osuna F., Hillaire-Marcel C., Soto-Jiménez M., Gheleb B. (2001). Principle component analysis applied to the assessment of metal pollution from urban wastes in the Culiacán river estuary. Bull Environ Contam Toxicol 67:741–8.

Sakai, H., Ichihashi H., Suganuma H., Tatsukawa R. (1995). Heavy metal monitoring in sea turtles using eggs. Mar PollutBull 30:347–53.

Sakai, H., Saeki K., Ichihashi H., Suganuma H., Tanabe S, Tatsukawa R. (2000). Species-specific distribution of heavy metals in tissues and organs of loggerhead turtle (Caretta caretta) and green turtle (*Chelonia mydas*) from Japanese coastal waters. Mar Pollut Bull 40:701–9.

Sánchez-Rodríguez, I, Huerta- Díaz MA, Choumiline E, Holguín-Quiñones O, Zertuche-Gonzáles JA (2001) Elemental concentration in different species of seaweeds from

Loreto Bay, Baja California Sur, Mexico: implications for the geochemical control of metals in algal tissue. Env Poll 114: 145-160.

Sañudo-Wihelmy , S.A., Flegal A.R. (1996).Trace metal concentrations in the surf zone and in coastal waters off Baja California, Mexico. Environ Sci Technol 30:1575–80.

Sawidis ,T., Brown M.T., Zachariadis G., Sratis I. (2001). Trace metal concentrations in marine macroalgae from different biotopes in the Aegean Sea. Env Int 27: 43-47.

Seminoff J.A., Resendiz A., Nichols W.J. (2002). Diet of the East Pacific green turtle, Chelonia mydas, in the central Gulf of California, Mexico. J Herpetol 36:447–53.

Seminoff, J. A. (2000). Biology of the East Pacific green turtle, *Chelonia mydas agassizii*, at a warm temperate feeding area in the Gulf of California, Mexico. Dissertation, University of Arizona.

Shumilin, E.N., Rodriguez-Figueroa G., Bermea O.M., Baturina E.L., Hernandez E., Rodríguez-Meza G.D. (2000). Anomalous Trace Element Composition of Coastal Sediments near the Copper Mining District of Santa Rosalia, Peninsula of Baja California, Mexico. Bull Environ Contam Toxicol 65:261–8.

Shumilin, E., Paez-Osuna F., Green-Ruiz C., Sapozhnikov D., Rodriguez- Meza G.D., Godinez-Orta L. (2001). Arsenic, antimony, selenium and other trace elements in sediments of the La Paz lagoon, Peninsula of Baja California, Mexico. Mar Pollut Bull 42:174–8.

Storelli, M.M., Marcotrigiano G.O. (2003). Heavy metal residues in tissues of marine turtles. Mar Pollut Bull 46:367–400.

Sparling, D., Bishop C., Linder G. (2000) Ecotoxicology of amphibians and reptiles. Pensacola FL: Society of Environmental Toxicology and Chemistry.

Szefer, P., Geldon J., Anis-Ahmed A., Paéz-Osuna F., Ruiz-Fernandez A.C., Guerrero-Galvan S.R. (1998). Distribution and association of trace metals in soft tissue and byssus of *Mytela strigata* and other benthal organisms from Mazatlan Harbour, Mangrove Lagoon of the northwest coast of México. Env Inter 24: 359-374.

Valiela, I. (2009) Ecology of Coastal Ecosystems, in Fundamental of Aquatic Ecology, Second Edition (eds R. S. K. Barnes and K. H. Mann), Blackwell Publishing Ltd., Oxford, UK. doi: 10.1002/9781444314113.ch3

Villares , R., Puente X., Carballeira A. (2002). Seasonal variation and background levels of heavy metals in two green seaweeds. Env Poll 119: 79-90.

Talavera-Saenz ,A.L., Gardner S.C., Riosmena-Rodríguez R., Acosta-Vargas B. (2007). Metal Profiles Used as Environmental Markers of Green Turtle (*Chelonia mydas*) Foraging Resources. Sci Tot Env 373: 94-102.

Thomas, P., Baer K.N., White R.B. (1994). Isolation and partial characterization of metallothionein in the liver of the red-eared turtle (*Trachemys scripta*) following intraperitoneal administration of cadmium. Comp Biochem Physiol C 107:221–6.

Work, T. M. Balazs, G. H., Rameyer, R. A., Chang, S. P., Berestecky, J. 2000. Assessing humoral and cell-mediated immune response in Hawaiian green turtles, Chelonia mydas. Veterinary Immunology and Immunopathology 74:179–194.

Work, T.M.; Balazs, G.H.; Schumacher, J.L.; Marie, A. 2005. Epizootiology of spirorchiid infection in green turtles (*Chelonia mydas*) in Hawaii. *J. Parasitol.* 91:871-876.

Zaytsev, O., Cervantes-Duarte R., Montante O., Gallegos-Garcia A. (2003): Coastal upwelling activity on the Pacific shelf of the Baja California Peninsula. J of Ocean 59, 489-502

Permissions

The contributors of this book come from diverse backgrounds, making this book a truly international effort. This book will bring forth new frontiers with its revolutionizing research information and detailed analysis of the nascent developments around the world.

We would like to thank Dr. Krzysztof Śmigórski, for lending his expertise to make the book truly unique. He has played a crucial role in the development of this book. Without his invaluable contribution this book wouldn't have been possible. He has made vital efforts to compile up to date information on the varied aspects of this subject to make this book a valuable addition to the collection of many professionals and students.

This book was conceptualized with the vision of imparting up-to-date information and advanced data in this field. To ensure the same, a matchless editorial board was set up. Every individual on the board went through rigorous rounds of assessment to prove their worth. After which they invested a large part of their time researching and compiling the most relevant data for our readers. Conferences and sessions were held from time to time between the editorial board and the contributing authors to present the data in the most comprehensible form. The editorial team has worked tirelessly to provide valuable and valid information to help people across the globe.

Every chapter published in this book has been scrutinized by our experts. Their significance has been extensively debated. The topics covered herein carry significant findings which will fuel the growth of the discipline. They may even be implemented as practical applications or may be referred to as a beginning point for another development.

The editorial board has been involved in producing this book since its inception. They have spent rigorous hours researching and exploring the diverse topics which have resulted in the successful publishing of this book. They have passed on their knowledge of decades through this book. To expedite this challenging task, the publisher supported the team at every step. A small team of assistant editors was also appointed to further simplify the editing procedure and attain best results for the readers.

Our editorial team has been hand-picked from every corner of the world. Their multi-ethnicity adds dynamic inputs to the discussions which result in innovative outcomes. These outcomes are then further discussed with the researchers and contributors who give their valuable feedback and opinion regarding the same. The feedback is then collaborated with the researches and they are edited in a comprehensive manner to aid the understanding of the subject.

Apart from the editorial board, the designing team has also invested a significant amount of their time in understanding the subject and creating the most relevant covers. They scrutinized every image to scout for the most suitable representation of the subject and create an appropriate cover for the book.

The publishing team has been involved in this book since its early stages. They were actively engaged in every process, be it collecting the data, connecting with the contributors or procuring relevant information. The team has been an ardent support to the editorial, designing and production team. Their endless efforts to recruit the best for this project, has resulted in the accomplishment of this book. They are a veteran in the field of academics and their pool of knowledge is as vast as their experience in printing. Their expertise and guidance has proved useful at every step. Their uncompromising quality standards have made this book an exceptional effort. Their encouragement from time to time has been an inspiration for everyone.

The publisher and the editorial board hope that this book will prove to be a valuable piece of knowledge for researchers, students, practitioners and scholars across the globe.

List of Contributors

Bofeng Zhang, Susu Jiang and Ke Yan
School of Computer Engineering and Science, Shanghai University, P.R. of China

Daming Wei
School of Computer Engineering and Science, Shanghai University, P.R. of China
Professor Emeritus, The University of Aizu, Fukushima, Japan

Yasutaka Chiba
Division of Biostatistics, Clinical Research Center, Kinki University School of Medicine, Japan

Paolo Barbini and Gabriele Cevenini
Department of Surgery and Bioengineering, University of Siena, Italy

Daniel Catalán-Matamoros
University of Almería, Spain

Sergio Eduardo Gonorazky
Hospital Privado de Comunidad de Mar del Plata, Argentina

Elisa Pieragostini, Elena Ciani, Giuseppe Rubino and Ferruccio Petazzi
University of Bari, Italy

Chris J. Bushe
Eli Lilly and Company Ltd, Basingstoke, UK

John Pendlebury
Ramsgate House, Manchester, UK

Rafael Riosmena-Rodriguez and Ana Luisa Talavera-Saenz
Programa de Investigación en Botánica Marina, Departamento de Biología Marina, Universidad Autónoma de Baja California Sur, La Paz Baja California Sur, México

Gustavo Hinojosa-Arango
The School for Field Studies, Puerto de Acapulco s/n, Puerto San Carlos, Baja California Sur, México

Mónica Lara-Uc
Depto. de Virología, Facultad de Medicina Veterinaria y Zootecnia, UADY, Mérida, Yucatán, México

Susan Gardner
Centro de Investigaciones Biológicas del Noroeste, La Paz Baja California Sur, México

Printed in the USA
CPSIA information can be obtained
at www.ICGtesting.com
JSHW011357221024
72173JS00003B/313